Religious Theories
of Personality and Psychotherapy
East Meets West

Religious Theories
of Personality and Psychotherapy
East Meets West

R. Paul Olson, MDiv, PhD
Editor

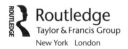
Routledge
Taylor & Francis Group
New York   London

First published by

The Haworth Press, Inc., 10 Alice Street, Binghamton, NY 13904-1580.

This edition published 2012 by Routledge

Routledge   Routledge
Taylor & Francis Group   Taylor & Francis Group
711 Third Avenue   2 Park Square, Milton Park
New York, NY 10017   Abingdon,Oxon OX14 4RN

Cover design by Anastasia Litwak.

Library of Congress Cataloging-in-Publication Data

Religious theories of personality and psychotherapy : East meets West / R. Paul Olson, editor.
  p. cm.
 Includes bibliographical references and index.
 ISBN 0-7890-1236-7 (alk. paper) — ISBN 0-7890-1237-5 (pbk. : alk. paper)
 1. Psychotherapy—Religious aspects. 2. Personality—Religious aspects. 3. Psychology, Religious. I. Olson, R. Paul.

RC489.R46 R45 2002
616.89'14—dc21

                    2001046326

We wish to dedicate this volume to our mentors who have
shared their spiritual wisdom and psychological insights,
and to all mental health professionals who are striving
to integrate science and religion into their clinical practice
for the well-being of their clients.

CONTENTS

About the Editor   xi

Contributors   xiii

Foreword   xv
P. Scott Richards

Preface   xix

Acknowledgments   xxi

Introduction   1
R. Paul Olson

Objectives of This Book   1
Underlying Assumptions   2
Separation of Psychology and Religion   4
Apologetic Function of Theology   6
Critical Theory and a Method of Critical Correlation   6
Organization of This Book   10

Chapter 1. Hindu Psychology and the *Bhagavad Gita*   19
Asha Mukherjee

Introduction   19
Personality Theory   28
Theory of Distress   38
Theory of Therapy   41
Practice of Therapy   47
Evaluation   50
Points of Dialogue   63
Case Study   70

Chapter 2. A Buddhist Psychology   85
Scott Kamilar

Introduction   85
Personality Theory   88

Theory of Distress   96
Theory of Therapy   99
Practice of Therapy   109
Evaluation   121
Points of Dialogue   123
Case Study   132

Chapter 3. Taoism and Psychology   141
Lynne Hagen

Introduction   141
Personality Theory   157
Theory of Distress   167
Theory of Therapy   173
Practice of Therapy   181
Evaluation   194
Points of Dialogue   195
Case Study   197

Chapter 4. Jewish Anthropology: The Stuff Between   211
Elaine E. Hartsman

Introduction   211
Personality Theory   216
Theory of Distress   227
Theory of Therapy   231
Practice of Therapy   236
Evaluation   236
Points of Dialogue   237
Case Study   239

Chapter 5. Christian Humanism   247
R. Paul Olson

Introduction   247
Personality Theory   250
Theory of Distress   259
Theory of Therapy   261
Practice of Therapy   271
Evaluation   278
Points of Dialogue   281
Case Study   290

Chapter 6. Islamic Psychology   **325**
Zehra Ansari

Introduction   325
Personality Theory   332
Theory of Distress   343
Theory of Therapy   343
Practice of Therapy   346
Evaluation   350
Points of Dialogue   351
Case Study   352

Chapter 7. Convergence and Divergence   **359**
R. Paul Olson
Bruce McBeath

Personality Theory   359
Theories of Psychotherapy   385

Index   **409**

ABOUT THE EDITOR

R. Paul Olson, MDiv, PhD, earned his BA in sociology from Carleton College, his master's degree in divinity from Yale Divinity School, and his doctorate in clinical psychology from the University of Illinois at Urbana. He worked as a clinical psychologist for fifteen years. For nine years Dr. Olson served as Dean of the Minnesota School of Professional Psychology. He is currently teaching at Argosy University–Twin Cities in Minneapolis in the areas of psychology and religion, professional ethics, integrative psychotherapy, health psychology, and experimental psychology. Dr. Olson lives with his wife Mary in Bloomington, MN. He is author or editor of numerous publications in his field.

CONTRIBUTORS

Zehra Ansari earned a master's specialist degree in school psychology from the University of Wisconsin, River Falls, after obtaining a master's degree in psychology and a bachelor's degree in journalism from Osmania University, Hyderabad, India. She is a licensed psychologist practicing currently at the Well Family Clinic, St. Paul, Minnesota, in addition to working as a school psychologist with learning disabled students at the Northeast Metro Intermediate School District #916 in White Bear Lake, Minnesota. An active member of the Islamic Center of Minnesota for over thirty years, Zehra is one of the founders of Al Birr Islamic Social Services. As a psychotherapist, Zehra strives to empower immigrants by including their own unique cultural strengths and religious values.

Lynne Hagen obtained a PsyD in clinical psychology from the Minnesota School of Professional Psychology. The focus of her clinical career has been serving Native American clients in community mental health agencies. She has worked with the Minnesota Indian Women's Resource Center, an outpatient substance abuse treatment facility, to provide mental health services to Native American clients and their families, and to assist in establishing their first mental health clinic. Presently, she is a staff psychologist with the Allina Medical Clinic in Hastings, Minnesota. Her interests include culturally sensitive psychotherapy and assessment, spirituality, grief, and trauma.

Elaine E. Hartsman received a PhD in educational psychology from the University of Minnesota. Her postdoctoral work includes completing a two-year program at the Gestalt Institute of the Twin Cities. She served on the Institute's faculty and then as director for three years. Currently she has a private psychotherapy practice and teaches at St. Mary's University of Minnesota and the Minnesota School of Professional Psychology. Elaine's present interest is exploring how the therapist's spiritual belief system affects the process and outcome of therapy.

Scott Kamilar obtained a MA and a PhD in clinical psychology from Wayne State University. He has been in private practice with Minnesota Human Development Consultants for the past eleven years and is on the adjunct faculty of the Minnesota School of Professional Psychology. His clinical and teaching interests include Buddhist Psychology, group therapy, family therapy, and hypnotherapy.

Bruce McBeath received an MSW from the University of Minnesota and a PhD in psychology from the Saybrook Graduate School in San Francisco, California. He co-founded the Psychosynthesis Institute of Minnesota in 1979, and since 1985 he has been an adjunct Associate Professor of Psychology and Human Development at St. Mary's University of Minnesota. His teaching and research interests emphasize existential-contemplative approaches to psychotherapy theory, practice, and research. He continues in private practice in St. Paul, Minnesota.

Asha Mukherjee was born in India and completed bachelor of science and master's degrees at the Maharaja Sayajirao University of Baroda, India, in human development, with minors in sociology, education, and psychology. She obtained a PhD in human development and clinical psychology from Iowa State University, Ames. She has worked as a clinician for nearly twenty years, with diverse populations in Canada and currently in Minneapolis. She has taught psychology part time at the university level in Florida, India, Jamaica, and Canada. Asha's clinical orientation is integrated and individualized to client cultural backgrounds.

Foreword

After more than a century of alienation between religion and mainstream psychology and psychotherapy, a new, more spiritually open, zeitgeist or "spirit of the times" is upon us. Many behavioral scientists have challenged psychology's long-standing adherence to exclusively naturalistic perspectives (e.g., Bergin, 1980; Jones, 1994; Richards and Bergin, 1997). During the past decade, an international, interdisciplinary, and ecumenical movement to incorporate spiritual perspectives and interventions into mainstream psychological theory, research, and practice has gained momentum and is having an impact on the profession (e.g., Benson, 1996; Kelly, 1995; Miller, 1999; Richards and Bergin, 1997, 2000; Shafranske, 1996; Worthington et al., 1996).

Religious Theories of Personality and Psychotherapy: East Meets West makes an important contribution to this movement. Most behavioral scientists to date have adopted a unilateral relationship between psychology and religion; that is, they have objectified religion and used "psychological findings or theories to revise, reinterpret, redefine, supplant, or dismiss established religious traditions" (Jones, 1994, p. 195). *Religious Theories of Personality and Psychotherapy* is one of the few books available today that adopts a truly dialogical relationship between psychology and religious tradition.

Jones (1994) suggested that if behavioral scientists will engage in a more constructive, dialogical relationship with religion, religious worldviews could contribute "positively to the progress of science by suggesting new modes of thought that transform an area of study by shaping new perceptions of the data and new theories" (p. 194). *Religious Theories of Personality and Psychotherapy* makes an outstanding contribution to the literature because it sheds much light on how religious worldviews might lead to new or revised theories of personality and psychotherapy. Each of the contributors begins with the assumption that there is truth and wisdom in the religious tradition that he or she writes about and then considers what implications the teachings of this tradition might have for personality theory and psychotherapy.

As I read, I found it fascinating to reflect on how the metaphysical teachings of the various religious traditions—Hinduism, Buddhism, Taoism, Judaism, Christianity, and Islam—might inform the way we think about human nature, personality development, psychopathology, therapeutic change, and the practice of psychotherapy. I found myself agreeing with Campbell (1975) who suggested that the principles and values of the great world religious traditions are "recipes for living that have been evolved, tested, and winnowed through hundreds of generations of human social history" (p. 1103). I was led to conclude again that perhaps there *is* much that behavioral scientists and psychotherapists can learn from the world's great religions.

I was also reminded as I read this book that the intellectual genealogy of many of the secular theories of psychology and psychotherapy can be traced, in part at least, to the teachings and philosophies of the world's great religious traditions. Unfortunately, the secular theorists of the past century have omitted what matters most in the teachings of the world religions; namely, that humans are spiritual beings. As expressed by my colleague Allen Bergin:

> the human spirit, under God, is vital to understanding personality and therapeutic change. If we omit such spiritual realities from our account of human behavior, it won't matter much what else we keep in, because we will have omitted the most fundamental aspect of human nature. With this dimension included, our ability to advance psychological science, professional practice, and human welfare can truly soar. (Richards and Bergin, 1997, p. xi)

I appreciated *Religious Theories of Personality and Psychotherapy* because it did not leave the spirit or soul out of the spiritual psychologies it described.

I appreciated that the book clearly illustrated the fact—often not recognized by clinicians—that psychotherapists' metaphysical worldviews and values have a major influence on how they do therapy. Psychotherapists' theoretical orientations, treatment goals, assessment methods, interventions, and evaluations of therapy outcome are all ultimately grounded in and influenced by nonempirical assumptions and values about the nature of the universe and deity, human beings, ethics, death and suffering, spirituality, and the purpose of life (Bergin, 1980; Browning, 1987; Jones and Butman, 1991; Richards and Bergin, 1997; Slife and Williams, 1995; Tjeltveit, 1989). *Religious Theories of Personality and Psychotherapy* made this clear by explicitly linking spiritual worldviews and values with implications for personality theory and the practice of psychotherapy. I hope that in the future more books about personality theory and psychotherapy will do this— including those based on naturalistic and atheistic assumptions.

In conclusion, I have long believed that as the implications of the various religious worldviews are more fully understood and appreciated by behavioral scientists, new theories and therapeutic approaches will emerge that will contribute to the progress of the science and practice of psychology. *Religious Theories of Personality and Psychotherapy* is valuable because it articulates new and revised views of personality theory and psychotherapy that are explicitly grounded in religious worldviews. I hope that the spiritual theories of psychology and psychotherapy described in this book will be applied, empirically tested, and further developed in the years ahead. I believe that as this occurs, these theories will contribute to the progress of science and practice and enhance the ability of behavioral scientists and psychotherapists to understand and work sensitively and effectively with all sectors of the human family.

P. Scott Richards, PhD
Professor of Counseling Psychology
Brigham Young University
Provo, Utah

REFERENCES

Benson, H. (1996). *Timeless healing: The power and biology of belief.* New York: Scribner.

Bergin, A. E. (1980). Psychotherapy and religious values. *Journal of Consulting and Clinical Psychology, 48,* 75-105.

Browning, D. S. (1987). *Religious thought and the modern psychologies: A critical conversation in the theology of culture.* Philadelphia: Fortress.

Campbell, D. T. (1975). On the conflicts between biological and social evolution and between psychology and moral tradition. *American Psychologist,* 1103-1126.

Jones, S. L. (1994). A constructive relationship for religion with the science and profession of psychology: Perhaps the boldest model yet. *American Psychologist, 49,* 184-199.

Jones, S. L., and Butman, R. E. (1991). *Modern psychotherapies: A comprehensive Christian appraisal.* Downers Grove, IL: InterVarsity.

Kelly, E. W. (1995). *Religion and spirituality in counseling and psychotherapy.* Richmond, VA: American Counseling Association.

Miller, W. R. (1999). *Integrating spirituality into treatment: Resources for practitioners.* Washington, DC: American Psychological Association.

Richards, P. S., and Bergin, A. E. (1997). *A spiritual strategy for counseling and psychotherapy.* Washington, DC: American Psychological Association.

Richards, P. S., and Bergin, A. E. (Eds). (2000). *Handbook of psychotherapy and religious diversity.* Washington, DC: American Psychological Association.

Shafranske, E. P. (Ed.). (1996). *Religion and the clinical practice of psychology.* Washington, DC: American Psychological Association.

Slife, B. D., and Williams, R. N. (1995). *What's behind the research? Discovering hidden assumptions in the behavioral sciences.* Thousand Oaks, CA: Sage Publications.

Tjeltveit, A. C. (1989). The ubiquity of models of human beings in psychotherapy: The need for rigorous reflection. *Psychotherapy, 26,* 1-10.

Worthington, E. L., Jr., Kurusu, T. A., McCullough, M. E., and Sanders, S. J. (1996). Empirical research on religion and psychotherapeutic processes and outcomes: A ten-year review and research prospectus. *Psychological Bulletin, 119,* 448-487.

Preface

Since the 1994 edition of the *Diagnostic and Statistical Manual* (DSM-IV), the American Psychiatric Association has regarded spiritual issues as distinct and legitimate concerns that may warrant the attention of mental health practitioners providing services, and particularly to religiously oriented clients. A number of books have appeared within the last decade to help clinicians address these issues respectfully and competently in the context of psychotherapy. The publication by the American Psychological Association of several of these books reflects a significant change in the Zeitgeist in the profession of clinical psychology in particular. It is no longer taboo to explore spiritual concerns and religious issues within psychotherapy, nor is being religious considered evidence of maladjustment either de facto or de jure.

Addressing spiritual concerns that emerge in psychotherapy is only one of the ways in which religion and psychology may be related. At a theoretical level, the psychology of religion has been a long-standing academic discipline devoted to understanding the psychological dimensions, origins, and consequences of religion and religious phenomena such as the experience of conversion. In this approach, religion is considered the object of psychological study, and the relationship is unidirectional—from psychological theory to religious topics.

Another kind of relationship between psychology and religion is to reverse the direction of dialogue, and to search for religious concepts and principles upon which to construct a psychological theory of personality and psychotherapy. This approach is also unidirectional, but in this instance, the movement is from religious perspectives to psychological topics. Some attempts have been made to derive a theory of psychotherapy from a single religious tradition. Few attempts have been made to place in dialogue theories of personality and psychotherapy derived from a variety of religious traditions. That is one of the general purposes of the present book. Six major religions are presented: Hinduism, Buddhism, Taoism, Judaism, Christianity, and Islam. The contributors were asked to comment on the relation they envision between their own tradition and other traditions in the context of psychotherapy. The book concludes with a chapter on the points of convergence and divergence among these approaches, not as a final comparison, but as an invitation to further dialogue that is vital in an increasingly heterogeneous population of both religiously committed clients and clinicians.

A second purpose of this book is to show how a religious theory of personality and psychotherapy can inform clinical practice. Contributors to this book were all invited to provide a case formulation of the identical clinical case, and to make recommendations about intervention strategies assuming the client was identified with the same spiritual tradition as the contributing author. Readers will find an enlightening array of spiritual and therapeutic strategies to consider in their work with individuals identified with any of these major spiritual traditions.

A third general purpose of this book has been to illustrate how professional psychologists have attempted to integrate their personal identity anchored in a particular religious tradition with their professional identity as a licensed psychologist. The contributors sought to answer the question of how they relate their spirituality or religion with their professional clinical practice. None of the contributors would describe themselves as either expert theologians within their tradition, nor as spokepersons for the singular way their tradition construes personality and psychotherapy. There is considerable variety in each of these traditions, just as there are numerous approaches to psychotherapy. All of the contributors have struggled with this issue, and much wisdom is to be gained by hearing their formulations, even though we might disagree with one or more of them on both religious and psychological grounds.

The general purposes of this book suggest that it is written primarily for mental health professionals and for clergy of various faith traditions who seek to relate religion and psychology, or spirituality and psychotherapy. A second audience is academic instructors and students in undergraduate and graduate courses on religion, cross-cultural studies, personality, counseling, and psychotherapy. If readers are awakened to the compassionate wisdom found in both their own and other spiritual traditions relevant to understanding what it means to be a person and how mental sufferance can be ameliorated, they will have taken a significant step toward the kind of ecumenical dialogue the contributors have illustrated in this book. Although there is no greater compliment than imitation, our readers are encouraged to formulate their own unique integration of religion and psychology as it pertains to personality theory and psychotherapy practice.

Acknowledgments

The contributors of this volume wish to thank their mentors, colleagues, families, students, and clients for the wisdom they have shared, and especially the inspiring mediators who founded the spiritual traditions that give meaning to both their personal lives and professional service. We are also grateful for the expert work done by the Haworth editorial staff, and particularly by our Senior Production Editors, Peg Marr and Dawn Krisko.

Introduction

R. Paul Olson

OBJECTIVES OF THIS BOOK

In addition to the general purposes stated in the preface, this book has four specific objectives. First, to encourage readers to explore religious traditions for constructs to use as building blocks in a theory of personality.[1] What are some of the ideas expressed in religious anthropologies that address personality structure, personality dynamics, human development, and individual differences? A second goal is to explore religious theories of transformation and healing relevant to the purpose, process, and practice of psychotherapy. What accounts for human suffering and maladjustment? What are the explicit or implicit views of health and the models of personal transformation? What is the religious vision of the good life toward which psychotherapy might be directed? A third goal is to indicate the variety of spiritual/religious interventions that can serve as therapeutic procedures to help ameliorate human suffering and to promote human growth. The fourth goal is to provide, in a single volume, a variety of views from diverse religious traditions, which are presented in a manner that facilitates comparisons and encourages respectful dialogue.

Many of the contributors to this book are in full-time clinical practice. They are clinicians committed to one of several spiritual traditions, but none claims the expertise of a professional theologian or spiritual director. All have selected from their spiritual traditions seminal ideas and guiding principles that make sense to them as practitioners dedicated to relieving psychological distress and to promoting personal growth in their clients. The selections are uniquely their own and should not be considered as either comprehensive or official representations of spiritual tradition, nor are the selected themes what other devotees might choose to emphasize. For example, this book is not a comparative study of the personal or social ethics advocated in various religious traditions, nor is this a book on either the philosophy or psychology of religion.

As practitioners, they share a desire to explore and express the ways in which spirituality or religion is relevant to their professional lives. Consequently, the selections of religious concepts have been motivated by practical concerns. All contributors have sought to illustrate resources within their own tradition for understanding the human suffering their clients have experienced, and to give meaning to both their professional experiences and personal journeys. Moreover, they have sought constructs within their own traditions, which help to understand the purpose and process of psychotherapy, and they have highlighted spiritual strategies that have therapeutic benefits. In short, they believe there is an important relationship between mental and spiritual health.

As practicing clinicians and/or educators, each contributor has articulated a pragmatic spirituality. They have related their spiritual psychologies to issues of human development, to coping with the stress of life, to mental health, and to ultimate concerns as they influence personal strivings and adaptive functioning. Each chapter expresses one form of what may be considered generically as a psychology of ultimate concerns.[2] Each is an application of spiritual wisdom and insights to both ultimate and practical questions that emerge in counseling and psychotherapy.

Although their paramount concerns are practical, the contributors affirm that in principle it is possible to construct a religious theory of personality and psychotherapy in such a manner that it leads to hypotheses that can be tested empirically. Researchers will find numerous hypotheses implicit within the discussions of concepts and principles. Thus, another reason for presenting these theories is to stimulate research in spiritual psychology by acquainting readers with the rich conceptual resources within a variety of spiritual traditions, East and West.[3] Just as Hood and colleagues (1996) encouraged researchers to examine constructs embedded within spiritual traditions in order "to enliven the psychology of religion,"[4] so the contributors to this book wish to encourage researchers to look to spiritual traditions for the development of theories of personality and psychotherapy in order to enrich clinical and counseling psychology. The primary focus, however, is upon the practical application of religious anthropologies to the assessment and treatment of clinical problems. It is this practical emphasis that led to the selection of a common clinical case to illustrate how respective religious theories of personality and psychotherapy might yield a heuristic case formulation, a valid explanation of therapeutic change, and relevant treatment strategies.[5]

UNDERLYING ASSUMPTIONS

There are several underlying assumptions evident in this book. First, spirituality is an integral and unifying dimension of human experience, not a realm limited to either special "spiritual" occasions or to particular "religious" locations. Second, psychological theories of personality and psychotherapy can be informed and guided by spiritual wisdom in such a way that the relevance of a spiritual principle to the psychosocial dimension of experience is demonstrated without compromising its truth or distorting the reality it references in the spiritual dimension. Third, spiritual insights can be related to psychological constructs and procedures without compromising the integrity of scientific psychology, either in terms of its content, methodology, and basic assumptions, or in its applications to clinical practice. In one way or another, the contributors have claimed the relevance of the spiritual dimension to their daily clinical practice while maintaining their loyalty to the scientific corpus of clinical and counseling psychology. Fourth, for religiously committed professionals, psychological theory may be evaluated in part according to the principles, concepts, and values expressed in their religious tradition. Moreover, a religiously oriented psychologist should not be expected or required to endorse concepts, values, principles, or procedures contrary to his or her deeply held religious convictions and ethics. Nor should religiously oriented students be forced underground in clinical training programs through the not-so-benign neglect of their agnostic or antireligious professors. Fifth, human experience is a multidimensional unity. People experience life in not only biopsychosocial dimensions, but also in spiritual, moral, and historical dimensions. Insofar as clinicians strive to understand their clients as unique individuals, they must appreciate the distinctiveness of each dimension and their interrelationships as they are unified dynamically within a whole personality structure and in a concrete personal life. The particular emphasis of this book is the spiritual dimension as it relates to personality theory and to the theory and practice of psychotherapy.

A basic conviction shared by the contributors is that in order to understand what it means to be a person and to comprehend the experience of human healing, a theologically informed model of personality and psychotherapy is needed, which is rooted in one or more of the world's spiritual traditions, in addition to being grounded in contemporary empirical research.[6] Collectively, the contributors present several forms of a spiritual psychology or *a religious-scientific psychology.* For individuals whose identity is anchored exclusively in either religion or science, it may seem like an oxymoron to speak of a spiritual psychology, and especially of a religious-scientific psychology. Theologians may object that it amounts to a reduction of religion to its therapeutic function, while psychologists may protest a compromise of scientific principles such as verifiability through experimental methods.

The contributors have dual allegiances to both scientific psychology and to their spiritual traditions, yet without the distressing conflict or compartmentalization one might expect. Each one has articulated a unique synthesis of his or her own spiritual tradition with psychological theory and clinical practice. These integrations have been created by professional psychologists who are both seasoned clinicians and practicing devotees of the spiritual tradition they represent. By agreeing to have their views published, the contributors have joined many other colleagues who have "come out of the closet" over the last decade—religiously committed professional psychologists, who refuse to be forced to choose between their religious worldview and spiritual life versus their commitment to scientific psychology and clinical practice. Eastern spiritual traditions have taught that dualistic thinking of this sort is one of the major causes of human problems, and has taught clinical experience that such "either/or" dichotomies lead to impaired problem solving.

SEPARATION OF PSYCHOLOGY AND RELIGION

Nonreligious psychologists will consider this whole approach as foreign to the secular, scientific orientation they learned in graduate school. Even more strange for them is the turn to ancient wisdom and spiritual sages for insights into the human condition to inform personality theory, and for principles of constructive change to inform psychotherapy. After all, neither Krishna, Gautama Buddha, Lao-tzu, Moses, Jesus, nor Muhammad was a graduate of an APA-approved program in either clinical, counseling, or educational psychology. Most of them had no advanced education beyond their own religious training, and were they living today, it is unlikely that they would be admitted to a psychology doctoral program because they lacked the prerequisite bachelor's degrees and basic courses in scientific psychology. Moreover, most of these spiritual geniuses spoke foreign languages, which would be an obstacle to obtaining an American education in psychology. Furthermore, these mediators of the spiritual dimension of life lacked the professional credentials expected of practitioners today. None of them ever took the EPPP exam, hence they would not be licensed to practice. Nor did any of them achieve diplomate status with the American Board of Professional Psychology. (But then, neither did Freud, Adler, or Jung.) The titles they did receive seem strange to agnostic and atheistic psychologists: prophet, seer, sage, lord, charismatic, holy man, *hasid,* spiritual teacher, master, guru, rabbi, miracle worker, exorcist, or healer.

By contemporary academic standards, these founders of religious movements had unsuccessful or unimpressive careers—no publications in refereed journals, no promotions to full professor, no academic honors as distinguished and tenured members in a research-based program at a prestigious university. Judged by contemporary professional criteria, these charismatic figures seem to be unlikely sources for psychological insights and concepts. Finally, the worldviews expressed by these prophetic sages are both religious and prescientific, and seem to be incompatible with the scientific, biopsychosocial model that dominates our post-Enlightenment, postmodern world of secular psychology.

In light of some of these criteria, and based on other principles and/or prejudices, it is understandable that at a theoretical level, psychology as a discipline has resisted relating with any religion except as the latter is an object of psychological investigation. After all, psychology defines itself as the science of behavior, not as a metaphysic of the soul. Neither is psychotherapy the same as spiritual direction.[7]

An implicit norm evident in these observations is that psychology and religion ought to be separate. This *separatist point of view* is expressed in two versions: dualistic and reductionistic.[8] In the first version, psychology and religion are considered separate, but equal in their respective domains; in the second version, they are viewed as separate and unequal, hence the authority of one is reduced by the dominance of the other. The psychoanalytic, behavioral, humanistic, and cognitive revolutions in psychology are characterized by a common tendency to reduce the spiritual dimension of experience to psychic derivatives, to behavior, feelings, or beliefs, or to ignore it altogether as irrelevant, if not superstitious or irrational. The recommendations for separation in both versions are usually grounded in an overemphasis on the points of divergence between psychology and religion. These are real differences in methods, content, sources, attitudes, and assumptions. We shall not foster genuine dialogue between psychology and religion by denying or ignoring their differences.

Convergence As a Basis for Dialogue

In addition to several differences, there are also several points of convergence,[9] and increasingly, psychologists are recognizing that the separation of the psychological and spiritual dimensions of life is neither possible nor desirable if the goal is to advance psychology as an authentic human science of the whole individual. The Achilles' heel of scientific psychology has been that the unity and uniqueness of the human individual has been fragmented or oversimplified in various specialties within the discipline.

In attempts to relate these two disciplines, neither the domination of psychology by theology (under the guise of "integration") nor the domination of theology by psychology (as in the psychology *of* religion) has proven satisfactory, any more than their continued separation and mutual indifference. A *dialectical relation of continual dialogue* is recommended here as an alternative mode of interaction. Stated another way, the points of both divergence and convergence between psychology and religion suggest that at a theoretical level (a) complete separation between these two disciplines is neither necessary nor possible, (b) they cannot and should not be unified into a single discipline, and (c) a greater degree of rapprochement between these disciplines is both possible and desirable. This dialogical relation between psychology and religion is illustrated in this book.

APOLOGETIC FUNCTION OF THEOLOGY

Implicit within each chapter is the common view that *theology must be engaging:* it must answer the questions raised by the contemporary situation. In the present period in which a therapeutic interpretation is salient,[10] a dialogue between theology and clinical psychology is crucial. Theology must be genuinely concerned with psychological interpretations of human experience, and insofar as these interpretations have implications for our understanding of self and the world, theology has both the right and responsibility to address them.

Among the psychological topics that theological anthropologies need to address are explanations of the structure and dynamics of personality, theories of human development, individual differences, psychopathology, and theories about the purpose and process of psychotherapy. Significant questions raised in the current situation by psychological theories of personality and psychotherapy include: What does it mean to be a person? What does it mean to say that an experience is therapeutic?

Theological anthropologies must attempt to answer these psychological questions if they are to fulfill their apologetic function and to avoid being judged as irrelevant by the professional, psychological community. Moreover, they must address these questions by providing normative descriptions that can inform and transform psychological understandings without dominating or controlling them. To encourage this mode of dialogue, each chapter has been structured by psychological categories or topics. The contributors have been asked to indicate how their own theological anthropology addresses each of these categories essential to a comprehensive theory of personality and psychotherapy.

CRITICAL THEORY AND A METHOD OF CRITICAL CORRELATION

Each contributor presents a *critical psychological theory* of personality and psychotherapy. A critical psychological theory recognizes that theories of psychotherapy assume and promote a basic vision of the nature of the world, the purpose of life, and principles by which life should be lived. By "critical" is meant that their theories are both descriptive and prescriptive, both objective and normative, both empirical and philosophical.[11] Clinical psychologies cannot avoid a philosophical and ethical horizon, and for this reason we need to be self-conscious and explicit about the ontological premises, epistemological assumptions, and principles of moral obligation that undergird and shape our theories of personality, psychopathology, and psychotherapy. Theories of psychotherapy serve counselors and clients alike as practical systems of moral philosophy. They are not simply detached, scientific theories grounded solely in objective, empirical research. A variety of religious traditions can broaden the philosophical horizons of clinical psychology and contribute to the development of integrative psychotherapy based on an interdisciplinary perspective.

The approach taken here illustrates one aspect of a *method of critical correlation*. In this method of relating psychology and theology, both disciplines are considered as credible sources of both relevant questions and meaningful answers.

> The conclusions expressed in psychological theories that are based on scientific research raise questions of a theological nature. And as expressions of religious experience and convictions, theological answers raise psychological questions. By ensuring that both disciplines perform both functions of raising questions and providing answers.[12]

This method encourages genuine dialogue between them as discrete disciplines without sacrifice of their unique sources, content, or methodologies. *Religious Theories of Personality and Psychotherapy* provides a variety of spiritual answers to psychological questions about the structure, dynamics, and development of personality, and about individual differences. In addition, psychological questions about the purpose and process of psychotherapy and mechanisms for producing constructive change are answered from diverse spiritual traditions. By providing theological answers to psychological questions, the contributors demonstrate the relevance of religious anthropologies to the disciplined inquiry of scientific psychology.

Religious anthropologies have implications for understanding the biological, psychological, and social dimensions of human experience. Both theological anthropologies and psychological theories of personality address the question of what it means to be fully human. Authentic personhood is a common focus, hence there is a basis for dialogue between psychology and religion in terms of personality theory. Moreover, both spiritual traditions and scientific psychology, especially clinical and counseling psychology, are cognizant of the diverse manifestations of human distress and alienation. Whether construed as mental disorders, problems in living, manifestations of sin, or as illusions of separateness, both disciplines provide theories about the etiology of human suffering. In addition, both address the nature and purpose of healing, articulate its processes, and recommend strategies for constructive change. Both spirituality and psychotherapy are concerned with personal transformation, and both function as effective media of change. Finally, both involve the transformation of personal goals and life meanings, and both can contribute to enhanced well-being through increased personal integration.

Pluralism and Constructive Relations

The religious anthropologies presented here are both diverse and enriching because of their unique content, illuminating constructs, and their visions of both human being and ultimate reality. Just as there are multiple theories of personality and psychotherapy in psychology, so it should not be surprising to discover *pluralism in religious anthropologies*. Each contributor has placed his or her spiritual tradition in dialogue with psychological topics addressed in theories of personality and psychotherapy. Each manifests a unique type of spiritual psychology. Implicit within all of them is the notion that an interdisciplinary approach is desirable and fruitful in an effort to understand what it means to be a person and why and how people suffer and change.

One type of *constructive relation* between these two disciplines and dimensions of experience is to utilize spiritual wisdom as a source for creating psychological theories from which one can deduce hypotheses to be tested using scientific-methodologies, both quantitative and qualitative in nature. The spiritual psychologies in this book illustrate a constructive relationship between psychology and religion as one of the modes of interaction that has been advocated.[13] The contributors have provided several heuristic concepts from their respective spiritual traditions to inform and reform psychology as a truly human science that appreciates the spiritual dimension of human experience. Nevertheless, by looking to their spiritual traditions for insights and strategies for personal change, none of the contributors has rejected his or her training in the science of psychology.

The contributors acknowledge their indebtedness to the growing number of individuals who have taken seriously this challenge of engaging psychology and religion in a dialogue within the context of psychotherapy in a manner that preserves the uniqueness and independence of each discipline, while fostering their *creative interdependence*. There has been a gradually increasing membership in Division 36 within the American Psychological Association for psychologists interested in religion, a division that was unfortunately renamed to reflect the academic subspecialty called the psychology *of* religion. A number of professional associations and journals have existed for some time, which are either interdisciplinary, such as the Society for the Scientific Study of Religion, or which encourage the integration of psychology with a particular religious tradition, such as the *Journal of Psychology and Theology, Psychology and Judaism, Tricycle: The Buddhist Review,* and *Islamic Social Sciences*. Within the last five years, the American Psychological Association has published four volumes devoted to models for relating psychology and religion in clinical applications, though primarily with Western religious traditions.[14] It would seem that the taboo of talking about the relationship between one's spirituality and professional life has been gradually eroding.

Clients As Teachers

Many clients suffering from mental disorders construe their experience in religious terms as a spiritual struggle for redemption, enlightenment, or union with ultimate reality. Americans in particular express an increasing influence of religion in their lives, and a heightened sensitivity to spiritual concerns. For many people, spiritual aspirations and religious practices make life meaningful and valuable, enjoyable and purposeful. Their spiritual disciplines contribute to their psychological well-being and enable them to cope with life's daily hassles and deeper tragedies. Their ultimate concerns give order to their personal strivings, transform their work into a calling, sanctify their family life, and motivate them to struggle for social justice.

Spiritual goals, beliefs, and practices are central in many people's lives. Although somewhat dated, a national survey in 1989 revealed that nearly two-thirds of Americans reported that religion plays either an important or very important role in their lives.[15] Moreover, empirical research on motivation and personality has revealed that spiritual strivings are the content of the personal goals for many individuals.[16] Spiritual convictions and religious affections can be, and often are, powerful influences on cognition, emotion, motivation, and behavior. Consequently, to understand their clients, clinicians need to appreciate the spiritual dimension of their clients' experiences.

An increasing openness to spirituality has been evident among clinicians who have become aware that while psychological explanations of human behavior and change provide answers to some questions, such as how thoughts influence behavior, nevertheless, psychological theories do not address other relevant questions that arise in psychotherapy. These other questions address religious issues of ultimate concern, that is, *spiritual concerns*. These include such questions as the meaning of one's suffering and the purpose of life, expressed poignantly by the depressed, suicidal patient, but also by many other clients as they reflect upon the relationship of their present condition to their values and personal strivings. Their struggles for psychological well-being raise questions about the nature of happiness, the good life, and what it means to live a purposeful life of real worth. Basic values and commitments are involved in ethical decisions such as whether or not to marry or divorce, to have or to end an affair, to relocate one's family for the sake of career advancement, to place one's child in a special education program or in a residential treatment center, to pursue aggressive treatment for one's cancer, and so forth. In their search for sources of courage and hope, many clients affirm the relevance to their lives of spiritual truths and insights grounded in both historical revelations affirmed by their faith community and in their personal religious experiences. These are all matters and questions of meaning and values, faith and hope, and involve the risk of personal decision. These types of questions are addressed in religious theories of personality and psychotherapy illustrated within this book.

ORGANIZATION OF THIS BOOK

Religious Theories of Personality and Psychotherapy begins with this introduction and ends with a chapter on divergence and convergence among these religious theories of personality and psychotherapy. Suggestions are provided for further dialogue, motivated by a genuine respect for religious pluralism and by the desire for a mutually enlightening reconciliation.

To facilitate comparisons among the religious anthropologies presented, all *chapters* consist of the following nine sections:

1. An introduction to the spiritual tradition including its historical context, major themes, sacred scriptures, and a summary statement of some of its defining characteristics.
2. The religious theory of personality, including concepts and metaphors related to personality structure, dynamics, and development, and individual differences.
3. The religious theory of the symptoms and etiology of distress, suffering, or pathology.
4. The religious theory of therapy, including the ultimate purpose recommended, and the mechanisms of change salient to its process.
5. The procedures and techniques recommended to facilitate change.
6. An evaluation of the religious theory based on both theoretical criteria and empirical studies.
7. Points of dialogue with other religious anthropologies and with other selected theories of personality and psychotherapy.
8. Reflections on an identical case.
9. Reference notes.

This common outline provides a structure that facilitates comparisons among theories in terms of both general areas and specific topics. As the chapter subheadings appear on the table of contents, the reader can find relevant sections in each chapter to compare and contrast theories on particular topics.

About the Contributors

A few words *about the contributors* are in order by way of introduction. They vary in their professional roles and work settings, in their theoretical orientations to personality and psychotherapy, in their preferences for treatment strategies and modalities, and especially in their personal perspectives on spirituality and religion. Although they find their root metaphors for life in different religious traditions, they share a common respect for the spiritual dimension of human experience, and a desire to relate the anthropological and therapeutic wisdom of their spiritual traditions to their psychological interpretations of personality and to psychotherapeutic practice. They have also shared a common struggle to articulate this relationship in a meaningful way.

Although spiritually oriented, none of the contributors can be labeled as "otherworldly." Neither are they soft-hearted as opposed to hard-headed. All are empirically oriented insofar as they take human experience as both a source of knowledge and wisdom, and the arena in which the truth and value of ideas are tested. But their primary laboratory is located in clinical settings, not in ivory towers nor in animal mazes. It is human experience and behavior they seek to understand and heal through their interdisciplinary inquiry. They believe that their religious anthropologies express empirical and practical approaches, and they strive for a reasonable faith to help them interpret and change human behavior.

The contributors all hold advanced degrees in the discipline of psychology, and they have prepared for their professions by being grounded in the corpus of scientific psychology. They acknowledge dependence upon psychological theories and research as sources to guide empirical approaches to clients and endorse the research methodologies of their discipline. They strive to apply an approach to their work with clients of the kind one would expect from a scientist-practitioner or from a professional psychologist, thus none of the contributors rejects the psychological moorings of his or her professional identity and clinical practice. They are decidedly psychologists by background, education, identity, and chosen profession.

Many clients construe their suffering in spiritual or religious terms. Their interpretations of their distress and its causes take a spiritual form and their personal strivings reflect ultimate concerns. Moreover, several clients seek resources within their faith tradition to help them cope with their distress. Confronted increasingly with religiously oriented clients, clinicians have concluded that while heuristic, the *biopsychosocial model* that informs their discipline and profession is incomplete. Attention to the spiritual dimension of a client's experience is not only relevant and fruitful; in some cases it is necessary to establish a therapeutic bond and to help the client cope and function with greater equanimity. Consequently, a common theme implicit in each chapter is that psychotherapy is not merely a secular, psychosocial experience. Nor can its nature or purpose be comprehended solely by the dominant biopsychosocial model. Rather, each contributor suggests that spiritual insights about the human condition and about processes of change are relevant to psychological theory and therapeutic practice.

Methodological Comments on the Clinical Case

A theory of personality and psychotherapy is related to clinical practice through the medium of a clinical case formulation. A case formulation organizes descriptive information coherently and comprehensively while leading to prescriptive recommendations tailored to the unique needs of an individual client. Thus, a case formulation serves as a bridge between theory and practice.

To ensure a practical application of their spiritual psychologies, each contributor agreed to provide a formulation of an identical published case. The only variation is that the client is presumed to be identified with the contributor's spiritual tradition in order to illustrate freely and fully the salient concepts and approaches derived from that tradition.

The case selected is the analysis published by Madill and Barkham (1997) of a forty-two-year-old, married, employed, Caucasian woman suffering from a major depressive episode.[17] Discourse analysis was applied to a particular theme identified by the authors from transcribed sessions of psychodynamic-interpersonal therapy.

The method of *discourse analysis* applied in this case formulation seems to be a variant of linguistic analysis.[18] In this approach, the central concern is the meaning of statements, which is determined by asking about their function in a particular linguistic and social context. The question addressed is not whether the statements are true, but what their functions are relative to accomplishing some specific human purpose. Consequently, a case formulation is commended primarily in terms of its usefulness ("fruitfulness"). A useful analysis also provides a coherent interpretation or explanation. Absent from the evaluation criteria for the validity of the discourse analysis is whether in fact the interpretation represents what really occurred in this case. Is the explanation of this woman's change a true interpretation? Is there another more accurate interpretation of why and how she improved?

Although rejection of any dogmatic claim to one true understanding of the process of change in psychotherapy is commendable, the author's pluralistic view of truth and reality does not prevent one from claiming that a particular interpretation may be relatively more true than another interpretation of the actual change experienced. In fact, Madill and Barkham (1997) commend discourse analysis over a developmental model of change based on stages of assimilation. Nor does a pluralistic view necessitate abandonment of the criterion of validity as a true or accurate representation of the reality described and interpreted. Stated negatively, an explanation may be both useful and coherent, but simultaneously a false account of the real processes of change in psychotherapy.

For example, the authors commend their discourse analysis on the grounds that it explains both broad patterns in, and microsequences of selected statements from the transcribed therapy interview. In particular they claim that "the pattern of *subject positioning* in the theme studied here offered a means of understanding variations in description identified across some of the sequences."[19] To wit, the concept of "dutiful daughter" helped to explain why the client's self-reference as a "damaged child" and her perception of her "bad mother" were alluded to obliquely in early therapy sessions but more directly later in therapy.

This analysis, however, seems no more useful or coherent than alternative explanations, nor does it necessarily reflect more accurately what the client actually experienced during the course of therapy. One alternative interpretation will illustrate this point. A phenomenological-humanistic theory of the therapeutic process provides an account for the movement from oblique references to more explicit self-references made by the client later in therapy. Based on their analyses of transcribed therapy sessions, humanistic psychologists such as Carl Rogers have noted that clients experience change in psychotherapy in terms of both their focus and the manner of their self-expression. The movement described is from an initial focus upon matters external to oneself, with feelings and personal meanings not owned or accepted, and construed as past objects or as experiences remote from the self. Thus it is predictable that a client would make oblique allusions to core issues at the beginning of therapy until a therapeutic relationship is established. As this relationship is experienced in the course of client-centered therapy, the client focuses more upon one's present experiences and communicates more directly, openly, and freely what one is feeling here and now. There is an increasing sense of one's self as a real subject and as a responsible and effective agent of action. In a therapeutic relationship, one explores, experiences, and expresses oneself more immediately by trusting one's changing feelings and personal meanings, and using them as a referent for effective choice of new ways of being. One's self-concept becomes more congruent with one's actual experience and/or with one's self-ideal.

This phenomenological and interpersonal interpretation of the change process seems more useful and at the same time more real and experiential than the interpretation provided by discourse analysis. The latter emphasizes the cognitive domain of meaning as the mechanism of change evident in the client's uses of language. Phenomenological theory appreciates the role of personal meanings in the change process and adds the affective domain experienced in an empathic, therapeutic relationship. This is not to say that the therapeutic condition of empathy is merely the reflection of feelings; rather, empathy is an accurate understanding of the client's perceived meanings *and* associated emotions.[20] Discourse analysis does not seem to grasp that meanings experienced by clients are *felt*-meanings, just as their emotions are meaningful feelings.

Moreover, phenomenological theory adds the unifying *concept of the self* viewed from the client's internal frame of reference, which appreciates the client's subjective experience as an intentional subject and agent of decision and action. A phenomenological analysis seems more true to the internal psychological processes as the client experiences and expresses them, but which discourse analysis seems to reject as "internal mechanisms of change hidden within the client's head."[21] In short, discourse analysis seems to be *unnecessarily abstract* and an *excessively cognitive* representation of the client's experience of change in therapy.

Even if one adopts a linguistic analysis as a basis for a clinical case formulation, the diverse uses of language allow one to include *religious language* as a way of construing the change this woman experienced in psychotherapy. Religious language has multiple functions, as the authors of the chapters in this book reveal. The *moral* function is emphasized in the view of religious statements as recommendations for a way of life. Religious language expresses the *conative* (volitional) domain as an intention to act in specific ways (with compassion) or it declares a commitment to a way of life. A *motivational* function is evident in religious language that functions to encourage commitment, to inspire hope and action, or to motivate one to alter one's existential orientation toward others, self, and God based on ultimate convictions and concerns. Religious language also functions to *express* and *evoke* feelings of awe and reverence, and *inspires* courageous acts of love and justice.

Several of these functions of religious language can be applied to describe changes in one's inner life in *noncognitive domains.* An appreciation for the affective and conative domains particularly would complement the more cognitive focus of discourse analysis upon the culturally available meanings adopted by the client and expressed in her "social positions" as a dutiful daughter or damaged child. Indeed, religious meanings and identities are among the culturally available meanings to clients, as subsequent chapters in this book will indicate. One may affirm the relevance of these noncognitive functions of religious language for understanding therapeutic change while also affirming the cognitive functions of religious language related to its claims about what is real and true.

Discourse analysis of clinical cases seems comparable to the procedure of *redaction criticism* in New Testament studies.[22] Both approaches attempt to determine the meaning intended by the one who writes or speaks, through careful attention to the structure and content of the language used. The approach amounts to a microanalysis of short, selected statements (an "extract" in discourse analysis) or biblical text (such as a "pericope") in the context of a more complete work understood in terms of the client's/author's purposes and the social-historical context in which it was produced.

A crucial question relates to the *method and criteria used for selection* of the short statements or text. The discourse analysis applied in this clinical case extracted dyads from taped interviews. In all cases, the dyad was defined as a therapist statement followed by a client statement,[23] although only five of the fifteen extracts reported actually included therapist statements. By contrast, a phenomenological analysis of the client's experience of change requires more than the selection of transcribed statements of therapist-client dyads as in discourse analysis; it requires the study of a whole sequence of transactions before, during, and after a change event occurring in therapy.[24] At the very least, an analysis of triplets (statements by the client-therapist-client) seems essential to assess changes in the client's processing level from the first to second client response as a function of the therapist's statement.[25] Apart from that sequential analysis, it seems difficult to incorporate therapist effects as an independent variable in a process analysis.

The final methodological observation relates to the outcome measures. Support for the validity of discourse analysis would have been more convincing if the changes in meaning analyzed from transcribed extracts were assessed and correlated with *appropriate outcome measures* of changes in the same cognitive domain of meaning. The major outcome measure reported was reduced severity of depressive symptoms on the Beck Depression Inventory. Moreover, of the ten presenting problems that constituted the Personal Questionnaire, weekly ratings assessed only the severity (the degree to which each problem bothered the client during each prior week). Finally, the scale used to measure severity was both a unidimensional and unidirectional scale with numerical anchor points of one ("not at all") to seven ("extremely severe").[26]

The criticism here is twofold: (1) the qualitative changes in meaning presumed to occur in the process of change were not assessed in pre-post measures to document change in this cognitive domain of meaning as the active ingredient or cause of change (or even as a correlate of change); (2) the measures of change in the client's perception (meanings) of her problems were unidimensional (severity) and unidirectional (linear). Many linguistic terms have several connotative as well as denotative meanings. The content of their meaning depends upon their usage and context. Moreover, human thinking is more aptly described as dialectical reasoning than demonstrative reasoning,[27] and the concepts employed are not simply unipolar, but often bipolar. Consequently, bipolar measures of changes in meaning seem more appropriate for assessing change using discourse analysis. A bipolar measure of meaning is the Semantic Differential.[28] Pretest and posttest administrations can be used to assess changes in meaning as function of therapeutic interventions. The Semantic Differential can be applied within sessions to assess client meanings prior to and after change episodes initiated by either the therapist or by the client.

These general methodological comments are intended to provide the reader with some sense of the diversity that is possible in clinical case formulations. The linguistic and phenomenological analyses cited in this introduction are illustrative of only two approaches. In the chapters that follow, the contributors will provide alternative case formulations that are also viable, persuasive, and relevant to understanding the nature and origins of clinical disorders (in this case depression) and that guide treatment planning.

NOTES

1. The terms "religious" and "spiritual" are used interchangeably as adjectives describing the spiritual dimension of human experience. While it is common to distinguish the two in terms of institutional versus individual expressions, most people express their spirituality through their religion (though not exclusively in an organized religion), and most religions include a spiritual theology and provide spiritual direction about ultimate concerns such as the meaning of being, the nature and purpose of life, and how it ought to be lived.

2. Emmons, R. (1999). *The psychology of ultimate concerns: Motivation and spirituality in personality.* New York: Guilford Press.

3. A few relevant resources for researchers are Corcoran, K. and Fischer, J. (1987). *Measures for clinical practice: A sourcebook.* New York: The Free Press; Hill, P. and Hood, R. (Eds.) (1999). *Measures of religiosity.* Birmingham, AL: Religious Education Press; Kazdin, A. (1998). *Research design in clinical psychology* (third edition). Boston: Allyn and Bacon; Ogles, B., Lambert, M., and Masters, I. (1996). *Assessing outcome in clinical practice.* Boston: Allyn and Bacon.

4. Hood, R. W., Jr., Spilka, B., Hunsberger, B., and Gorsuch, R. (1996). *The psychology of religion: An empirical approach* (Second edition). New York: Guilford Press, p. 198.

5. The published case was presented and conceptualized from the perspective of discourse analysis by Madill, A. and Barkham, M. (1997). Discourse analysis of a theme in one successful case of psychodynamic-interpersonal psychotherapy. *Journal of Counseling Psychology, 44* (2), 232-244.

6. The term "theological" is used generically here to refer to the intellectual reflections and formulations within any given spiritual traditions. Consequently, we may refer both to nontheistic theologies (Buddhist and Taoist) and to theistic theologies (Jewish, Christian, and Muslim). In this usage, the term does not presuppose a theistic worldview.

7. To help draw the distinction, the following definition is offered: spiritual direction is (a) a professional helping *relationship* in which (b) one person provides spiritual *guidance* (c) to enhance and encourage the spiritual *healing* and spiritual *formation* (growth) of another (d) through the experiential learning process of spiritual *discernment* of ultimate concerns, and (e) through the practice of spiritual *disciplines,* (f) which lead to a more reconciled life with self, others, and ultimate reality, experienced and expressed in wisdom, courage, compassion, and gratitude.

8. For discussion of the rationales for these separatist positions, see Olson, R. (1997). *The reconciled life: A critical theory of counseling.* Westport, CT: Praeger, pp. 31-38.

9. See Jones, S. L. (1994). A constructive relationship for religion with the science and profession of psychology. *American Psychologist, 49* (3), 184-197; Olson, *The reconciled life,* pp. 38-43.

10. Reiff, P. (1987). *Triumph of the therapeutic: Uses of faith after Freud.* Chicago: University of Chicago Press.

11. Browning, D. (1987). *Religious thought and the modern psychologies: A critical conversation in the theology of culture.* Philadelphia: Fortress Press, pp. xi, 5, 238, 242-245. As a basis for a normative theory of psychotherapy, Browning advocates a "limited theism" and "ethic of mutuality."

12. Olson, *The reconciled life,* p. 54.

13. Jones, S. L. (1994). A constructive relationship for religion with the science and profession of psychology. *American Psychologist, 49* (3), pp. 184-197. Jones observed there was a relative dearth of psychological theories constructed from religious concepts and principles. This volume is one attempt to help fill the gap and to illustrate a constructive relationship between psychology and religion.

14. Shafranske, E. P. (Ed.) (1996). *Religion and the clinical practice of psychology.* Washington, DC: American Psychological Association; Richards, P. S., and Bergin, A. E. (1997). *A spiritual strategy for counseling and psychotherapy.* Washington, DC: American Psychological Association; Miller, W. R. (1999). *Integrating spirituality into treatment.* Washington, DC: American Psychological Association; Richards, P. S. and Bergin, A. (Eds.). (2000). *Handbook of psychotherapy and religious diversity.* Washington, DC: American Psychological Association.

15. Gallup, G. H., Jr. and Castelli, J. (1989). *The people's religion: American faith in the 90's.* New York: Macmillan. A more recent reference is Balmer, R. (2001). *Religion in Twentieth-Century America.* Cary, NC: Oxford University Press.

16. For a summary of this research, see Emmons, R. (1999). *The psychology of ultimate concerns: Motivation and spirituality in personality.* New York: Guilford Press.

17. Madill and Barkham, Discourse analysis of a theme . . ., pp. 232-244.

18. For a discussion and critique of linguistic analysis as applied to religious language, see Barbour, I. (1966). *Issues in science and religion.* New York: Harper Torchbook, (pp. 243-252).

19. Madill and Barkham, Discourse analysis of a theme . . ., p. 241.

20. In his theoretical article, Carl Rogers defined empathy as an ability to "perceive the internal frame of reference of another with accuracy and with the emotional components and meanings which pertain thereto as if one were the person, but without ever losing the 'as if' condition" (p. 210). Rogers, C. (1959). A theory of therapy, personality and interpersonal relationships as developed in the client-centered framework. In S. Koch (Ed.) (1959). *Psychology: A study of a science* (Vol. 3). New York: McGraw-Hill, pp. 184-256. Another book on this topic is Bohart, A. and Greenberg, L. (1997). *Empathy reconsidered: New directions in psychotherapy.* Washington, DC: American Psychological Association.

21. Madill and Barkham, Discourse analysis of a theme . . ., pp. 242, 243.

22. Redaction criticism is distinct from both form criticism and literary criticism by virtue of its focus on the relationship between form and content, the significance of structure or form for meaning, and its appreciation for the capacity of language to direct and to mold experience. Perrin, N. (1969). *What is redaction criticism?* Philadelphia: Fortress Press, p. vi.

23. Madill and Barkham, Discourse analysis of a theme . . ., p. 233.

24. Rice, L. and Greenberg, L. (1984). *Patterns of change.* New York: Guilford Press, p. 20.

25. See Sachse, R. (1990). Concrete interventions are crucial: The influence of the therapist's processing proposals on the client's intrapersonal exploration in client-centered therapy. In G. Lietaer, J. Rombauts, and R. Van Balen (Eds.), *Client-centered and experiential psychotherapy in the nineties.* Louvain, Belgium: Leuven University Press, p. 297. The author presents three options and two scales for assessing client-therapist-client triads.

26. Madill and Barkham, Discourse analysis of a theme . . ., p. 233.

27. Ryclak, J. (1981). *Introduction to personality and psychotherapy: A theory-construction approach.* Boston: Houghton Mifflin, pp. 6-9.

28. Osgood, C., Suci, G., and Tannenbaum, P. (1967). *The measurement of meaning.* Champaign, IL: University of Illinois Press.

Chapter 1

Hindu Psychology and the *Bhagavad Gita*

Asha Mukherjee

INTRODUCTION

Basics and Philosophy of Hinduism

The origin of Hindu religion dates back to at least 6,000 years ago when the Aryan race first immigrated to India through the Himalayas. Another controversial view strongly supported by many scholars, on the basis of excavated evidence (mentioning the *Vedas*) from two ancient cities *(Harappa* and *Mohanjodaro),* dates the origin at 31,000 years ago.[1]

Despite some confusion that Hindus appear to worship many different Gods, it is clear to Hindus that all of them are not gods but *devatas* (deities),[2] and understood to be aspects or roles of the "one Absolute" or God.[3] The Hindu trinity are *Brahma*, the creator; *Vishnu*, the sustainer; and *Shiva*, the destroyer of evil and the agent of positive change. Any of the trinitarian deity's names are often used to refer to the one God. The context determines the reference to either the Almighty or to one specific deity.

Hinduism affirms a monistic worldview of one universal reality. The Supreme Soul *(Param-Atman* or *Brahman)* is the one absolute. *Brahman* dwells within all individuals as *atman.*[4] All souls originate from the Supreme, consist of the same divine substance, and eventually reunite with their original source. The "right" time for such spiritual merger varies for each individual soul.

Brahman (the Almighty or the Supreme Spirit), conceptualized as the ideal image in human mind of a possible superior being, includes the culmination of all human values and denial of all human frailties. Scriptures have defined *Brahman* as the cause and fate of all creation.

The highest level of spiritual purification or "perfection" (perfection here means enhancement, not the abnormal obsessive-compulsive notion of perfection) is a definite qualification for such blissful union. When a soul has become spiritually cleansed almost to the level of the Supreme Soul, it is rewarded by eternal freedom from pain and troubles of life on earth as it reunites with God. This eternal merger leads to ultimate, unimaginable bliss and peace and the person is free from the struggles of the physical life governed by karma. Karma denotes the principle that each soul reaps what it has sown in its past through many different lifetimes or rebirths.[5]

Karma is actions as related to consequences. The term can be understood in literal and broad ways. Literally, it means that good and bad actions of the present lifetime of an individual bring him or her good and bad experiences in the next life upon rebirth. A second scientific meaning is that a cumulative log of all each person does in a lifetime is automatically influential, due to universal natural laws, in determining what is deserved in the future. The idea is similar to "one gets out of life what one gives to it" or "what goes around comes around." A third possible and psychological meaning can be that selfish actions have the automatic probability of regret, grief due to loss of control over circumstances, depression, and guilt provided the individual has a conscience. A fourth, much broader meaning is that the society reaps the results of its people's actions over a much longer period. Actions of religious and social reform leaders create better patterns and new laws in a society. Further, if all humans were to perceive a unity of the universe and identify with each other strongly, the birth of a person in the future would be as good as a person's own symbolic rebirth.

Removal of all past bad *karma* leads to purification and the individual soul attains *nirvana* or *moksha,* which is eternal freedom from the pains and anxieties of cycles of rebirths.[6] A second meaning is purely psychological, i.e., appropriate detachment from the worldly temptations and a divine connection (attachment) with the Almighty while living in the human form. Such a human being is known as *Jeevan-mukta* (liberated during life).

"Sense enjoyments" are enjoyments through the five physical senses well beyond the physical needs of the body, for instance, addictions. "Material pleasures" are due to tendencies to dwell on concrete and monetary gains at the cost of mental and spiritual accomplishments, e.g., obsession about collecting money. These pleasures based on physical and material aspects are seen as obstruction in the path of development and enhancement of spirituality in the Hindu perspective. Therefore, those with physical and material focus lose out in the spiritual area and those with spiritual focus experience little interest in the physical and material aspects of life.

Heaven is conceptualized as the first place between this world and the ultimate blissful union with *Brahman.*[7] It is a place for souls who are spiritual but still wish the pleasures more than ultimate freedom. Their wish is granted as reward for good karma. They go to heaven after death due to accumulation of good karma.[8] They go to heaven after death due to good karma but return to earth when such good karma is exhausted, in a manner analogous to depleted funds in a bank account. Reborn in a new body and family, one must collect a new account of good and bad karma all over again.[9]

Brahma-loka is the second abode for the souls who no longer have a wish for sense enjoyments/material pleasures. They do not return to earth; instead they remain in *Brahma-loka* undergoing further spiritual enhancement needed to merit the divine merger with the Supreme Soul *(Brahman)*. It is not possible for any soul to have no bad karma at all due to the natural human tendency for attachment and emotional dependence. The temptations of the senses are immense in earthly life; even an accomplished *yogin* (a soul at the stage of highly advanced purification) can at times succumb to them.[10] The symbolic *Jeevan-mukta* view holds that one suffers during one's life on earth for bad karma. This constitutes an answer to the question "Why do the good suffer." This view does not accept the theory of reincarnation or physical rebirth.

The process of spiritual purification and enhancement is called yoga.[11] Yoga entails a clear understanding and diligent effort. Believing that he or she had accomplished complete mastery over all his or her senses and mind, the *yogin* may be involved in self-deception. This is a trap of overconfidence and a sign of "egoism," the enemy of spirituality. A popular illustration is the story of the devout soul who had almost reached the divine merger point when, on his deathbed, he was caught unaware by the sight of a luscious berry on a tree branch, and experienced the long forgotten desire for the pleasure of its taste. It is noteworthy that this *yogin* was neither hungry nor thirsty nor in need of any nutrition, but he experienced a pure desire for the pleasure of its taste. The sage did not go to *Brahma-loka,* was reborn to enjoy the fruit, and his merger took place only then. The story suggests that one ends up getting one's wish, until sufficient fulfillment of the sense occurs. One can be detached only after basic satisfaction of the physical needs. All needs must be satisfied and after that one must rise above undue attachment to substances not truly needed.

The sincere wish, genuine effort, and renunciation of physical and material temptations in a wholehearted manner, bring about eternal freedom.[12] Slacking, pretending, and trickery do not work with the all-pervading and all-knowing[13] *Brahman. Brahman* is kind in the sense of rewarding quality effort but also is the pure principle of truth and justice, hence is uncompromising in terms of concessions for inappropriate attitudes and conduct.[14] This is the "firm" discipline of a "well-wisher" rather than a harsh, punitive attitude.

Yoga expresses the concept of the union of the finite with the infinite or the union of the human being in his or her physical form with the formless God. The significant belief of yoga is revealed as the supreme secret in the thought that man is tomorrow's God and God is today's man. Further, yoga is simultaneously humanized and "divinized" because it creates a connection between human and divine aspects. The literal meaning of the word yoga is (to "yoke") to unite the soul with God.

Any constructive action harmless to others and helpful to at least some people or some human cause can qualify as yoga. Therefore functioning in the appropriate role as a wife or parent is yoga. Popularly recognized types of yoga are work, knowledge, devotion, meditation, practice, renunciation, service to others, doing one's duty or dharma, sharing wealth, and actions honoring and supporting "truth" and "justice." Thus ethics are built into dharma and yoga.[15]

Of the previous *yogas,* four are most popular, namely, work or *Karma-yoga,* knowledge or *Jnana-yoga,* meditation or *Dhyan-yoga,* and devotion or *Bhakti-yoga.*[16] All four condone the practice of charity and involve renunciation of the fruit of one's actions.[17]

All types of yoga are different paths to Self-realization.[18] Spiritual achievement through yoga is like trying to reach the mountain peak: travel from any direction, by any method, and, eventually, one arrives at the peak, as long as movement is upwards and forward. People can begin with a preferable type of yoga and later add on several others for greater benefits.[19]

Central to the *yogas* is the concept of the self. The self is not another term for the conscious ego, "self-image," or "self-concept"; rather self refers to the *atman* in the *jiva,* which is perpetually connected with the universal Self (*Brahman,* the Absolute or the Supreme Soul).[20] The essence of the Self is already in every self or being in its pure, natural form.[21] The usual worldly attachment makes it tarnished as silver is, with lack of use and impact of the environment. Removal of "tarnish" of attachment and ignorance shows the clean shiny metal of the self, the essence of *Brahman* in its true glorious form.

In each being, the self is separate from both body and mind. The Self is present in all life forms and in inert objects and matter. Inert matter is a latent, potential energy form of *Brahman.* This is supported by the scientific fact that matter merely changes form (is not destroyed), in the transformation or conservation of energy.[22]

The term "Self-realization" expresses the awareness of the identification with *Brahman* and the understanding that the higher spiritual values and principles are inherently present in humans, i.e., they are there as potential waiting to be realized.[23] Another name for Self or *Brahman* is *Sat-chit-anandam.* It translates as a combination of *sat* or good, *chit* or mind and *anandam* or joy.[24] The *yogas* connect directly with these three aspects in the form of *Karma-yoga* (yoga of work) for *sat* or good; *Jnana-yoga* (yoga of knowledge) and *Dhyana-yoga* (yoga of meditation) for *chit* or mind; and *Bhakti-yoga* (yoga of devotion) for *anandam* or joy of attachment with *Brahman* or the Almighty. The balance of all three is spirituality. Thus yoga constitutes the bridge between the Almighty and humans.

The concept of the abstract Self involves the notion of the formless Supreme Spirit.[25] It may be conceptualized as a set of principles of cosmic organizations that comprise *Brahman,* not one being in a specific form, such as a deity. These principles are in operation all the time, sometimes visible and sometimes not. They are not to be perceived by the senses but to be realized internally and experientially through peaceful inner-concentration (meditation).[26] This is the primary goal of meditation. The resulting fulfillment involves peace, bliss, and contentment. It appears as though removing attention from the "details" and "major parts" is a prerequisite to focusing on the "whole." Rorschach's perceptual test of inkblots is based, in part at least, on this principle. It is the balance of all three that is necessary.

Background of the Bhagavad Gita *Message*

The *Bhagavad Gita* is a portion of the *Mahabharata.* It enjoys a very special identity and existence as an independent volume of sacred scripture. Translations of the original Sanskrit version have been made in many languages all over the world attempting to clarify the vital message of a harmonious philosophy of life that benefits the individual and the society simultaneously. A brief account of the historical background of the *Bhagavad Gita* follows to clarify the context.

Prior to 800 B.C., India was not one united country. Instead there were many territories, each ruled by a king. The oldest son of a king was always the automatic heir to the throne. One such territory in northern India faced a challenge when the oldest son happened to be blind. An exception to the rule became necessary and therefore the oldest son, *Dhritrashtra,* was passed over in favor of his younger brother, *Pandu.* However, *Pandu* passed away early in life, when his sons were still too young to take over the rule. The kingdom had to be managed by their grand uncle until the oldest prince came of age.

When *Pandu's* first born grew to adulthood and the community began to prepare for the coronation of *Pandu's* oldest son, an objection arose from *Dhritrashtra's* sons who claimed the throne due to a feeling of rivalry, on the premise that their father had been the original rightful heir. There was confusion among the leaders as to which firstborn prince was the true inheritor of the royal throne. *Pandu* and his sons (the *Pandavas*) were known to be kind, adequate, appropriate, and noble principles, hence viewed by spiritual leaders as more suitable for the benefit of the community. By contrast, *Dhritrashtra's* sons (the *Kauravas*) were disliked for their selfish conduct.

This was a conflict between the preservation of moral and spiritual values versus the rigid and antisocial misuse of the tradition of hereditary succession to gain inappropriate power over the kingdom. Peaceful negotiations initiated by Lord Krishna and other nonviolent leaders failed, the conflict escalated because of the *Kauravas'* unreasonable resistance, and eventually war became unavoidable.

At the onset of war, *Pandu's* son *Arjuna,* a renowned, brave warrior with many past victories, discovered that all of the enemy army included his teachers, friends, cousins, and relatives. His attachment to them, based on many positive memories, brought about feelings of guilt about harming them in battle. Experiencing doubts about his role in the war, *Arjuna* felt guilt, anxiety, and panic, and viewed the war as unethical. He announced to his charioteer, friend, and guide, Lord Krishna, "I will not engage in battle!"

Lord Krishna discussed with *Arjuna* his confusion, his needs, society's needs, and the necessity for him to broaden his outlook to consider the benefit of the whole society, not just his own personal feelings. This discourse, recorded in the *Bhagavad Gita* states ways to (1) achieve an objective and spiritual view of life generally, and (2) attain equilibrium to make appropriate decisions in crises. As a result of his dialogue with Lord Krishna, *Arjuna's* confusion based in spiritual ignorance was removed. He became much more aware of the spiritual aspect of reality, and gained clarity of vision and conviction that not only was the war necessary but that his role in it was vital as both a warrior and a righteous man of his times. Thus, he was able to participate in the war with clarified goals, motivation, and undivided focus. His victory led to the establishment of good over evil at that juncture. The positive effects of this lasted for several hundred years in the society's conduct.

Cosmic/Universal Time Cycle

A *kalpa* is a very large unit of time including 10,000 cycles of four *yugas* each. The cycle of *yugas* is repeated only because conditions on earth deteriorate from the righteous days of *Sat-yuga* to the corrupt, violent times of *Kali-yuga.* A description of the ten divine incarnations and the four *yugas,* appearing within a cycle clarifies how this occurs.

Each creation or *kalpa,* including millions of years, is seen as creator *Brahma's* one day and each dissolution is equal to one night for Lord *Brahma.* Each *kalpa* has 10,000 cycles and every cycle consists of four *yugas* known as *Sat-yuga, Treta-yuga, Dwapar-yuga,* and *Kali-yuga.* Each cycle is completed in 4,320,000 years and within each cycle, Lord Vishnu, the sustaining deity, appears several times in mortal form to regulate the disrupted balance of good and evil in the world.[27]

Divine Incarnations

Through the cycle, from the beginning of *Sat-yuga* to the end of *Kali-yuga,* whenever spiritual deterioration reaches a peak, God appeared in the form of an earthly being to destroy evil and to establish righteousness. As a result life went well for a time; but when it deteriorated again, God needed to reappear in order to reestablish a higher level of spirituality in human life.

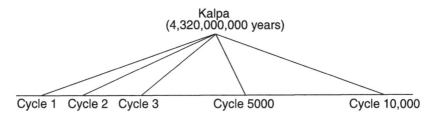

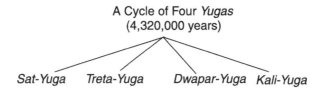

FIGURE 1.1. The Cosmic Time Cycle

Each such appearance of the divine spirit in physical form is known as a divine incarnation. This is the role of the sustaining deity Lord *Vishnu* and often these incarnations are called *Vishnu's* incarnations. The consistent goal of the divine incarnations is to give humans every possible chance to prevent total destruction of life itself.

Sat-Yuga

Humans first came into being on earth at a time of truth and goodness *(Sat)*. Conflict, tensions, and behavioral deviations from values were minimal. The individual and society were in a congenial balance; with needs of the majority being met, everyone was happy. The population was small and resources were abundant. It was an idyllic time suggested by the myth of paradise. Brahmins were the leaders of society during this era.

Treta-Yuga

Brahmin leadership was relinquished to Kshatriya leadership due to lack of physical and financial power among the Brahmins. Although they could preach great ideals and set examples with their own conduct, the vegetarian Brahmins lacked the physical capacity to enforce appropriate consequences for the inappropriate conduct of the deviant. The Kshatriyas were a muscular, hunting, and meat-eating group, with physical and financial powers. Conquering other territories through battles to increase their own prosperity was the norm for the kings. King Dasharatha was famous for his subjects' happiness and prosperity during his reign. High ideals were practiced, such as "truth at any cost," "honor a promise even at the cost of own life," and "justice for all."

Dwapar-Yuga

This is the Era during which Lord Krishna ruled. By this time, moral-social deterioration had reached a low enough point that unborn Krishna's parents were imprisoned by an evil king so that the newborn could be destroyed at once. The goal was to prevent materialization of religious forecasts that he would be the one to overcome the evil use of power. During this time the great war, *Mahabharata,* occurred due to the conflict about the rightful heir to the throne. Selfishness, greed, anger, deceit, and hurtful manipulations of others had become prevalent. The spiritual aspect was still present in a minority, but social life was under the physical control of the Kshatriya rulers. This was the righteous war to support the good against the evil.

Kali-Yuga

This is the last of the four eras. Lord Buddha is the divine incarnation of this era. He has set the first example of nonviolent and compassionate assertiveness. The previous eight incarnations were unable to escape use of violence when they worked for human welfare. Their ventures to great ends were not always through good means and their violence had to be justified by their goal to win against the evil. Although Krishna resisted it for a long time and improved the civilization's value to using violence only as a last resort, he could not avoid it. Buddha was the first incarnation that did not use

---

TABLE 1.1. The Ten Divine Incarnations *(Dash Avtar)*

1. *Matsya avatara* or Fish incarnation
2. *Kurma avatara* or Turtle incarnation
3. *Varaha avatara* or boar incarnation
4. *Vamana avatara* or dwarf incarnation
5. *Narasimha avatara* or incarnation as a being who was half human and half man
6. *Parashurama* in human form
7. *Rama* in human form Human
8. *Krishna* in human form
9. *Buddha* in human form Human (Buddha)
10. *Kalki* expected in Superhuman form in the future in the present *yuga* (*Kali-yuga*)

---

violence but instead used patience, tolerance, and compassion with those who acted against him. His own father could not understand his views and pressured him. However, Buddha was nurturant to all opponents while staying firm on his stand. He was able to emphasize the value of self-assertion in the most positive and therapeutic sense through the conduct of the monks who were his disciples. Violence was totally absent from their conduct. He was the most recent and the ninth incarnation.

However, leadership in this era is assumed by businessmen *(Vaishyas),* the group with focus on materials, and this is also the era of maximum spiritual decline. Material and nonspiritual ways are not only tolerated more; they are accepted as justified ways of practical living for personal advantage and material gain. Corruption is prevalent and selfishness is the norm rather than an exception. Violence is common, pain and suffering abound for the few spiritual folk, both physical and mental deteriorations occur in many to disrupt appropriate role function. Spirituality is reduced and humanity suffers with poverty, crime, violence, and disease.

The evolution pattern of the animal kingdom is represented in the divine incarnations.[28] Of the ten incarnations in each cycle of four *yugas,* the earlier animal incarnations were situational: they miraculously appeared at a time of crisis, remained for only moments necessary to complete intervention, and disappeared after their work was done. The appearance of each form was in response to the desperate crisis of the time and therefore the incarnation was appropriate for those needs. The later human incarnations lived a whole lifetime on earth, set appropriate examples of role function for all ages and aspects of life, acted as spiritual teachers and therapists, and also took care of crises.

The last of the divine incarnations, *Kalki,* is yet to occur in the future and is expected within the current era *(Kali-yuga).* He or she is anticipated to be the timely and super power to deal with evil in its mightiest form. *Kali-yuga*—the dark age: when spiritual illumination or awareness is lowest and evil ways at the peak. It is also foretold that this incarnation would be superior to the previous incarnations.

When all ten incarnations have completed their efforts and there is still evil in the world to make the good suffer, God acknowledges that the only way to eradicate evil and restore good, truth, peace, and congenial living, is to destroy the whole world. Since *Brahman* stands by the good, the victory of evil is prevented because it is simply not permissible.[29]

Sacred Scriptures and Primary Sources

The most important sacred scriptures include four *Vedas,* eighteen *Puranas,* and two classic historical epics, the *Ramayana* and the *Mahabharata.*

The *Vedas* were written first, with *Riga-Veda* being the oldest. All of the *Vedas* have supplements added at various times in history. The early portions contain concrete, academic information, collectively known as the Human Law. A second type of knowledge is abstract and philosophical, contained in the added-on portions called the *Upanishad* (all collectively called *Vedanta*). This is the Science of Life or the Divine Law.

The *Puranas* include eighteen main volumes and eighteen subsidiary ones, each telling short simplified stories to convey the values, ideals of social conduct, beliefs, standards of conduct, and rules.

The *Ramayana* written by *Valmiki* and the *Mahabharata* by *Vyasa* are two famous epics.[30] A portion of the *Mahabharata* is the *Bhagavadgit,* consisting of Lord Krishna's guidance to confused *Arjuna.* The *Bhagavad Gita* expresses the essence of the *Upanishads,* hence it is called "the fifth *Veda*" with reverence.

All scriptures and traditions of Hinduism emphasize a sense of unity among followers.[31] A Hindu living anywhere in the world would understand connection of all aspects of life with dharma. It is seen as a grand unity of worship, love, language, science, the arts, music, life, and religion: "religion is all of life, and life is all of religion. Hence the intensely intertwined mosaic of religion, music, poetry, dance, sculpture, architecture, and living itself in the Indian tradition."[32]

PERSONALITY THEORY

The *Bhagavad Gita* is a theory of psychotherapy. It assumes the personality theory described in the *Upanishads.*

Personality Structure

The individual is known as the *jiva* and the Almighty as *Brahman.* The human structure of personality involves three major layers: (1) the Gross layer, (2) the Subtle layer, and (3) the Causal layer.

The Gross layer is concrete, and is the result of nourishment consumed for survival. The physical body, sense organs, and motor activity mechanisms are included in this layer. It is as susceptible to environment as it is dependent on it due to vulnerability to damage (by poisons, disease germs, carnivorous beings, natural disasters, and developmental degeneration).

The Subtle layer includes the vital air sheath (connected with breathing, circulation, and utilization of oxygen for brain function), the mind (all natural mental actions and reactions), and the intellect (organized thought in connection with identity as in beliefs, values, and attitudes). The dynamics of the Subtle layer of personality are more abstract (attitudes, opinions, feelings, thoughts, ideals, and values), but it is dependent on the brain for cognitive operations, and on other physical features for communication with the environment.

The Causal layer is the deepest and the most subtle in human personality. It is universal and above the reach of all types of individual differences. Attachment and *maya* have no impact on it.[33] Further the Causal layer is purely spiritual and invisible to others, while the gross and subtle layers are observable either in form or action (thought, behavior, and speech are included as aspects of action).

The Causal aspect is representative of the Supreme Spirit that is eternal, omniscient, and omnipotent *Brahman.* "Consciousness" (meaning here is limited to spiritual awareness) is the universal soul or Self (in the form of *atman*) within the individual person *(jiva)*. Each being thus shares a constant bond or union with *Brahman,* the self or *Param-Atman.* Therefore the Supreme Soul/Self/*Param-Atman* or *Brahman* is the ocean and the individual soul/self/atman/*jiva* is similar to the drop of water within the ocean, in constant connection with its origin, Source, and permanent abode. The drop may jump up in the air once in a while, due to wind and wave formation but it soon drops back in the ocean where it belongs. Although momentarily up in the air, it is still a full-fledged representative of the ocean. We humans have a similar connection to the Supreme Spirit. The lifetime of the human being, in proportion to the universe, is akin to the relatively brief time the drop is up in the air. However, in contrast to the drop of water, the human has a capacity for awareness of own identity as similar to and in connection with the Supreme Spirit. The awareness of the Almighty and the connection with own self jointly form the concept of Consciousness or Self-realization.[34]

Self-realization or Consciousness is the awareness of the connection or unity of own self with *Brahman.* Without such recognition or awareness, there is little spiritual benefit of the divine affiliation. Although the presence of such Consciousness is subjective, the resulting higher level of spirituality is sensed and noted by others in compassion, selflessness, broad vision of welfare of all, and in positive leadership of peers.

The causal layer is also transcendental across many lives of the same individual. It is the only constant part of a soul that remains upon physical death and is reborn with a new body. Figure 1.2 shows the personality of the *jiva* in part "a," with connection to *Brahman* in part "b." The Gross layer is the largest signifying high quantity and low spiritual quality and the Causal layer is smallest in size but signifies enormous spiritual quality as it culminates in the life center. This is the spiritual aspect of the personality where *Brahman (O-U-M),* is in connection with *jiva's* life center (small but high in quality).[35]

These were derived from an adaptation. Therefore earlier references in the actual *Upanishad* (as shown in Table 1.2) are slightly different. Taitriya Upanishad includes only the food sheath *(Anna-maya)* in the Gross layer. The Subtle layer includes the vital air sheath *(Prana-maya),* the mental sheath *(Mano-maya),* and the intellect sheath *(Vijnana-maya);* and, the

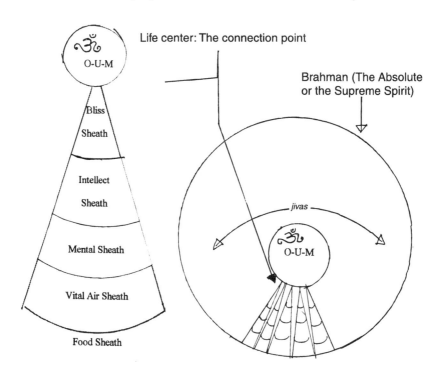

a. The internal structure
of an individual *(jiva)*

b. The view of Brahman's
connection with all *jivas*

Life center: The connection point

O-U-M

Brahman (The Absolute
or the Supreme Spirit)

Bliss
Sheath

Intellect
Sheath

Mental Sheath

Vital Air Sheath

Food Sheath

jivas

O-U-M

FIGURE 1.2. (a. and b.): The Basic Structure of Personality. *Note:* O-U-M
signifies *Brahman.*

causal layer includes only the bliss sheath *(Ananda-maya)*. Each sheath represents an area in which there is potential for attachment and illusions
(maya).[36] For instance, the food sheath *Anna-maya* is the potential for illusion or attachment related to physical nourishment.

The life center, in either interpretation, is not included in any sheaths or
layers of the body because it is *atman* (not a part of the body). But, it is in
close proximity to the body as a detached observer and immune to all
maya.[37]

The Gross and Causal layers are mutually exclusive, and the subtle layer
is "the middle man" trying to negotiate a balance between the others. For
physical survival, a minimum of material use is essential and this is spiri-

TABLE 1.2. Personality Layers and the Sheaths

1. The Gross Layer	a. The food sheath: the physical body including all its systems and the various physiological functions.
	b. Vital air sheath: the respiratory and the circulatory systems.
2. The Subtle Layer	a. The mental sheath: all reactions and tendencies of the mind and its potential for reactions.
	b. The intellect sheath: the organized thinking, memory, cognition, and evaluation (i.e., executive abilities).
3. The Causal Layer	a. The bliss sheath: the subjective experience of spiritual bliss attained through *yoga/s*.

THE LIFE CENTER: The *atman* in connection with *Brahman*.

tual, especially if it aids in role function, in leading others to spirituality, and in serving others. The sages and monks deny the gross sheath to a high degree for the enhancement of the Causal layer.

Personality Dynamics and Motivation

Instinctive motivation for basic survival belongs to the Gross layer of personality and the psychological motivation to the Subtle layer of personality. As components of the Subtle layer, the mental and intellect sheaths are implicated in personality dynamics.[38]

In the mental or mind sheath, thoughts and emotions are reactive, spontaneous, undisciplined, and constant. They occur automatically and continuously, similar to the flow of a turbulent with little inner stability. In addition, the mind has a strong inborn tendency to attach itself without discrimination.[39] The mental sheath of the younger child and infant has little organization. It is expressed in short attention span, distractibility, and fleeting emotions. By contrast, as a higher aspect of the subtle body, the intellect is regulated and focused. The intellect is connected to goals, guidelines, and values. Resolved issues create conclusions, decisions, and commitments, which help to settle a sense of identity by early adulthood. The older child, adolescent, and the adult all have an intellect developed to varying degrees. The infant may be viewed as having the inborn capacity to develop an intellect.

In optimal growth, the intellect of the healthy person is organized in a realistic, flexible, and meaningful balance of mental activities such as memory, emotions, thoughts, and a variety of cognitive abilities. These aspects are both stable and capable of being change consciously if further need of adjustment arises. This concept of mental organization for adjustment is akin to Piaget's notion of accommodation.[40]

The guiding principles of the personality become the source of motivation for change.[41] One who is at a low stage of development, is more likely to be motivated by the mind sheath. A person advanced in development motivated by self-regulating intellect.[42] When we notice exceptions to this pattern, we speak of a child "mature for her or his age" or an "immature older person."[43]

In Hindu philosophy, motivation is related to the following four human aspects: (1) the stage of intellect development, (2) identification with a sheath in self-concept, (3) inner positive self-control issues, and (4) awareness of the Causal body.[44]

Stage of Intellect Development

In the adult with a secure identity, motivation leads to more organized action, with "good reasons" (a rationale) behind it, and results in a sense of success and/or accomplishment. The success here is defined by the awareness and fulfillment of being "true to the values of one's own inner-self."

Identification with a Sheath in Self-Concept

One's self confidence or identity is a second motivational factor. The spiritually unaware individual's identity can be with the gross or mental sheath and the attraction to material wealth would define success as making money. With an Intellect-sheath identification, a person would focus on goals determined by different values.

Inner Positive Self-Control Issues

Despite good plans and noble intentions, when an individual is unable to follow through due to temptations, the problem may be of deficiency in inner control and/or a very low level of frustration tolerance. The socialization process provides opportunity and demands to develop frustration tolerance. It is not only desirable but almost essential to reduce the random mental activity and develop an intellect sheath. A child's motivation for parental affection, peer approval, and learning thus leads to the side effect of more mature interactions.

Awareness of the Causal Body

Awareness of the spiritual aspect within oneself, namely the bliss sheath, is another source of motivation. For example, a person aware of more creative and satisfying hobbies is likely to engage in such fulfilling activities. The lack of awareness focuses the person onto the lower level involvements, which can generate fear of failure/loss, and, after the fact, regrets and despondency.[45]

Personality Development

In Hindu anthropology, the personality development of the individual is governed by the joint impact of prevalent religious beliefs and cultural practices expressing these beliefs. Three important features with a strong influence are *Varna-dharma, Ashrama-dharma,* and *Kala,* the concept of time as per the cosmic time cycles and human-life time cycles.

The Sanskrit word *dharma* is from the root *"dhr,"* which literally means "to bear," "to carry," "that which supports," "that which upholds." Hence, *dharma* in broad sense is the cause of the maintenance of a society through law and order. In another personal way, it is the essential human nature, character, and need of affiliation to the group so that *dharma* determines the individual's duties to the society. Thus moral standards become working principles.[46]

Dharma is broad and inclusive, with laws applicable to "all that there is."[47] Recognition, acceptance, and respect for "all that there is" determined laws for how humans should think, emote, act; what they should believe, value, and decide; and how they should structure their personal and collective lives for meaningful survival. *Dharma* is the very foundation for human lifestyle. The *dharma* for various aspects is stated with a descriptive prefix and named *Samaj-dharma* (social religion), *Sva-dharma* (personal religion), *Ashrama-dharma* (life-span stage religion), and *Varna-dharma* (work-group religion). Religion is fully interwoven into all aspects of Hindu life at all times. A view of *Varna-dharma* and *Ashrama-dharma* in Tables 1.3 and 1.4, respectively, reveals their impact on personality development.

Varna-dharma has its source in tradition. Originally, the society's division of labor was structured in these terms. The boundaries were considered sacred but flexible and the groups intermingled, depending upon need. Kshatriyas included the kings and special higher level education Brahmin teachers were closely involved with the royal families. It was understood, believed, accepted, and encouraged that flexibility could meet individual as well as group-needs better. Later, social and political pressures resulted in a rigid caste system replacing *Varna-dharma.*[48]

The years in Table 1.4. for each stage are to be seen as flexible and approximate, allowing for individual variation, rather than rigid. At each stage, a person should have the appropriate attitudes, activities, and goals for the involved developmental tasks.

TABLE 1.3. *Varna-dharma* (Work Group Culture and Roles)

Brahmins:	(The priests, teachers, counselors/therapists): This group primarily worked with the human mind and spirituality through worship, learning, teaching, guidance, therapy, and enhancing own spirituality. Such work was seen as the noblest and the closest to *Brahman* (hence the name Brahmin), and they were the highest in the social-respect hierarchy. They were quiet, subdued, idealistic folk, with minimum material needs to exemplify "simple living and high thinking" in values and conduct.
Kshatriyas:	(The warrior and protection/guard group): Second only to Brahmins, this group was the physical power of the society, with protection/enhancement of the territory and protecting vulnerable individuals as basic responsibilities. Their mastery of battle skills was supported by their stronger, bigger builds. Their ideals were righteous battles and rewards in material enjoyment.
Vaishya:	(Trade/business group): Manufacture, sales, and development of industry for all utility items was their work area. This meant production of all non-natural materials and refinement and dispensing of natural materials.
Shudras:	(Physical labor/hygiene work group): This was the group responsible for all cleaning and hygiene-promoting duties and due to the nature of their work, alienated from higher-level mental activities.

Individual Differences

A product of many different factors, individual variations define the unique personality of each individual. Several features account for individual differences: heredity, environment, stage of life, highest-developed sheath level of the personality, current personality traits, application of aspects of *dharma,* and the individual's level of conscious effort. In turn, the individual's unique personality impacts future feelings, thoughts, actions, decisions, and accumulation of new karma. Despite these differences, the universal soul *(atman)* in all persons and at all stages, is the same because it is part of the one Supreme Soul, *Brahman.* Figure 1.3 lists several hereditary and sociocultural factors in relation to tendencies, differences, and combined impact.

Hindu psychology accepts many determinants of individual differences are a result of the interaction of two significant factors, heredity and environment. These factors are believed to take equal roles in the creation of individual differences. Life itself is viewed as a result of the creative union of nature and life force. Nature includes both heredity and environment and life force consists of motivation, energy, and creative action.

TABLE 1.4. *Ashrama-dharma:* Developmental Stages, Goals, Tasks, and Focus of Action

Time Span	Stage of Life	Goals/Tasks	Focus of Action
0 to 25 years	*Brahmacharya-Ashrama*	Grow, learn, and prepare future adult role as per own caste group	Get educated, develop and master skills, serve the *Guru* and exercise self-restraint
26 to 50 years	*Grihastha-Ashrama*	Marry, start family, and raise family	Attend to all aspects of the role of a spouse, parent, adult, and citizen
51 to 75 years	*Vanaprastha-Ashrama*	Gradually begin to detach self from family and get involved in society and spirituality	Give of own time and mental energy to the community in the form of help and guidance
76 to 100 years	*Sanyasa-Ashrama*	Withdraw totally from the material world, perform many *yogas,* and prepare for end of the physical life	Practice spirituality with serious efforts at Self-realization, meditate, and pray for divine merger

Individual temperaments are believed to occur with various combinations of three basic tendencies ranging from most to least spiritual: *Sattva* (good and truth), *Rajasa* (energy and activity), and *Tamasa* (ignorance and delusion). Although humans have all three basic tendencies, there is special affinity in each human for one of the three, i.e., the person's prominent tendency. Therefore, a person with primarily *Sattva* tendencies would have some *Rajasa* and *Tamasa,* but the last two would be smaller and with minimal focus.

The "ignorance" prior to spirituality is not of facts but about appropriate understanding and the right attitude by which to live life. The ancient Indian thinkers laid down four ideals for a moral life. These are, *artha* (material/financial prosperity), *kama* (desire for various enjoyment experiences),[49] *dharma* (satisfaction in righteousness), and *moksha* (the final liberation from the cycle of life). The spiritual progressive order of these ideals is from the grossest to the subtlest. These correspond with stages of human life as described in *ashramas* in Table 1.4. Known as "usual motives of human beings," the first is most important in the earliest developmental stage of growth and the last become meaningful in the senior years.

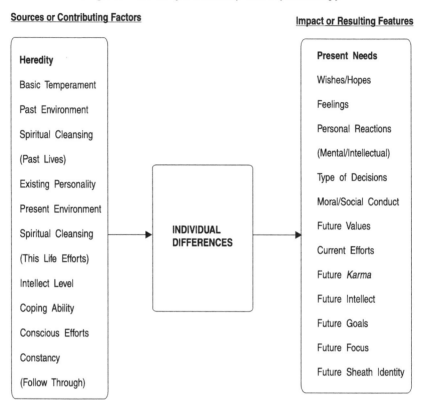

Sources or Contributing Factors   **Impact or Resulting Features**

FIGURE 1.3. Individual Differences: Source and Impact

The application of the meaning of "ignorance" to the adult population in general indicates that those lower in spirituality focus on the first two (financial prosperity and experiences of sense-related enjoyments) much more than those high in spirituality because they are the ones ready for *moksha* and have little interest in anything else. At this stage they renounce the world almost completely. Therefore, "ignorance" means lack of awareness of the higher-level human values. According to this definition, it is possible for an illiterate person to have such knowledge while a very learned (in terms of formal degrees and books) person may still be "ignorant" if his general behavior, beliefs and values reveal lack of awareness, absorption, and utilization of spirituality. This can be seen as a parallel to what we call "psychological sophistication" in those outside the profession of psychology.

Spiritual cleansing is a form of purification that occurs through sincere and conscious efforts and the practice of *yogas,* through the study of the scriptures and Saint's lives, and through *satsang* (company of serene, spiritual folk). *Yogas* are available, ranging from simple to complex, for all personality types and levels of intelligence.

In an abstract sense, "spiritual cleansing" involves getting rid of inappropriate conclusions and beliefs based on notions that are nonspiritual in terms of the unity of humankind (faulty and impractical cognitions, narrowness of perspective, limited to personal experience only, selfish, greedy, violent, noncompassionate, and personal attachment-based attitudes that limit empathy, team work, and perception of unity). The rules of cleansing recommended are physical cleanliness or *saucha,* general contentment or *santosha* (freedom from greed and hoarding materials), purifying action or *tapas,* individual study or *svadhyaya,* and focus on *Brahman* or *Isvara-pranidhana.*

In conclusion, many determinants play there, but the most important spiritual determinant is insight, upon which the role of all other factors becomes smaller in terms of impact. With insight and awareness, all enhancement follows naturally. Two stories illustrate the life changing aspects of spiritual insight. Due to a forecast in his horoscope that he might become either a mighty emperor or a world-renouncing saint, Prince *Siddhartha* was raised in a very sheltered royal environment. His father, being a full-fledged Kshatriya, had naturally preferred his son to be the future emperor. So from infancy, the prince was completely protected and kept ignorant of any unhappy or negative aspects of life. In early adulthood, he encountered by accident, the reality of others' illness, disabilities of old age, and death. Along with the experience of shock and confusion, he perceived the pleasures offered by wealth and youth as temporary illusions beyond human control. He developed compassion for human vulnerability and detachment for material goods. These experiences prompted a long spiritual search which led to enlightenment about the nature, causes, and remedy of human suffering. Due to his nonviolent and compassionate wisdom, in time Prince *Siddhartha* came to be known as the Buddha, founder of Buddhism. The title "Buddha" is derived from the Sanskrit words *"boadh"* (clear and appropriate awareness) and *"buddhi"* (wisdom).

The second story is of *Ratnagiri,* a highway robber, who killed for material wealth and was extremely insensitive.[50] Once as he shot a male bird, the intense, painful lamentations of the female bird awakened compassion in him that society had failed to uncover. With the sudden insight, he vowed to never hurt another being in any way. *Ratnagiri* became a religious devotee and sought spiritual counsel. As a result of his guru's guidance and spiritual practices, he later became Saint *Valmiki.* These stories of both *Siddhartha* and *Ratnagiri* illustrate that no matter how the person has lived before, once insight appears, no personality determinant or individual feature blocks

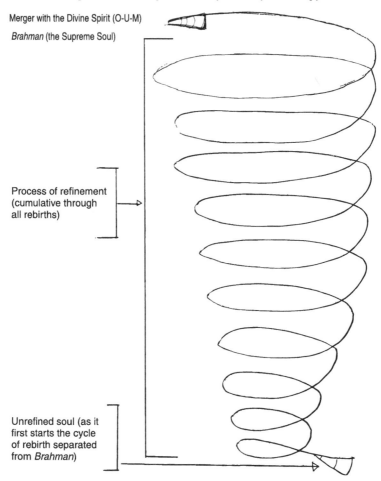

Merger with the Divine Spirit (O-U-M)

Brahman (the Supreme Soul)

Process of refinement
(cumulative through
all rebirths)

Unrefined soul (as it
first starts the cycle
of rebirth separated
from *Brahman*)

FIGURE 1.4. The Spiritual Evolution of a Soul Through Rebirths

spiritual growth and fundamental change. Such insight includes immunity
to illusions or maya as well as immunity to inappropriate attachments or
tendencies.

THEORY OF DISTRESS

The chief cause of distress in human life is ignorance or *avidya*. Lack of
education leads to inappropriate thoughts as well as inappropriate psycholog-

ical and perceptual sets. Ignorance leads to poor personal management of internal and external affairs. Rendered inactive and hidden by ignorance are three vital areas of life that promote health, happiness, and adjustment. These are truth *(satya),* nonviolence *(ahimsa),* and self-restraint *(brahmacharya).* Whenever the balance of these three important principles of conduct is absent or disrupted in a human mind, chaos occurs, resulting in distress.

The three major blocks to awareness are the three knots of the heart. "Knots" is a symbolic term meaning non-straightforward, complicated issues that cause tension, turmoil and lack of peace in the person. They represent conflict of instinct-based personal emotion with broader spirituality-based values of the intellect and higher level civilization. The conflict progresses, and sooner or later, causes distress. These knots of the heart are ignorance *(avidya),* desire *(kama),* and, action *(karma).* Ignorance leads to involvement and identification with lower level sheaths. Desire is a result of such identification, leading to a narrow outlook (related only to the senses of the body). When motivated by desire of an ignorant person, action is selfish, greedy, and contrary to the teachings of the scriptures about an appropriate balance between individual and societal needs. The result is distress because that is the only outcome they can yield.

Moreover, it is a natural function of desire to create attachment with sense experiences. This attachment creates illusions *(maya),* which denotes ideas and experiences divorced from "supreme reality." The net result is that desire, naturally insatiable, continually increases as one makes efforts to satisfy it and creating thereby more and more bad karma, the accumulation of negative merit from inappropriate actions. It is ignorance that designates satisfaction of desire as the ultimate goal; the goal leads to related actions; actions to temporary satisfaction and attachment so that the whole cycle must be repeated in order to become "happy." This is how one gets bound (addicted) to sense-related experiences. The sense experiences are not to be shunned or renounced but they are to be managed in an appropriate way and at appropriate times. Actions without spiritual rationale/intent are self-defeating behaviors and cause distress.

A person with a low level of intellect development is more vulnerable to turmoil of life's distractions and temptations. Conflicts and stress are common because one does not accept limitations, delays, or defeats. In modern terminology, the level of frustration tolerance and the ability to postpone gratification, to achieve long-term goals, is low in one with an underdeveloped intellect.

Being a part of *Brahman,* humans are naturally and essentially spiritual. The ignorance, desire, and inappropriate action are build-up of the material illusion that hides our own true spiritual self. Being confused, humans hunt for spirituality in books, religious institutions, and gurus when the potential for it is within us, right in our soul. Such behavior is very similar to a species of deer called *Kasturi mriga,* which wanders around looking for the source of the lovely fragrance everywhere while it carries the fragrance right in its own navel. Other metaphors are (1) a mirror covered with a dark cloth, and (2) tarnished silver. The illusion (dark cloth) must be removed in order for us to see our true image in the mirror. The silver dulled with tarnish does not shine even though its basic tendency is to reflect light in a brilliant manner. However, it has the potential to shine upon the removal of tarnish just as we have the potential to be spiritual upon spiritual cleansing and removal of ignorance.

Humans are vulnerable to distress when they are not in a state similar to that of the Supreme Soul. This occurs within the bliss sheath of experience The bliss sheath provides fulfillment because we are in our true form when in contact with own spirituality. The point is that removal of tarnish on the silver of our souls can free us from distress. Dualistic thinking is an example of such tarnish, the result of an ignorant (unhealthy) viewpoint, and cause of distress. Dualistic thinking is the rigid focus on the poles of a continuum as definitely separate and totally unrelated aspects. It completely ignores the shades of the gray variations in between the black and the white ends of the large continuum.

Dualistic thinking is opposite to the perception of unity. The totality or "oneness" of the continuum gets forgotten when the focus is on either end of the continuum. As a result, dualistic thinking obstructs the path of Self-realization, wherein the oneness of the human and the divine qualities are two ends of the continuum. The most important goal of Self-realization is against egoism. It is emphasized in the *Bahagavad Gita* that "I-ness" needs to perpetually reduce in a seeker until he or she perceives only *Brahman* in the identity of everyone else, her or his own self, and everything. Such identification counteracts dualistic thinking.

The nondualistic focus should be broad, that is, on the overall continuum rather than on polarities. Examples of dualities are good/bad, happy/unhappy, within/without, high status/low status, ugly/beautiful (based on physical appearance). If we alter these to make an effort to see the unity in any two seemingly opposite ideas, we would experience less distress. Analytical, dichotomous thinking needs to replaced by synthesizing, dialectic in order to make good decisions. In general, the practices of truth, nonviolence and self-restraint reduces distress. The recognition of the totality, unity, and universality of the all-pervading Supreme Spirit in every aspect of creation is encouraged by the scriptures: first, through an effort to see the Lord in all beings; second, to accept basic laws of nature in unity; and third, by promoting harmony with the universe. These strategies prevent and remove distress, give peace and bliss, and are harmlessly applicable in different cultures as well as over time. Without such Self-realization, distress is inevitable.

THEORY OF THERAPY

Purpose of Therapy

The goal of therapy is the removal of distress, confusion, and pathology. This requires a change in thought content, style, and process. Changes in thinking may occur as sudden insight due to an experience of intense impact, or slowly with the help of/exposure to a more enlightened human being, namely the therapist/the saint. In the absence of sudden insight, removal of distress becomes necessary through spiritual guidance.

Principles of Therapeutic Change

Five important principles of change are: (1) an emphasis on changes through awareness (spirituality), (2) awareness of unity for mental health, (3) awareness of environmental limits and impacts on human life, (4) the value of congeniality and cooperation, and (5) spiritual guidance toward a higher level of human civilization.

Emphasis on Changes Through Awareness (Spirituality)

The emphasis of Hindu psychology on changes in content, process, and style of thinking is even stronger than that of cognitively oriented forms of psychotherapy. Hindu psychology demands a more profound change in thinking beyond the intellect. It is within the spiritual realm that changes must occur. These changes involve a movement away from the conventional, dualistic, and superficial style and content, toward the deeper fundamental unity of all humanity, all experience and all reality, including the unknown, hard-to-accept parts of reality.[51]

Awareness of Unity for Mental Health

In the spiritually aware individual, other people are not viewed as separate entities, but as manifestations of the one being. The relationship of individual humans to ultimate reality *(Brahman)* is analogous to the millions of cells in the physical body all related to the living organism as a whole. Each individual cell may have different functions, areas, biological compositions, but in the last analysis, they are united in the organism as one whole entity. In a similar manner, each and every human being is a part of the one God, even though each one differs in many ways, and appears to be separate. Hence the statement: "You and I are not 'we,' you and I are one." This expression of unity applies to both one's relationship with God, and to relationships with others. This perception of unity and the associated universality in attitude and thinking foster cooperation, acceptance of mutual differences and rights, team spirit, unity, cohesiveness, congeniality, empathy, and compassion. Many of these features are indicative of progress in group psychotherapy for goals of both "growth" and "mental" treatment.

Awareness of Environmental Limits and Impact on Human Life

Early in human civilization, it was naturally possible to have the attitude of "live and let live," because we had not yet experienced the limits of our natural resources, and we could survive without conservation. Today, we have reached a point when the balance of supply and demand is the opposite. It took us "by surprise" because we did not know to watch for this before things went out of control. Competing for scarce resources, our adjustment has been to "divide and conquer." Such competitive attitudes are less conducive to mental health than cooperativeness, respect for mutual rights, and self-restraint.[52] The universal connection of all life is clear in the physical aspect, in terms of our environmental interdependence. The food chain, global warming, and a depleting ozone atmosphere are examples that threaten the survival of life on earth. At the psychological level, we are well aware that changes in one person have an impact on the other members of the family or group due to their relationships involving mutual dependencies and influences. When we overlook this, we create stress and conflict for ourselves and others.

Values of Congeniality and Cooperation

For mental health, a more universally responsible and positive adjustment seems to be needed to replace aggressive competition. We can deal with problems cooperatively and peacefully if most people make an attempt to perceive the totality, think of its survival and progress rather than a narrow view determined by the value of personal advantages. We can anticipate less discord, less violence, less tension and more cooperation with a broad concern for the welfare of all. A more egoistic perspective based on self-interests overlooks that if everyone is made secure, the individual is not neglected because he or she is included in the all.[53]

Spirituality As Guidance Toward a Higher Level of Human Civilization

With nothing constant in nature, a secure and stable context is provided for all those who must share the universe. Most forces of nature operate mechanically and cannot possibly act at cross purposes with other definite natural laws. Many animal species with less developed brains cannot go wrong either because of their natural, mostly instinct-dependent functioning. By contrast, humans have the complex problem of the freedom of decision, because the highly developed brain of this species depends the least on automated instinctual physical systems for regulating behavior. With the capacity to imagine as well as manipulate, humans have the capacity to disrupt the balance in the overall situation and act in self-defeating ways for their planet, their species, their particular national group, their community, family, and in their personal lives.

Therapeutic intervention illustrated in the *Bhagavad Gita* aims toward an unity and universality, which leads to consistent guidelines for decisions and actions. We can make a positive and creative difference in terms of social development, benevolence, and brotherhood through Self-realization. The *Bhagavad Gita* provides a yardstick for the creative, beneficial, and appropriate conduct. The author of the *Bhagavad Gita,* Lord Krishna, whether as the divine incarnation, or as the imaginative human leader, knew this wisdom a long time ago. However, it has been only understood and applied primarily at the individual level by very few people. Nor has a nonspiritual method been found to solve the problem. This is why saints, once they have the insight, take trouble to make others see the light. The goal of therapy is to gain such insight in order to restore understand this and restore intrapersonal and interpersonal states of mental health.

Therapeutic Principles Revealed in the Original Content of the Bhagavad Gita

Lord Krishna revealed to *Arjuna* the distinction between the lower sheaths and upper sheaths in a simplified form. He called the body, the senses, and the mind (gross sheath and the mind sheath) "the field" *(kshetra),* and the spirit or the soul (the Causal body) "the knower of the field" *(kshetrajna).* The goal was to help *Arjuna* perceive the "whole" and align with the spiritual through modification in his perceptions, beliefs, and attitudes.

Process of Therapy

The therapeutic process is an experience of heightened awareness brought about in the interpersonal context. The *Bhagavad Gita* describes *Arjuna's* distress and Lord Krishna's insight that the real cause of the predicament was *Arjuna's* ignorance of Supreme Reality. Today we believe that the therapist, who is one step ahead of the patient, facilitates the process of problem resolution. Lord Krishna's broader perception of reality appreciated both *Arjuna's* personal needs and the gravity of the impending war. Based on his greater perception of unity of personal and societal aspects, Lord Krishna sought to make *Arjuna* aware that the victory of evil would result in a society unacceptable to *Arjuna* and others. The holistic view included the negative impact of *Arjuna's* reactions on his army. Both the content of the therapeutic discourse and the therapeutic process were important.

Five elements of the therapeutic process can be inferred from the therapeutic encounter between Lord Krishna and *Arjuna.* These are: (1) stages of the process, (2) therapeutic attitudes, (3) therapeutic values, (4) fice considerations relevant to action, and (5) the value of flexibility.

Stages of the Process

Prince *Arjuna,* depressed, totally alienated from current social, moral, and spiritual realities but still in touch with objective physical and personal emotional realities, was in shock. His spiritual alienation had kept him from the reality that events had been leading to such a conclusion over many months, if not years. Although idealistic in attitude and tendency, he was staggered at the role-function dilemma posed by reality. Unable to face and attack reality, he gave up through withdrawal, avoidance, and in his depression, passively and unhealthily accepted prospects of self-destruction.

Lord Krishna seized the opportunity to help *Arjuna* address the reality of the situation before *Arjuna* left the battlefield. As a dejected, vulnerable warrior, *Arjuna* listened passively, and disinterestedly at first. Then he became more resistant, dogmatic, and argumentative. Lord Krishna engaged *Arjuna* in a discussion gently, yet firmly and confronted him with the demands of current reality in the context of his work-group ethics and his personal strengths. Krishna reminded him that an attitude of weakness did not become a brave warrior *(Kshatriya).* Arjuna's self-esteem was strengthened as his therapist made him more aware of his own strengths repeatedly.

Still far from awareness, *Arjuna* progressed from a stage of apathy to more active but negative participation, namely arguments. He resisted the change through a persistent "inability to understand" and repeatedly questioned the content despite his above-average intelligence. Lord Krishna patiently answered questions, but realizing that awareness had not come yet, he continued their dialogue.

Next, *Arjuna's* resistance involved anger as he expressed sarcasm and challenged Krishna's statements more directly. *Arjuna* expressed disbelief and criticism of apparent inconsistencies in Krishna's ideas, for which *Arjuna's* basis was superficial.

Finally, *Arjuna* made demands on the therapist for immediate and empirical demonstration of the truth of the imparted information. When proof was given, the fear of the magnitude and complexity of the "whole" overwhelmed him. Thereafter, he experienced humility and became aware of his own narrow perceptions and focus. His emotional reactions of fear and awe were overwhelming enough to interfere with his cognitions and inner balance. He graduated from recognition of what "should be" To "what is." But he was dazzled and threatened. *Arjuna's* therapist replaced pressure with gentleness, reassurance, sensitivity, and support, and provided relevant information to aid the cognitive reorganization and stability.

Throughout the three stages of the change, *Arjuna's* autonomy was respected by his therapist and he was permitted to return to his myopic view of life. *Arjuna* needed to find an appropriate balance of circumstances and values in order to adjust. The therapist practiced about required time for *Arjuna's* own pace. Although Lord Krishna was earlier urging *Arjuna* to "rise and engage in battle," he stopped being directive once *Arjuna* developed insight. Having shared the divine knowledge *(Brahma-vidya),* he respected *Arjuna's* decision as to whether or not to engage in the war. *Arjuna* revealed that his confusion and depression had lifted revealing important connections so that he was now ready, without doubts and conflicts, to participate in the righteous war of human values. There was a change in his perspective.

At this point, *Arjuna* had progressed because he no longer needed to deny or avoid important aspects of reality or resist his benefactor. As he became aware, open, and receptive to the requirements of his circumstances, he felt relief and found it easy to make a decision without undue concern and guilt. There was now congruence between his personal religion and his workgroup ethic. Actions and personal values were now in harmony as a result of Lord Krishna's counsel. In the therapy contact, *Arjuna* felt comfort, trust, and emotional security. His self-esteem remained intact even when he freely expressed negative feelings. As a result of a broadening of his perspective, *Arjuna's* resistance, hostility, conflict, pain, and distress melted away.

Therapeutic Attitudes

Lord Krishna was nurturing, reassuring, and fostered self-esteem through various ways of addressing *Arjuna.* These reminded him of his identity, duties, expected role, skills as a warrior, basic goodness, knowledge, and other strengths through a variety of positive addresses used by Lord Krishna. These being more subtle reminders than direct compliments, Lord Krishna managed to be more encouraging and insight producing. The divine therapist led the warrior to spiritual enlightenment with acceptance, respect, and brotherly affection.

Therapeutic Values

The therapist was accepting, patient, and "giving" in terms of time and efforts as long as the receiver needed more. The therapist was committed to the goal of resolving the conflict between personal and societal concerns. Other values implicit in Lord Krishna's therapeutic role included not losing sight of the big picture, and making sincere efforts to create awareness without damage to *Arjuna's* self-esteem and the therapeutic relationship. The therapist stated the harsh truth but remained a supportive and emotional ally in order to increase *Arjuna's* ability to take reality in his stride.

The role flexibility of the therapist is shown by Krishna in various other informal situations. Although his therapist role with *Arjuna* was that of a peer, he also acted as a young therapist for his father at a time of devastating permanent separation. Krishna's adoptive father of many years had difficulty coping with the fact that as a young adult, Krishna needed to return to his kingdom and take charge as a king. For the father this meant separation from the adopted son whom he had raised from very early infancy. The attachment had been strong and the father was so overwhelmed with pain and anxiety that he broke down with depression and could not function at all. Krishna's own appropriate detachment and empathic discourse on inappropriate and overly dependent attachment helped his father regain his composure and the father was able to cope. Similarly, Krishna helped female friends who were extremely attached to him and became depressed at the news of his departure. Acceptance of reality is a major milestone of therapeutic activity and makes room for active positive changes. Hindu therapy is a very gentle form of reality therapy.

Five Considerations Relevant to Action

To view action in a spiritual way, five aspects of action need to be considered: (1) the actor, (2) the action itself, (3) the field of action, (4) the efforts and skills required, and (5) *prarabdha* (providence/the unforeseen). Of particular relevance is an appreciation of *prarabdha.* The value people place upon their own role in the success or accomplishments is exaggerated, and leads them to take full credit for the outcome of their actions. As a consequence, they build a false sense of "ego," unrealistic expectations of themselves, and a lack of acceptance of the unforeseen blocks in the process. On the other hand, an appreciation of *prarabdha* and the other components of action realistically protects the actor from assuming undue responsibility and also frees the actor from unrealistic self-blame, when action does not bring about desired results. It is a mental health asset to be tolerant and forgiving of self and others when plans do not succeed and hopes are thwarted. Basically, action should be guided by a strategic rationale, not merely by an anticipated outcome. In the *Bhagavad Gita,* this is stated as "dedicating action to the Lord" or renouncing the fruit of action. Intent and plans for action need to be based on principles. This way we protect the totality of existence: environment, other people, and ourselves, because all aspects are informed by inclusive principles and a perspective of appropriate detachment from the outcome. Whereas the welfare of family and relatives can be viewed as the limit of concern by some, others extend their concern to the neighborhood, city, state, and humanity. The broader our definition of the whole, the less selfish and materialistic we can become in our attitudes and actions. The subtle aspect of the personality is related to the broad perspective and brings us increasingly into the spiritual realm.

Value of Flexibility

Those who are unable to identify with an abstract principle have the option of identifying with concrete images of God in one form of deity or another. If it is difficult for one to identify with both the principle and a deity, he or she can follow a spiritual leader to learn and practice a spiritual path. If this is also difficult, one can simply become a devotee or learn to act without desire for the result of actions. In the event that a person cannot achieve even this, there is the option of simply performing required actions and dedicating them mentally to *Brahman*. Consequently, a variety of pathways are acceptable to achieve the goal of spiritual enhancement. These are summarized in Table 1.5.

PRACTICE OF THERAPY

The practice of therapy is either informal or formal, and involves such considerations as therapist attributes, client readiness, and assessment of both progress and outcomes.

TABLE 1.5. Options for Spiritual Enhancement

Abstract Mental Activity	Concrete Ritual Activity	Emotional Devotional Actions	Practical Simple Daily Actions
1. Identification with the abstract principle of God: Highest level of workship of the formless.	5. Worship of a diety.	9. Become a devotee and workship.	12. Sing hymns.
2. Renunciation of "Doership."	6. Follow a spiritual leader.	10. Reduce other attachments.	13. Chant names.
3. Dedication of all action to the Supreme Spirit.	7. Act without a desire for results.	11. View all beings sacred and share.	14. Act within roles.
4. Renunciation of the fruit of action.	8. Perform actions based on principles and verbally dedicate them to God.		15. Nonviolence. 16. Truthfulness. 17. Equanimity. 18. Give to needy.

Informal Practice of Therapy

Therapeutic intervention occurs informally outside a professional therapeutic relationship. According to Hindu philosophy and spiritual ideals, whenever any person becomes aware of distress in a fellow being and believes that his or her own insights or skills might be helpful, he or she wants to make an effort to help.

This spontaneous therapeutic role is based on the ideals of universal brotherhood and unity and can be assumed by anyone regardless of status and role. Informal help of this kind is beyond the ideal of unconditional compassion because it is perceived as an honor and an opportunity for fulfillment through service to others.

The fulfillment from service is in terms of spirituality. The joy of another person's relief from pain or a restricted state is a rewarding experience. This is an aspect of the bliss sheath of personality, in which we experience unselfish joy and satisfaction, through identification with others at a nonmaterial level, as opposed to pleasure based on personal agenda. Further, the ability for such emotions is the by-product of the high spiritual progress of the person and it is also secondary to the goal of spiritual progress. In such situations, people do the selfless thing because they cannot refrain from doing it because of their values, and not with the goal of the anticipated fulfillment or reward. A good example is the rescue of another drowning individual at risk to a person's own life. The spiritual values bring forth the motivation and urgency to do the needful rather than a wish to "do kind deeds to others in order to accumulate good karma." In such emergency situations, fulfillment of the bliss sheath is not preplanned, arranged, or goal oriented, but it is an incidental outcome of the services provided, without regard for anything else except a need to do the utmost for another's well-being at that moment. All material and nonmaterial rewards are far from a person's mind when he or she runs into a burning building to save a baby. Service to others is of an even higher priority than unconditional compassion. Lord Buddha expressed this as the most important feature of his philosophy for humankind.

The individual who is helped informally acquires awareness and a greater ability to manage his or her problem independently. Lord Krishna's help to *Arjuna* illustrates an informal therapeutic practice similar to his help to his sad foster father at his own departure form the foster home.

Formal Practice of Therapy

In ancient India, the teachers and priests were seen as primarily responsible for guidance of people of all ages on a regular basis. Their task was a formalized service, part and parcel of the total process of education of the individual. These cultural "therapists" rendered their service without a fee, as per needs, with or without crises. The community, viewing education as highly valuable, met the teachers' basic needs eagerly and reverently. Today, the priests share the task of formal therapy with a variety of mental health professionals.

Therapist's Attributes

The therapist's own spiritual enlightenment and unselfish dedication to spiritual growth is a prerequisite attribute in order to help others toward awareness of the divine Self in all beings. Specific qualities of the therapist include compassion, a nonjudgmental attitude, patience, persistence, and a selfless interest in all others' well being and spiritual progress. In the past a Hindu priest preferred gain of insight in the person through direct experience prior to therapeutic discussion. This is similar to John Dewey's educational philosophy of "learning by doing." Adjusting to the person's pace is expressed in acceptance of the client's resistance, procrastination, complaints, anger, and in imparting patient, calm, enlightening, and appropriate explanations in a respectful and caring manner. Everyone is worthy to receive therapy solely because one exists as an individual soul *(jiva)*. The therapist functions as a provider of unconditional spiritual services with equanimity. This is compatible with values of universal and unconditional positive regard for the welfare of all beings as extensions of the Almighty.

Readiness and Resistance

An individual who was uninterested in receiving guidance from another was described as lacking in readiness. This lack of readiness was accepted as a temporary block in the path of spiritual development, i.e., one's level of readiness was viewed respectfully as an unavoidable reality. The teacher or priest would either wait or foster readiness through assignment of suitable tasks and responsibilities related to needed changes so that such experiences would promote readiness gradually. Today, therapists hold similar values with due attention to societal welfare.

Therapeutic Progress

Invariably, the overall goal of therapy is the feature of increased acceptance of demands of the situation through the awareness of the Causal layer. This entails the removal of illusions about material reality. The human mind has a tendency to give much more importance to material matters because they are visible, concrete, and sources of sense-related pleasures.

Therapeutic progress results from awareness of the Subtle layer of existence and the awareness of the Causal layer. Problem solving, peace, contentment, and role functioning become easier and more rewarding in comparison with material gains or accumulation as "everything falls into place" spiritually for the person who needed a level of detachment from the material aspects of life.

Outcome of Therapy

With the acquired perception of a direct relationship between awareness of the totality of spiritual reality, one experiences less confusion, emergence of clearer goals, and an increase in motivation, efforts, and success. The outcomes may be significant or small depending on the situation and the developmental level of the individual.

Figure 1.5 illustrates these connections, suggesting that regardless of the individual's initial goals, therapeutic awareness brings about a new perspective and consequently a new set of goals. The goal is no longer to "win the race" or "gain the wealth," but to play the game in a spiritually appropriate manner because it is more satisfying than any material gains. The definition of "success" or "gain" is transformed. When this level of insight is achieved, the process of change is automatic, the therapeutic agent's work is almost done. Most problems of resistance occur prior to the spiritual insight. The individual becomes more process-oriented as a result of such awareness or insight. In any one situation, spiritual success for a person means some degree of progress toward a higher level of spirituality, and therefore one step closer to the eventual goal of "salvation."

It is understood, in the literal meaning of the word, that the saving awareness or knowledge for actual salvation is acquired only after efforts of many lifetimes. The symbolic interpreters, however, would see the meaning of "many lifetimes" as "many experiences," and "salvation" as leading to an optimum balance of insight and optimal spiritual function in the person.

EVALUATION

Scientific evaluation of a good theory requires it to be comprehensive, coherent, integrative, practical, parsimonious, precise, operational, empirically verifiable, and heuristic. Theories that meet the majority of the criteria are judged as better. Failure to meet all criteria is not, however, a reason for discarding a theory. The scope for utility and constructive values involved in a theory may outweigh some of its limitations. Ultimately, a good theory can be improved.

The *Bhagavad Gita* was not written as either a theory of personality or as a theory of psychotherapy. Its intent was to impart education to specific leaders about a philosophy of existence.[54] Nevertheless, assumptions about personality and implications for psychotherapy based on values of Hindu psychology and philosophy are implicit within the *Bhagavad Gita.*

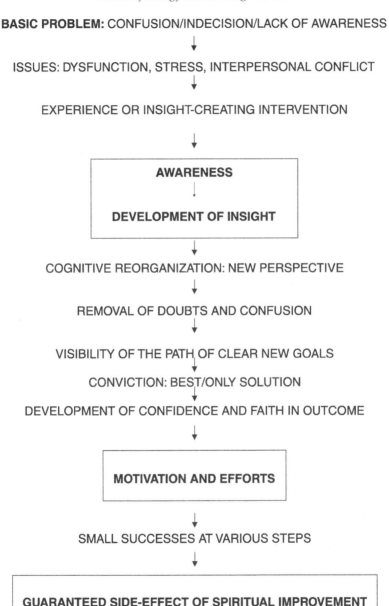

BASIC PROBLEM: CONFUSION/INDECISION/LACK OF AWARENESS

↓

ISSUES: DYSFUNCTION, STRESS, INTERPERSONAL CONFLICT

↓

EXPERIENCE OR INSIGHT-CREATING INTERVENTION

↓

AWARENESS

↓

DEVELOPMENT OF INSIGHT

↓

COGNITIVE REORGANIZATION: NEW PERSPECTIVE

↓

REMOVAL OF DOUBTS AND CONFUSION

↓

VISIBILITY OF THE PATH OF CLEAR NEW GOALS

↓

CONVICTION: BEST/ONLY SOLUTION

↓

DEVELOPMENT OF CONFIDENCE AND FAITH IN OUTCOME

↓

MOTIVATION AND EFFORTS

↓

SMALL SUCCESSES AT VARIOUS STEPS

↓

GUARANTEED SIDE-EFFECT OF SPIRITUAL IMPROVEMENT

FIGURE 1.5. Process of Change from Ignorance to Awareness

Personality Theory of the Upanishads

The Hindu personality theory has considerable strengths and some limitations. It is comprehensive and inclusive as well as internally consistent with respect to the concepts, facts, and processes it describes. However, although it has coherence of ideas that are clearly defined, some of its concepts have been derived from case studies, and have not been empirically validated by current methods of cross-sectional and experimental research. For scientists today, historical accounts not open to empirical investigation in the present may remain an enigma. Nevertheless, some aspects of spirituality (such as empathy) and their connections to behavior (e.g., tendency to nonviolence) can still be studied in the current population. The theory is particularly convincing to those who have faith and pride in the ancient scriptures, and to those with a deeper grasp of authenticity of concepts. Its utility depends on an objective grasp of concepts, appropriate application, and freedom from cultural traditions. There is a very wide acceptance of it among Hindus and many others because of its applicability to diverse cultures.

The personality theory is outlined in a simple manner, and most people can understand the description of sheaths or layers of personality. The distinctions between the Subtle and the Gross layers are tangible and verifiable through the bodily senses and measures of density. Based on principles of physics, any substance is in its gross form in the solid state when its density is greatest. Thus, ice is the gross form of the same compound (made of hydrogen and oxygen) that is water in its liquid state; water is subtler than ice; steam is the subtlest form of the identical substance. A second basis for subtle-gross distinction is the pervasiveness of the substances. The most subtle form is the most pervasive. Ice holds its shape and occupies a specific space. When melted into water, it will spread only to fit the container or in a downward direction due to gravity, and in the gas form, it spreads in all dimensions freely.

Of the five basic elements, defined by Hindu scriptures, "earth" (all the rock forms, minerals, and habitual solid materials) is dense, compact, and gross, hence least pervasive in the atmosphere. All solid materials can be experienced through the five senses. As we move from the gross to subtle forms, "water" is next as it has verification by all senses except one and is more pervasive than solids. "Fire" and "wind" come next, losing three and two sense experiences respectively. The last element, "space," permits only the perception of sound. The systematic aspect places each element at its own subtle or gross level based on the criteria of (1) rigidity and pervasiveness, and (2) the number of senses involved in its perception. The classification is based on facts, it is verifiable and authentic.

The *Upanishadic* theory has a parallel with the previous dimensions in the psychological area. An actual experience is more gross, relatively concrete, and verifiable as compared to a dream, daydream, fantasy, an aspect of imagination, a plan, or a hallucination. In a real experience, the presence of a person in a particular place is verifiable through the senses and other concrete measures, whereas fantasy, imagery, dreams, hallucinations, and ideas are not. However, the impact of the latter experiences on a person can sometimes be observable, as in rapid eye movement associated with stages of sleep, or in a person's verbal or facial expression during a dream or fantasy. Beyond this, scientific inquiry in this area depends on self-reports.

The spiritual application of this theory is a level higher beyond the psychological realm. This most unique and important aspect of the Hindu theory is the presence of the causal body of the personality based on the subtle-gross distinctions. The human Causal body is more subtle than space, and it is the essential life force within all people. Although it is an essence of *Brahman,* it is weighted down by its connection to the body. Therefore without a cumbersome physical body, *Brahman* is even more subtle than the *jiva's* causal body. As the most subtle, *Brahman* is pervasive enough to be in every aspect of the universe at all times, but neither *Brahman* nor the life essence *atman* can be experienced by any of the senses. It can be experienced in the *jiva's* deep-sleep state (peaceful temporary union with the all pervasive supreme spirit), because all other more gross functions of the physical system (the body, the mind, and intellect) are minimal and at rest. One of the ways in which humans can initiate a conscious connection with *Brahman* is through the use of special spiritual skills called *yogas.* Among all forms of life, humans are privileged enough in genetic heritage to be able to do this. Consequently, the humans have the greatest potential for progress and evolution in the "subtle" or spiritual aspects of existence. Such concepts make the mystery of the unknown positive and within grasp as they support and encourage human initiative toward a higher level of civilization that includes more compassion and unity on the one hand, and less competition, violence, and self defeating actions on the other. Abraham Maslow speaks of common values basic to humanity that transcend culture.[55] He sees components of such a civilization in the form of personality traits of self-actualized Persons as empirically verifiable and as scientific information.

There is no point in intellectually trying to grasp *Brahman,* because the subtlety involved is beyond the capacity of all human intellect except in brief mergers of Consciousness with *Brahman.* The all-pervasive concept of *Brahman* is empirically impossible to verify with the scientific measures available to date, but this concept is useful if believed as a symbol of positive potential for growth and improvement of human civilization. Belief in *Brahman* generates both (a) the internal therapeutic and rejuvenating opportunity for the individual, and (b) the notions of universality and unity that encourage cooperation and team spirit.

Brahman is present in each of us, just as the essence of the ocean is equally and fully present in every drop of the water it contains. The ocean is in each drop and all drops are in the ocean. As a symbol of creative energy and potential, *Brahman* is in each of us, and we are a part of its much larger overall Self (potential). However, just as a drop must join with millions of other drops to create a wave, we humans must unite to bring about effective positive changes for humanity. Such changes could raise human life to a higher level of spirituality. Despite being simple and obvious, these ideas can create a new and positive focus and are very influential due to their poetic and serene nature of presentation.

There is further elegance and utility in the description of recommended levels of attachment as that of "the lotus (a flower in the water-lily family) leaf" constantly in contact with water and yet "untouched" by water (its damaging effects).[56] The lotus leaf is large, round, deep green, shiny, and beautiful. Its wax-like surface makes water form in drops and slip off it. However, the round leaf always lies flat on the water with its underside in constant contact with water. The upper side is never wet, and always shows diamond-like drops shining on it. It is only the lower level of the leaf that is in contact with water all the time; the higher level stays unaffected and it is saved from the detrimental effects of water, just as the Causal layer of the human being or *jiva* can remain spiritual because of the appropriate level and kind of attachment despite the contact of the Gross layer with the material aspect.

The human use of materials for survival, sustenance, and good health is analogous to the lower-level contact of the lotus leaf with water, but attachment to these very materials must be permitted very discriminatingly by the higher level processes of our being, to make sure it is appropriate, and to guard against the addictive potential and related loss of control, disruption, and chaos in functioning. The clinical psychology concepts of inappropriate and self-defeating are very similar to the Hindu idea of living with non-spiritual, inappropriate attachment to materials, individuals, relationships, and one's own state of emotional satisfaction.[57]

The existence of each individual, separate from *Brahman* is merely temporary and fragile. One well-known example is that the physical body that separates the individual soul *(jiva)* from *Brahman* is similar to the thinly stretched membrane of an inflated balloon dividing the air inside outside the balloon. When the balloon bursts and collapses (the death of the physical body), the two areas of space reunite naturally. A similar clarification of the meaning of death is in another example. The space within a clay pot is the same as the space outside it. When the pot breaks (as when the *jiva's* body dies), the two spaces combine naturally and effortlessly.[58] Physical death becomes a nonthreatening natural process when viewed in terms of a merger with the divine in contrast to the view of death as separation, end and final destruction, or to the view that death is merely a process as natural as birth. The awareness of differences between birth and death keeps existential-anxiety alive and reassurance is difficult. It is clear to most individuals that birth is a beginning with tremendous scope and death is an end with unknowns pending. Further, the awareness of the aspect of "not being" prior to birth is either not known or not remembered by us during life, although the anticipation of death is a very real, long lasting, and existential-anxiety producing experience. The *Bhagavad Gita* provides spiritual reassurances about the inevitable unknowns, such as death, which threaten personal integrity and emotional security.

The causal aspect of a Self-realized personality is characterized by unconditional compassion, acceptance, brotherly love, and personal sacrifice for the benefit of the larger group. Further, there is optimism, constructive attitudes, and nonjudgmental care of peers even at their lowest levels of Self-realization. Lord Krishna, the king, not only gave material help generously to his helpless and poverty-ridden childhood friend *Sudama* but also rose above all status consciousness in relation to the poverty-stricken friend's "nonpresentable" physical condition.[59] He received his friend in the palace with humility, courtesy, and compassion because he was a friend and a guest. The Buddha easily resisted the overtures of the kingdom's famous and exceptionally beautiful dancer *(Vasavadatta)* but he came to her aid when she was unattractive, afflicted with illnesses, contagious, and discarded by society to die a lonely death.[60] Jesus accepted slow death by crucifixion without complaint on his own behalf, and with requests of forgiveness for his ignorant tormentors. Mahatma Gandhi accepted both brutal assaults[61] and imprisonment by the British police during his nonviolent movement.[62] Characterized by apparent frailty, saints and *yogins* have mental strength as well as forbearance, and they practice the ideal of simple living and high thinking. Spiritual research today can study traits of the causal body, such as sensitivity, compassion, determination, dedication, strength, and the person's ability to stand firm and alone for values. The *Upanishadic* personality theory recognizes and honors these traits of Self-realizing personalities, who have discovered their own causal body, and who manifest the causal body through spiritual actions that benefit both individuals and society.[63]

The personality traits of Maslow's healthy self-actualizing people were derived inductively from case studies.[64] Similar traits are affirmed in sacred Hindu teachings *(dharma)* by the original "law-giver," *Manu:*

> Steadfastness, forgiveness, control of the mind, non-taking of others' possessions, restraint of senses, [cultivation of] intellect, learning, truth, freedom from anger . . . this is the tenfold characteristic of *Dharma.*[65]

A celebrated author of Hindu religion and culture, S. D. Kulkarni commented in 1995 on the thoughts of *Swayambhu Manu:*

> *Manu*, in prescribing these virtues, qualities, attributes to be acquired and practiced by all, anticipates C. G. Jung and Abraham Maslow by at least twenty three centuries. These are the qualities which lead a man to sublimate his personality to a higher level of development and fulfillment, and help him maintain good relations with his fellow beings in a human society.[66]

The values of compassion, cooperation, and nonviolence make this personality theory relevant, meaningful, and applicable to modern times.

The Bhagavad Gita *As a Theory of Psychotherapy*

As a basic philosophy of life, the *Bhagavad Gita* was intended primarily to enable human beings to lead a peaceful life in harmony with the environment. The practical goal was to find ways to help most humans learn how to manage their lives well, here and now, rather than to establish a scientific theory. Solutions for problem situations were found as they occurred and took priority over formulating conclusions on the basis of formal research.

Scholars and authors of the ancient past have come to very authentic conclusions about life and human nature. They have interpreted and modified the *Vedas* so that they could be applied in a proper and flexible manner by a large variety of individuals to serve an extended portion of the population. The *Bhagavad Gita,* as the essence of the *Vedas,* is a theory of personal growth, personality change, spiritual enhancement, and is a guide to spiritual practice. An important goal is to achieve equilibrium among the three levels of personal, social, and cosmic functioning.[67] The *Bhagavad Gita* provides a formula for prevention as well as coping with distress. It acknowledges need for individualized interpretations depending upon the mental tendency and level of the individual.

This author's conjecture based on the knowledge of the culture and history is that in ancient times, the physical aspect of life had impressive face validity due to its concreteness and its relevance to human survival. The authors of Hindu scriptures, especially the *Bhagavad Gita,* seemed to have feared neglect of the intellectual and spiritual aspect of life to the point of their possible extinction. A visionary, born much before his time, the author of the *Bhagavad Gita* may have been aware that the chances of peer support for his views were slim on this matter. To the goal of saving humans from neglecting the species' spiritual potential, the leader may have chosen to tie the ideas and principles to religion in terms of "the word of the Almighty" so that people would adopt them.

Further, the writers of the *Upanishads* may have noted that humans had the advantage compared to less evolved animals, but the disadvantage of higher mental capacities to remember the past and imagine the future. The cognitive capacities of logical anticipation and expectation based on observations and experience created anxiety, fears, and worries due to the basic conflict between the survival instinct and the awareness of the fact of eventual death. Fear of one's personal demise has not been easy to handle, as is evidenced even now, in individual struggles and by every culture's efforts to promote health, longevity, and to affirm eternal life.[68]

The observation that everyone dies regardless of power, possessions, virtue, and status might have led to reactions of distress evident in symptoms of mental illness such as anhedonia, the loss of one's will to live, and mental withdrawal. The necessity to accept the inevitability of death could create anxiety. In addition, in those days many life threatening diseases and little scope of immunization, caused earlier and higher mortality rates. Symptoms of such Axis I disorders as anxiety and depression could interfere with one's ability to function in necessary roles.[69] Distress is exacerbated by experience of loss, and by the fear of the unknown quality of afterlife. As a result, at least in some, there would be the sociopsychological withdrawal and dysfunctional alienation although their participation was still needed by the family and society.

The experience of helplessness and feelings of loss of control might have caused a different reaction in some other humans, making them belligerent, hostile and purposefully self-centered in attitude.[70] Lowered altruism and the risk of conduct-problems may have made matters urgent for the needs of the overall community. The *Kauravas* and their allies fit the description of the conduct disorders (Axis I). When such individuals also had power as well as social and legal authority as princes or leaders, it became a very dangerous combination for the well-being of other folk. To deter development of such characters, the *Bhagavad Gita* philosophy may have been developed.

A reasonable hypothesis is that the authors of Hindu Scriptures observed existential anxiety, low morale, and insecurity among the masses and made many efforts to help people to cope with less personal distress and role disruption. They found a common solution for anxiety and depression in some, and to human aggression in antisocial personalities so that healthy patterns could be encouraged to protect both individual and universal interests. These hypotheses seem compatible with the therapeutic perspective of the *Bhagavad Gita*, which provides emotional support, reassurance, and encouragement, with the aid of stable and important long-term values to both individuals and society. The complete trust in the compassionate divine organization, despite the mystery of never knowing where life is headed, encourages harmony with nature, protection of human welfare, and long-range interests over immediate personal pleasures. The basic existential trust, despite the mystery about the Almighty's ways, is expressed in proverbs that translate: (1) "Divine wheels turn slowly but always with good results," (2) "There may be delay but not darkness in the Divine Spirit's courthouse," and (3) "Whatever the Almighty brings about, is for the best in the long run" (because it eventually creates a balance for all beings even if it is individual wishes in the short term). These proverbs imply a sense of trust and unity within the universe, and a need for patience with the course of inevitable events in a predetermined cycle of existence for the universe. Hindu spiritual wisdom discourages a self-absorbed view of personal life as contrary to the natural order.

The struggle of life as depicted in the *Bhagavad Gita's* story of *Arjuna* is an internal struggle for all humans, at various junctures of life, between polarities (material/mental; personal/interpersonal; convenience/principles). Consequently, as with *Arjuna,* most humans are perplexed with indecision as to the appropriate action. When unable to resolve the situation, the person needs external help. Not all of us are lucky enough to have a personal guide (Lord Krishna); however, his spiritual wisdom is expressed in the *Bhagavad Gita.* As a summary of the *Upanishads,* it is available to all of us as an encyclopedia of spirituality. The application of its principles is believed to be possible to all circumstances, if the principles are first grasped correctly. As preventive education, it tells us to be prepared to cope with a variety of situations that must be faced to avert disaster. Each one of us needs to develop an inner Lord Krishna, as the representative of our inner Self/*Brahman,* to guide us from time to time in our internal struggles and indecisions as well as with stressful events.

The appropriate human conduct ideas of the *Bhagavad Gita* require consistent efforts of regularity, conservation, equanimity, honor of role-adherence to maintain general predictability, maintenance of the social organization for appropriate function, and the overall balance of all natural and human aspects (intrapersonal, interpersonal, societal, ecological and cosmic) of life and humans. Mere logic does not elicit such constant effort and dedication, nor such strong motivation as to overcome the pull of instincts and natural pleasures. Therefore the variety of *yogas* respect individual temperament and personality differences and allow and are each suitable to various personal inclination and aspects of experience. *Bhakti-yoga* engages the emotional aspect; *Jnana-yoga* addresses the intellectual aspect; *Karma-yoga* addresses motivation and actions; *Dhyana-yoga* focuses on one's ability for attention and concentration and so forth.

As the peak of devotion, *Bhakti-yoga* makes it possible to mobilize one's self—for fulfilling emotional expression through useful actions, and, promotes one's self-esteem although appreciating simultaneously concern for societal welfare. As a possible side effect of the ideas of the *Bhagavad Gita,*

Bhakti-yoga provides a personal and spiritual meaning of life as an antidote to emptiness and boredom, and to a lack of goals and direction. Devotion is clearly seen in the emotion expressed in the religious congregations today and also in the need of youth for membership in newer cults.

Karma-yoga appreciates and intends the impact of behavior and role-functioning on the psychology of the individual akin to a behavioral approach to psychotherapy. However, in Hinduism human actions and attitudes about roles performance are viewed as connected to spirituality. The individual is encouraged to renounce the credit for self-focused actions, and to Act on principles without thought of results in order to reduce anxiety and selfish interests; also repeated dedication of specific fruit of action to the Supreme Spirit are methods to stabilize the person. Reverently dedicating one's actions and their fruits to *Brahman* yields a beneficial impact on the human mind due to the focus on values and traits connected with *Brahman*. It is a parallel to reading good books or listening to good thoughts. The same focus and calming effect occur in the practices of chanting the name of one's favored representation or symbol of the Supreme Spirit. These practices bring about incorporation of divine values, beliefs, and attitudes in the devotee. A side effect may be that they give the mind a rest and reduce stress of the brain-overtime needed to cope with the role juggling and the "rat race" of modern society.

Although the primary and ultimate goal of all the *yogas* is union with *Brahman,* they yield many other beneficial effects for the business of living a healthy life, as in the Gestalt therapy's "here and now," in harmony with the natural environment. These practical benefits contribute to the popularity of the *yogas* both with The ultimate purpose and the outcome is spiritual growth and enhancement, and the short-term benefits are experienced as restored calm, stability, confidence, physical exercise, and better use of inner and outer resources. In terms of psychological growth and personality enhancement, the benefit is a more mature and constructive outlook due to a broader understanding of one's self, world, existence, and its laws, often leading to greater life satisfaction and to realistic pride in successful coping, in addition to more positive modeling for the younger generations.

The concept of the Supreme Spirit (unaffected by human weaknesses, and accepting of all) encourages a perception of strength, dependability, and reliability in harmless ways. Purification opportunities are equally available to all. The *Bhagavad Gita* concepts and values can be useful in both psychotherapy and self-help.

Major Features of Bhagavad Gita *As a Theory of Psychotherapy*

- Liberation or freedom is both the ultimate and penultimate goal of Hindu psychotherapy.

- It provides specific techniques for paths of spiritual enhancement.
- These pathways *(yogas)* recognize individual differences and a variety of needs and styles.
- It permits flexibility of interpretation of its wisdom in both literal and symbolic ways.
- The therapist adopts a flexible approach, which begins with the client's needs.
- Individual enhancement is promoted in conjunction with the welfare of society. Disapproval of antisocial conduct and attitudes ensures the survival of the whole group (always goes hand in hand with) from the welfare of the totality of the society and the cosmos. Greater acceptance of the "a-social" and disapproval of antisocial ensures survival of the whole group.
- An inner detachment from the physical aspect of being is not only desirable but necessary. The objects of sense pleasures may be used and enjoyed, but in a nonaddictive manner and without loss of inner control on the healthy balance.
- A therapeutic outcome is the person who is more patient, forgiving, tolerant, accepting, reassuring, gentle, warm, emotionally secure, and self accepting with positive self-assertion ability. One is encouraged to move toward goals of greater self-awareness, and to take specific actions and steps toward appropriate and constructive role functioning.

The goal of *jeevan-mukta* (liberated while living) encourages improvement in conduct "here and now" and helps to reduce the tendency to procrastinate, and fear of failure and avoidance. It lends itself to the dual interpretation of the theory of rebirth. Whether interpreted literally or symbolically, this concept provides for general life goals, guidelines to meaningful experiences, and to ward off existential anxiety.

The therapeutic approach of the *Bhagavad Gita* can be characterized as a system of guidance varied to suit different human groups. For individuals capable of philosophical understanding and intellectual meaning, it provides the requisite education for leadership roles in their society. For those of average intelligence, it provides general guidance for achieving balance between personal and societal needs. Finally, the *Bhagavad Gita* provides moral guidance to those who cannot evaluate situations based on moral, socially acceptable, or spiritual criteria. For this wider population, it provides prescriptions for a moral life in the form of dharma, the prescribing system of religious conduct.

The *Bhagavad Gita* addresses all three groups just noted. Those of the highest mental level understand and interpret it in a symbolic sense. The middle level enjoys the social-emotional aspect of it through celebrations and ceremonies, sometimes taking its word literally about rituals and austerity. The third group consists of the largest number of people who remember some important basic rules connected to religion, and follow them regularly because it is a basis for their social identity and social image as "good, decent, and God-fearing people."

The application of the *Bhagavad Gita* today honors the individual right of freedom of choice in spiritual practices. Complete autonomy of the individual is expected and respected. The stage of personal spiritual development is respected and not judged. Sincere interest and effort are viewed as more important than facade by the truly spiritual. Finally, quality is valued and honored above quantity. Constancy of effort and appropriate psychological state is very important.

It is believed that important decisions can be made and conflicts resolved with the application of the values endorsed by the *Bhagavad Gita*. At times, the formal help of a guru is also required. Even the Hindu scholar, Sage Narada, after studying all scriptures, was unhappy because he could not really "know the Self." It was the therapeutic interaction with his guru that enabled him to achieve the ultimate realization of the Self. Such confusion is seen as human, because for some, the grasp is possible only in therapeutic relationships with the enlightened guru. It is possible that the spirituality of basically good humans may remain latent due to ignorance, which means a lack of development of appropriate attitudes, efforts, and actions. Removal of ignorance (yoga of knowledge), dedication to principles (yoga of devotion), practice at concentration (yoga of meditation), appropriate self restraint and conservation of materials, and equanimity of perception are valued. Equanimity means an integration of democratic perception of all individuals as equals, a nonjudgmental attitude and nonattachment with specific individuals and experiences.[71]

There is no one particular or "right" way to reach a higher spiritual level, nor to make a decision in a dilemma. Flexibility with a view to reality is most strongly advocated by Lord Krishna himself. In conflict situations prior to the *Mahabharata* war, efforts were made to negotiate and compromise to prevent it, but they failed because the *Kauravas* wanted the war. During the meetings with the *Pandavas* and their allies, Lord Krishna described four levels of coping with difficult, antisocial personalities, who not only neglected their own spirituality but also had no qualms about destruction of the whole society. To deal with such people, a hierarchy of practical techniques was recommended: (1) *sama* (communication) is the strategy of respectful communication, reasoning, and persuasion to help one appreciate human values; (2) *dama* (payment) is the provision of material compensation to bring about appropriate behaviors; (3) *danda* (physical force and/or restriction) refers to more forceful and punitive measures when the first two fail; (4) *bhaida* (spying and manipulations) is the use of deceit or trickery as a last resort to deal with the most destructive and antisocial individuals or groups.

These four ideas were developed in service of nonviolence (permitting offenders to live but to protect others from their harmful efforts). These are extremely realistic and practical solutions for a complex situation involving a balance of individual and total-group welfare. As compared to the very idealistic principles of the *Treta-yuga*, this era (the *Dwapar-yuga*) advocated going beyond the naive and overly "good" unrealistic perceptions. These ideas seem consistent with research on psychotherapy with antisocial personalities, the results of which are not very positive and hopeful even now.

Knowledge of *Bhagavad Gita* is believed to be "evergreen," as it has been useful whenever it is brought back into focus for both the preparatory education of leaders for life, and at a moment of tremendous crisis. Its values relate to the human need for personal meaning, as well to promote global welfare. It employs spiritual identification and principles to guide personal conduct and to individuals attain peace and harmony through spiritual contentment. The revival of its principles may help human mental evolution in its current stage. Though most humans are aware of self-defeating actions such as violence, wars, and the abuse of power, as a species, they seem unable to refrain from them! Any reasonable ideas that can contribute toward positive changes would be very welcome, regardless of their origin or scientific rigor. The *Bhagavad Gita* envisions a hopeful future provided humans put forth the requisite efforts. At this stage of human evolution, the required efforts are spiritual in nature, not primarily physical, technological, or even intellectual. The *Bhagavad Gita* tells us that we need not remain captive in a violent and material stage of evolution. We can go beyond this stage through spiritual efforts.

In conclusion, the *Bhagavad Gita* is at once a theory of education, guidance, philosophy, psychotherapy, and cosmic life with clear specification of the human role. It is an open system that presents ideas through exposure rather than coercion. Total freedom without exclusive demands on one's loyalty make up the entity of *dharma* as sacred teachings about religion, philosophy, social ideals, and an ethical lifestyle. The person determines the path based on one's readiness and level of inner discipline. One is free to explore or join other faith traditions and to worship in the temple or at home according to personal preferences. This respect for personal autonomy permits relaxed exploration and self-development. The encouragement for this is expressed in a policy similar to that of a public library, but even more open, with an "all welcome" and "no fines" situation. The knowledge and ideas are available to anyone with interest and sufficient initiative to make use of the spiritual resources. Thus Hindu psychology practices what it preaches: acceptance and respect, universality, unity, and nonviolence. Spiritual progress is seen as vertical, rather than horizontal, that is, each religion aims to improve spirituality, hence there is no need to change from one religion to another. Instead the need is of the grasp of spiritual and regular practice of a spiritual lifestyle. All spiritual paths are respected because all lead to *Brahman* or the Almighty, even if recognized by another name.

POINTS OF DIALOGUE

With Other Religions

Some of the points of dialogue among religions concern their respective beliefs, value systems, and related practices. The beliefs and values expressed in the *Bhagavad Gita* are found in many other religions. These beliefs, values, and practices include union with the divine spirit, a life of devotion and service, knowledge, compassion, nonviolence, the truth and human dignity, moral virtue, wisdom, afterlife and liberation, nonattachment, respect, unity, and attainment of universal happiness.

Union with the divine spirit is a value in the *Bhagavad Gita* and is also found in mystical forms of Judaism and Christianity. The same is true of the expression of religious devotion expressed in private and public rituals and worship. The devotional path of *Bhakti-yoga* was chosen by large numbers in the lifetime of Lord Krishna (and Lord Rama). A boatman *(kevata)* used humorous expressions to be able to serve Lord Rama. An uneducated rural woman *Shabri* tasted each berry before offering it to Lord Rama so that he would not get a single sour berry. The subjective pain of separation from the Lord was expressed by some in beautiful songs of devotion, and by others in courageous detachment from pressures to conform, form peer approval, and from the threats of established social authority. These pathways are not unique to the *Bhagavad Gita,* but the latter advocates the intrinsic reward of fulfillment in devotion itself as a pathway to reach the Lord.

In addition to the values of devotion and service, the *Bhagavad Gita* values knowledge *(Jnana-yoga).* Similarly, Jesus Christ's last words "Father, forgive them, for they know not what they do," imply that at least some inappropriate and destructive acts are due to ignorance.[72] His nonjudgmental attitude and tolerance are visible in the gentle acceptance he showed of ignorant and immature people as "children." In his sermon on the Mount, Jesus is reported to have said: "Pity them for their ignorance and teach them that they may know."[73] In the *Bhagavad Gita, Jnana-yoga* is the conscious effort to obtain an intellectual understanding of the spiritual aspect of life. Mercy, righteousness, justice, loving kindness, and peace are all related to such knowledge. Truth is explicitly endorsed as a primary value by Zoroaster as in "He who utters a falsehood is of all men the most despised," and " For he wounds not only the ear but the soul of his neighbor."[74] In the *Bhagavad Gita, Sat* means "truth" and "good" combined.

Confucius taught a connection between scholarship and goodness. His belief was that the study of wisdom resulted in becoming good. Through his words and action, Lord Buddha emphasized service to the world as the prime commitment of the "enlightened" monk community. Knowledge is thus connected to "good action" in many major religions, as it is in the *Bhagavad Gita's Jnana Yoga*.[75] In *Karma-yoga*, words are actions of speech and thought.[76]

Buddhism, Christianity, Judaism, and the Bhagavad Gita all discourage elaborate ritualism that neglects attention to human need and suffering.[77] In most religions, the values related to this admonition are compassion and concern for justice. There is explicit and repeated mention of compassion in the *Bhagavad Gita,* Buddhism, Christianity, Confucianism, and Zorastrianism. Nonviolence is stressed by the *Bhagavad Gita,* Buddhism, Christianity, Confucius and Jainism.

The *Bhagavad Gita,* Buddhism, and Christianity approve of "harmony in living" as a mutually cooperative lifestyle so that no one's needs are neglected. Honoring the dignity of peers through respect and courtesy is another ideal for the *Bhagavad Gita,* Buddhism, and Zorastrianism.

Although heaven and hell are visualized by Christ, Confucius, Muhammad, and Zoroaster, the *Bhagavad Gita,* sees heaven *(swarga-loka)* as one of the two positive stations. The second is *Brahma-loka,* superior to heaven and closer to the ultimate bliss of merger with *Brahman* along with complete liberation from the suffering associated with the cycles of birth, death, and rebirth governed by the law of karma. Consistent with the values of rising above the material world, the material reward station *(swarga-loka)* occupies a lower place as compared to *(Brahma-loka)* for those wishing nonmaterial spirituality. See Figure 1.4 for a visual portrayal of this process.

Eternal life is described in terms of *moksha* (liberation), a parallel to Buddhism's *nirvana*. The Buddha taught "… each living soul is like a torch whose flame is handed down in turn to another torch, and so on, through the ages until at last it melts into the universal flame of immortal life."

The concept of liberation of the *Bhagavad Gita* can mean either to shed the rebirth cycle and its hassles, or to mentally rise above worldly attachments within this life, as *jeevan-mukta*. This is a parallel to Lord Buddha's nirvana at the end of the one and only human lifetime. Confucius believed in immortality and a positive path to salvation.

Virtue and vice are contrasted in the *Bhagavad Gita* as *sura* (the virtuous people) and *asura* (the evil people), personified in ancient Christianity by angels and demons, and in Zoroastrian religion as *Ahura Mazda* (the divine spirit) and *Ahriman* (the evil spirit). Further, the moral aspect is evident in Zoraster's statement: "Our duty is to teach friendliness to the enemy, righteousness to the wicked, and wisdom to the ignorant."

The notion of a Supreme Spirit in *Ahura Mazda* represents seven principles (eternal light, omniscient wisdom, righteousness, power, piety, benevolence, and eternal life). The ideal human being of the *Bhagavad Gita* is a stable, impartial, compassionate, forgiving, and nonattached (appropriate on the attachment/detachment dimension) *yogin,* although Confucius talks of the "Superior man" and Zoroaster of the "righteous man."

In the *Bhagavad Gita,* wisdom is illumination, experienced specially through the practice of meditation as a high-standard pathway *(Dhyana-yoga* or *Raja-yoga).* Meditations with exclusive concentration and dedication brings about enlightenment and wisdom in the form of new and creative awareness about the meaning of Life.[78] The ultimate goal and hope of all religions and saints is universal happiness by transcending suffering. The dream of an ideal world for many religions seems to be of one in which human life has unity, compassion, harmony, peace, mutual respect, wisdom, and eternal bliss. The emphasis of the *Bhagavad Gita* is to achieve this internally, even in materially difficult circumstances, not merely through environmental control. This emphasis encourages the focus of human efforts in their own personalities rather than the correction of environment or other individuals.[79]

Nonviolence is stressed by the *Bhagavad Gita,* Buddhism, Christianity, Confucius, and Jainism. The *Bhagavad Gita,* Buddhism, and Christianity approve of harmony in living as a mutually cooperative lifestyle so that no one's needs are neglected.

In conclusion, there are several common features and parallels among the world's religions that serve as points of dialogue despite their divergent spiritual practices. Ancient religious leaders of distant regions agree on many of the fundamentals of an authentic spirituality, though cross-cultural communication in those days was almost impossible. Their common views seem to point to universal human nature, needs, failings, behaviors, and psychological features involved in the evolution of human nature. The similarities among the different philosophies are of much greater value and importance rather than variations. The consensus among the wise in different sectors of the world, without mutual awareness, includes spiritual notions vital to humanity as a whole and points to a basic human unity despite diversity in environment, resources, and cultures.

With Other Theories of Personality and Psychotherapy

The structure of personality implied in the *Bhagavad Gita* (and described in *Upanishads)* represents a hierarchy of levels contrasted as superficial versus deep, and as levels based on instinctual physical functions. The hierarchical principle is similar to Kurt Lewin's graphic presentation of field theory[80] and Abraham Maslow's hierarchy of basic human needs.[81] In both Maslow's and the *Bhagavad Gita* hierarchies, the lowest levels are physical aspects. Maslow's characteristics of the self-actualized individual are similar to the assets of the *yogin* in the *Bhagavad Gita,* who is successful and advanced in spiritual progress.

Arjuna asked Lord Krishna what the characteristics of a *yogin* were. Although the question was in terms of external behavioral traits, Krishna's reply included the higher, psychological and spiritual aspect of development and maturity. Krishna described value-related, attitudinal, subjective, interpersonal, and interactional aspects of the *yogin's* personality.

The *yogin* is one who is above selfish attachments to actions and to their results, yet still performs role-related actions and actions helpful to others. A *yogin* is more liberated from personal desires and cravings because he or she is no longer dependent on any aspect of the physical world for his or her happiness, satisfaction, or joy. The *yogin* is "ever content" (content in outlook) because he or she is free from dualities (grief-joy, good-bad, yours-mine, friend-enemy, etc.); his or her mind is stable, established in knowledge (spiritual understanding), and he or she radiates the glow of inner peace and bliss. He or she has equanimity of perception and feelings, for all objects, people, and experiences.

The image of the *yogin* seems similar to Maslow's description of the self-actualizing individual.[82] The latter are characterized by a superior perception of reality, increased self-acceptance, and identification with humanity, improved interpersonal relations, a more democratic character structure and value system, greater spontaneity and creativity, a problem-centered focus, increased detachment and desire for privacy, increased autonomy and resistance to acculturation, a fresh appreciation of life and range of emotional reactions, and more frequent peak experiences.

Maslow characterizes the self actualizing attributes as "Being values" (B-values). These contrast with D-values (deficiency-motivated perception). The values of being are very much the same as Robert Hartman's intrinsic values that include wholeness, perfection, completion, justice, aliveness, richness, simplicity, beauty, goodness, uniqueness, effortlessness, playfulness, truth, honesty, reality, and self-sufficiency.[83]

All of these values are endorsed either explicitly or implicitly in the *Bhagavad Gita's* portraits of saints, divine incarnations, and the Supreme Spirit.[84] For example, the description of the *yogin* who rises above dualities of thought is similar to the transcendence of dichotomies associated with Hartman's concept of "wholeness." The *yogin's* detachment from the material world and external experiences is comparable to Hartman's "self-sufficiency." The Subtle bliss sheath of the personality is comparable to the values of aliveness, and the subtle nature of the spirit is comparable to the concept of richness.

According to the *Bhagavad Gita,* the divine incarnations and saint are very similar to the Supreme Spirit. They are human links to God, who is the unfailing "significant other," and a constant source of emotional security, strength, and guidance.[85]

An essential feature of our reality includes the element of time. Whatever begins, must have an end. The stress of being and living leads to striving for security. For the *yogin,* God is the unfailing significant other who provides emotional security and guidance to degrees not possible from any other living being or from any human experiences of material gain, achievement, pleasure, or relationships. All of these change over time. Wealth is known to be unstable; achievement is impossible to keep at the same level through different stages of life; changes in persons and/or circumstances impact the qualities of human relationships; pleasure varies with personality changes of beliefs, attitudes, and values. For the needs of human emotional security, nothing else could be as stable and foolproof as the all-pervading, omnipotent, and compassionate *Brahman* who cares unconditionally for all alike. Such a universal concept of God provides for optimal emotional security and relief from avoidable life stress. The divine incarnations and the enlightened *yogins* play the role of mediators between God and humans and therefore convey some of the divine capacity to provide emotional security to humans. The *yogin's* practice of *Jnana-yoga* brings about acceptance of realities in all aspects, and in the practice of *Bhakti-yoga,* one learns to love the "significant other" even in absentia, just as we learn to love our heroes without direct interactions with them, but by emulating their values.

The *Bhagavad Gita* idea of the "whole" being more important than each of its components is similar to the idea from Gestalt theory that the whole is more than the sum of all its parts. Likewise, the Gestalt idea of being responsible for one's self and to the "whole" is similar to the *Bhagavad Gita* idea of universality, unity, and of good and bad karma.[86] Unity applies to the relationship of an individual to God (the whole) and with other beings and environment (the parts). Even if "prior karma" determines one's fate (the given features of a situation in the Gestalt perspective), one must take responsibility for one's decisions and actions "here and now" to effect deliberate change. While carrying out such responsibility of living and acting, a *yogin* manages to remain united with the universe (other parts) and with *Brahman,* as the whole.

In the *Bhagavad Gita,* even fate can be changed by very clear and sudden awareness and a high degree of sincerity, or through proper channels of yoga. The parallel in Gestalt theory encourages tolerance for present frustrations so that one can persists toward even if one does not see immediate consequences. Patience (frustration-tolerance in the present is encouraged in Gestalt theory) to maintain persistence toward cherished long-term goals, remain responsible, and achieve better overall adjustment.

Just as the "adult ego-state" of Transactional Analysis must work toward practical compromises between the "parent" and the "child" ego-states, in the *Bhagavad Gita* spirituality works to create a balance between the fulfillment of personal needs and societal welfare.[87] Further, healthy interpersonal model the Transactional Analysis perspective of "I am okay-you are okay" finds a parallel in the *Bhagavad Gita's* assertion of all humans being basically good because all have the divine essence of *Brahman* within them. Personal satisfaction through self-acceptance as well as harmonious social life through acceptance of other people and disliked events as parts of "all that there is." This is grounded in the basic spiritual truth of existence that "all is He and He is all." A literal translation of the Sanskrit phrase, *"Tat Tvam Asi"* is "That Thou Art." The divine is found within all that exists— "you are what That is." This notion expresses an acceptance and regard for all beings in the universe as well as the environment exactly as it exists. It discourages a negative attitude, depression, acts of criticism, and the imposition of change upon others by pressure or force.

The universal acceptance can lead to the practical strategy of accepting the inevitable in the time dimension. This is similar to the phrase in the prayer: "Give me the serenity to accept what I cannot change." Having reached such a point of universal acceptance and equanimity in many aspects besides the time dimension, Lord Buddha became aware of a change in his own perspective as he looked at a rock and found it "beautiful" because "it is itself" rather than his earlier perception of its beauty based on sense-perceptions (because it was smooth and had a nice color). In his new spiritual perception, it was a unique part of creation to be appreciated in its own right. Such appreciation can extend to the interpersonal aspect for an optimal state of production and consumption, creating and maintaining balance in the environment. These values are foundational to democracy and human rights advocacy.

The *yogin's* appreciation and acceptance is similar to the psychological concept of positive regard. Positive regard is seen by the *yogin* as the only way to view and deal with others. It also happens to be the most promising way to maintain and improve mental health in self and others, both within and outside of the context of therapy. Carl Rogers has conceptualized "unconditional positive regard" as vital in the valued therapeutic relationship, necessary to promote autonomy, self-acceptance, self-respect, along with creative, responsible, self-direction.[88] Such unconditional regard also facilitates positive communication and mediation in conflict situations and it is the feature that discriminates between positive and negative self assertions. Carl Rogers relates the self-concept with components of the "ideal self" and the "real self." The greater the congruence between the two, the higher the mental health and personal adjustment level of the individual. In other words, in our civilization a person feels comfortable as their actions and behavior become similar to values. In the *Bhagavad Gita,* the "ideal self" is the Causal layer and the "real self" is the area of action.

In the early years of human life when identity is not yet fully developed, the ideal self, as defined by Carl Rogers, can be an interpretation of values (standards) deemed vital by significant others, along with appropriate regard for societal expectations concerning the current stage of the individual's life. The real-self is grounded experientially on own evaluations of more direct observations of one's feelings, thoughts, and actions they actually occur. The "Self" or *Brahman* as the divine spirit in the *Bhagavad Gita,* is analogous to the ideal self in Rogers' self-concept theory with the exception that the former is both universal and identical within all individuals. The "Self" may be perceived and/or experienced either in abstract or personified form by different person. The individual self *(jiva)* depicted in the *Bhagavad Gita* is closer to the real self in Rogers' experiential theory.[89] Hindu psychology affirms, through the *Bhagavad Gita,* common ideals for all individuals to be equally valued with the understanding and acceptance that actual individual applications will vary, and further advocates mutual unconditional positive regard as essential for harmonious survival and beneficial growth of individuals and humanity.[90]

The *Bhagavad Gita* values include aspects of many different theories of personality and psychotherapy, though it may seem to focus exclusively on the internal, subjective aspects of the human mind. The internal focus is similar to cognitive theories in psychology and *Jnana-yoga* is an appropriate path for intellectually oriented people. The more effective and relational pathway is the practice of *Bhakti-yoga.* People who need to utilize concentration may select *Dhyana-yoga.* The prescribed action-exercises in *Karma-yoga* constitute a form of behavior modification the impact of behavioral roles on one's identity is as important as the influence of thoughts and feelings on behavior.

The *Bhagavad Gita's* own pattern seems to have already included an integration of various ways of many theories of psychotherapy, which developed subsequently in western countries and received empirically support. Therapeutic progress occurred by including many suitable method tailored to clients. Interventions were developed relevant to the unique characteristics of the individual, including their specific needs, personality type, age, gender, culture, values, and readiness to change. Further, due attention was paid to the cultural environment and the need of the individual to cope with it.

Attention to the unique needs of the individual in the *Bhagavad Gita* philosophy is similar to The respect for the person in Carl Rogers' person-centered psychotherapy. A genuine centering on the person depends on the therapist's empathic understanding; the assessment of the particular client's perceptions and experiences; the assessments of client's capacity for autonomy, creativity, and self-direction. Insight and growth develop due to the therapist's reception, sensitivity, positive anticipations, and reflection of feelings providing feedback to the client.

Improved self-esteem eventually leads to development of greater autonomy, self-direction, and creativity, and, at the same time the need of direction from the therapist is reduced. Similarly, ancient Hindu gurus determined the type and degree of direction necessary for each individual in a very client-centered manner along with an eye to the nature of current circumstance.[91] Today, we refer to the total process in formal terms and parts or stages of intake interview, initial assessment/diagnostic interview, a treatment plan, and the development of the therapeutic relationship.

In the *Bhagavad Gita,* Lord Krishna's dialogue with *Arjuna* was based on an awareness of the nature of their preexisting relationship, knowledge of *Arjuna's* personality, cultural and family background, the present situation of the war, as well as the estimation of future needs and possibilities. Lord Krishna, in his therapist role, kept track of the practical aspect of the societal need/function as well as the aspect of individual growth and mental health. Lord Krishna was able to vary the level of direction with *Arjuna* from time to time within the therapeutic dialogue. He deviated from the client's pace and employed challenges and confrontations to jolt *Arjuna* into awareness only because of the emergency situation. However, this was balanced with positive personal feedback, gentle acceptance, reassurance, and support. Thus *Arjuna* was saved from slipping from his dharma or role in the battlefield as well as from future distress caused by guilt and regret about his own inappropriate conduct. The value of satisfaction with one's own life is a part of Erik Erikson's concept of "personal integrity," which is a major achievement of the last adult stage of life.[92] Taking stock of one's own life in terms of values and past actions occurs as a developmental task at his stage. Personal integrity includes congruence between "ideal self" and "real self," and thus promotes mental health. The therapist role of Lord Krishna included a unified approach with many criteria for overall welfare of *Arjuna* in the present and personal integrity in the future.

Presence of mind, sense of proportion, and sensitivity to a variety of related aspects in determining a treatment plan for a patient are recognized as features of a good therapist today. In addition, he or she keeps in mind available information to apply wherever it may fit to promote adjustment and mental health. These values, goals, and methods were included in Lord Krishna's integrated approach to help *Arjuna.*

CASE STUDY*

Principles from the *Bhagavad Gita* can be applied in both formal professional psychotherapy, and in the context of daily living. The case study presented here may seem informal but in the Hindu culture, it is still one of the

---

*The case selected is the analysis of a forty-two-year-old, married, employed, Caucasian woman suffering from a major depressive episode. Madill and Barkham (1997). From "Discourse analysis of a theme in one successful case of brief psychodynamic-interpersonal psychotherapy," *Journal of Counseling Psychology, 44* (2), 232-244.

formal modes of psychotherapy. A priest is permanently in the role of a therapist, has no personal interest in the situation, is seen only at the temple, people go to him deliberately to seek advice, there is no fee but anyone can dedicate gifts to the temple at any time, as per their capacity. The difference in this system and the current notion of formality are sessions by prior appointments, fee as personal income for the therapist, and special litigation for protection of boundaries and third-party management of health care.

The case is a single major depressive episode in a forty-two-year-old, married woman, who was revisiting her relationship issues with her live-in, aging mother. Mona is a mother of two children and is employed full time. She is of average intelligence, with no history of any major psychiatric problems or a personality disorder. She was born and raised a Hindu and is modern enough to doubt traditions. In this particular situation, because of her own age level, the priest is not a peer but someone belonging to her parents' generation. A transference of viewing him as a father figure is not a surprise. However, if she had been an older woman, the priest would have been a peer and would be viewed as a brother. It is typical in the Hindu culture to see close relationships as parallels based on consanguinity. At the same time, friends are in an acceptable status as well, just as Lord Krishna, as a cousin and a friend, was in a therapeutic role toward *Arjuna*.

The therapist is a priest at the temple in her community, who is dedicated to promoting God's will through service to humanity. His lifestyle is unique in that he does not own a home, lives in a small back room of the temple, eats whatever is donated by the community members, dresses simply, is available at any time, spends most of his spare time in prayer, and does not get involved in worldly activities such as buying, selling, hobbies, parties, personal and social relationships, social activities, or social visits. His role is to provide regular formal educational talks on spirituality to the congregation, and personal guidance to individual seekers on a "needs" basis. He remains at the temple twenty-four hours a day. The therapeutic approach will be described as a series of eight contacts, each time initiated by the client, Mona, in which the priest provides personal guidance to her.

Narrative Description of the Therapeutic Process

First Contact

Following the priest's usual discourse, Mona was one of the audience that approached the priest to speak to him but she hung back hesitatingly because she needed to discuss her problem in privacy. As the others departed, the priest noticed her. Seeing the expectant look in his eyes, she moved forward, bowed, and received the unconditional blessing the priest gave to everyone. His keen eyes, having taken in her sad expression and somber mood, waited quietly. She was unable to speak. The priest eased her task by acknowledging his awareness of her distress and made the inquiry about the cause of her concerns in a calm, compassionate voice. Mona nodded, choking back tears. Seeing that she was unable to talk, he stated soothingly and reassuringly that the all-pervasive *Brahman* is in everything and resided in her as well. With focus on and trust in the Lord "Within and Without" all would come out right.

Mona felt reassured and encouraged. She described taking her aging mother into her home and finding it frustrating that despite her sacrifices and hard work, her mother seemed to be displeased with her. As the priest listened attentively and nodded thoughtfully, she found herself opening up more and more and giving more details. Mona began to feel some emotional relief and to believe that the priest would understand and would be able to help her.

She asked the priest for suggestions. He recommended meditations so that an answer would emerge from the Self within her. Mona had heard this elsewhere before and did not know that if she believed in the traditional religious teachings. However, at this point she was ready to try anything. So Mona asked for instruction and was given some practical suggestions.

Second Contact

Mona arrived at the temple earlier than usual so as to not miss the early part of the discourse. The topic was need of human Identification with *Param-Atman* or atman or the Causal layer, in contrast with the physical body. The importance of this was discussed with examples of actual issues of current lifestyle for average humans. Impressed, Mona decided to come regularly to attend these talks. She wished her mother could also benefit from the discourse but knew her mother had been refusing all activities. She was puzzled about her mother's resistance.

After the discourse, Mona waited eagerly until the priest was alone. He greeted her warmly and inquired about how she was. Mona responded morosely that she wished her mother would attend the discourse at the temple. She explained that her mother had been avoidant of all social contact and that any efforts to change this caused her great irritation. The priest focused on her own understanding of the discourse and her efforts at meditation. Mona expressed disappointment that she had trouble in freeing her mind of worries and concerns about mother. She was assured that most beginners had similar experiences and with time and practice she would get better at it. She decided to not give up on it just yet. Her request for permission to speak with him again the following week was acknowledged with a reassuring, warm, and welcoming reply.

Third Contact

Mona realized that despite feeling hopeless all week, this particular morning she had felt a surge of hope and had wanted to listen to the next discourse. The day's topic was "Looking Within for Guidance." Mona was so preoccupied with worries about her mother that she was somewhat inattentive. She wondered if her mother could learn to ignore pain. Mona was unaware that her arena of change was in herself. Later, she shared her thoughts about her mother with the priest. His gentle focus remained on her own growth, her understanding of the discourse, and her progress with meditation. She revealed that her preoccupation with her own thoughts and her mother's needs interfered with meditation. The priest supplied no solution, and Mona felt disappointed. She began to have doubts about getting help with her domestic problems.

At home, she asked her mother to come to the temple with her. The mother declined. Mona felt frustrated and decided that if her mother could not care less, she would not bother to go to the temple in order to solve her mother's problems.

Mona missed the next discourse but felt miserable about it because she was aware that she had probably missed hearing something important. However, more than everything else, she missed the priest's fatherly and nurturing interactions with her. Somehow, speaking to him made her feel serene and calm afterward.

Fourth Contact

Now aware that even if the priest could not solve her mother's problems, there were some gains for her in the discourse and contact (a sense of relaxation, peace, and well-being), Mona resumed going to the temple on Sundays for her own needs. This time the discourse was on "Ignorance and the Personality Sheaths." She was amazed that it all made sense. She expressed regrets to the priest about her mother's refusal to come with her. Mona was reassured that this was not cause for concern. Perhaps the time was not "ripe yet." He stated that everything acceptable to *Brahman* will occur at its proper time, including her mother's readiness. He reverted focus to her meditation progress and status. Mona admitted ability to meditate for longer than a couple of moments without interference from own thoughts or mother's speaking to her. The priest suggested meditating either away from home or when her mother slept. He made two further recommendations: (1) To try to see *Brahman* in her own mother, and (2) to try to hand over mother's welfare to *Brahman's* capable "good hands." Mona had become more aware of overwhelming guilt over her own family's needs competing with her mother's needs, and now she felt a sense of relief in the sanction from the priest to "let go" and to trust *Brahman*.

Fifth Contact

Mona felt, and seemed, particularly excited. A meditation exercise at the end of the discourse made her discover that she was able to concentrate much better than ever at home. She experienced feeling refreshed, rejuvenated and hopeful that she might develop the skill of meditation after all. Later, as she spoke to the priest about this, he suggested that she meditate at the temple more often until she can get similar outcomes at home. Mona thought this would be a great idea because (1) she lived close to the temple, and (2) it would be outside the reach of her mother's voice! Mona smiled at her mother's "funny ways" and became aware of a feeling of affection for mother. She also noted that she felt less pressure from mother's reactions on this matter. She felt like an adult in her own right rather than a child resenting having to do everything as her mother wished. She was not sure if this was good or if she was slipping into an uncaring attitude toward her mother.

Sixth Contact

Mona was very unhappy. The previous evening she was interrupted by her mother just as she was starting to get absorbed in meditation. She had been relaxed and felt so completely off guard that even before she knew it, she snapped at her mother. Her offended mother said a few critical things in response. Mona was disappointed in the negative interchange and since then, the two had not spoken to each other. Later in the day she had felt envy and hurt as she saw her mother having a happy conversation with her visitor. Mona had arrived early today in order to meditate at the temple before the discourse. She felt calmer and enjoyed the discourse on "Compassion" and "Selflessness." At the end of it she began to feel that she had been selfish with her mother and had not tried to understand the older woman's perspective. Before she could speak to the priest, she saw her mother in the group with her visitor of the other day. Her mother had not seen her yet. Mona felt hurt that her mother refused to come with her but chose to come with someone else. Soon the two women approached her laughing and asking if she had liked their surprise. Seeing their delight in the little plan of surprising her, Mona became aware how isolated her mother was and how little it took to please her. She began to laugh with them. Today she did not have a chance to speak to the priest alone but all three ladies went to him for a couple of minutes to express thanks for the discourse.

Mona invited the two ladies to lunch, which went well for all three of them. She also discovered that her mother had known the same priest earlier and liked him. Further, her mother approved of the temple as the preferred place for meditation because it is "God's place."

Seventh Contact

Mona discussed with the priest the "surprise" from her mother the previous week, and her feeling that her mother did not need to be sheltered from social life in the name of "rest." Her mother needed some sense of pleasant and lively involvement. The priest called it a part of the "awareness" that was gradually awakening in Mona.

Eighth Contact

Mona felt content. She was aware that her mother would be coming to the temple too. She described to the priest that she and mother had had a long talk. Recently, Mona had felt calm, positive and brave enough, to initiate a conversation with her mother about their communication. Mother had responded positively. Each had apologized to the other for mutual insensitivity and clarified own perspectives. Mona had discovered that her mother thought of her as capable and efficient and most negativism was from her frustrations with her having to disrupt Mona's life. Mona had assured mother that it was her choice to have her mother live with her and she had looked forward to it eagerly. For her, there was fulfillment in serving her mother in addition to benefitting from her mother's advice. If they could have some more times similar to the last two days, Mona would be a very happy person. The mother and daughter felt close to each other for the first time since her mother had come to live with her. Mother felt relaxed because she knew she was not a burden and could contribute something. Mona said to the priest that awareness of each other's perspectives had helped them both. The priest was pleased and blessed her as usual. He asked her to continue meditation for spirituality and even if the crisis was over. Mona wanted to do this anyway because she felt definite gains from the practice of meditation.

The priest's discourse that day was about the performance of appropriate action, without focus on the fruit or the results of the action. Mona was impressed and made a decision that she would put forth her best efforts and leave the rest to *Brahman*. She became aware that this would make for a healthier and adult-to-adult relationship with her mother. She also began to understand the meaning of "ignorance is the root of all problems." She and her mother had been "ignorant" in that they had not understood each other's perspective and it had affected communication in a negative way. In addition, she realized the meaning of the word "awareness" more deeply and broadly as insight a person develops into the situation as a whole.

Therapeutic Values and Highlights of the Process

There are several parallels between the spiritual values of the *Bhagavad Gita* and the modern values, styles, and techniques basic to therapeutic intervention. There is no intent here to compare them in terms of one being better than the other. Both are useful depending upon the situation, and the recipient's personality, beliefs, faith, and culture.

First Contact

The therapist functions in ways similar to the values of Carl Rogers' Client-Centered Therapy and Abraham Maslow's respect for and acceptance of the state of "being." His attitude is calm, quiet and peaceful as he waits for the individual to take initiative. Being sensitive to distress, he sets the process of therapy in motion because he believes in being flexible. The initial session can be the most difficult one for the client due to emotional risks in sharing vulnerable personal aspects. The therapist puts the client at ease, listens warmly and patiently, reassures, and creates hope.

Second Contact

The client now has some eagerness, motivation, and hope mingled with helplessness and hopelessness. The therapeutic intervention for depression has begun. Even though her focus is on "changing mother," the therapist focuses on the client because that is the real arena of change through awareness. The therapist encourages patience and persistence with nurturance, support, and warmth, as the client complains of difficulties with meditation. His attitude generates confidence in the vulnerable, emotionally insecure person.

Third Contact

The attendance of the discourse from the same therapist is useful as it imparts information about the therapist's beliefs, values, philosophies at a time other than the one-on-one therapeutic contact. The consistencies between the therapist thoughts and actions reassure the patient, reinforce trust, and promote positive motivation for change.

Returning to focus on the client during their individual talk, the therapist compares meditating state of mind as the calm and turmoil-free water of the pond wherein the reflection of the surrounding scene can be viewed. The client views herself as a "good" woman doing her best for mother despite other commitments, but she is unaware of her own turmoil and insensitivity to her mother as a person. Her frustration with demand of extra pressures to care for her mother, is in conflict with her own resentments about her mother's power over her as an offspring. She is unaware of her latent expectation of gratitude and appreciation from mother for her efforts. The therapist aids her self-esteem and calmness, refrains from any premature interpretations, permits effects to play out in their own good time, again leaving all to the Lord once his best efforts are made in reassuring the client.

The client misses the next session but as a result becomes aware of what she missed. She manages to continue beyond a risk of "premature termination" as stated in modern psychology.

Fourth Contact

The improved self-esteem and confidence due to the reassurance from the therapist lead to a greater awareness of own rights, and the client is closer to greater self-assertion. Asking her to "see *Brahman* in mother" (see the good in her mother), is an effort toward greater objectivity in her perception of the mother's positive and negative personality traits. "Hand over the mother to the Lord" is a parallel to "letting go" that is essential for people when appropriate boundaries need to be developed.

Fifth Contact

With lack of success in meditation, the client is advised to make some practical adjustments. Before she has put this into practice, a showdown with her mother occurs and the conflict has come out in the open. The client asserts herself, although not positively, and the resulting pattern is new in which they stop speaking to each other (the old pattern was that mother cried and client apologized out of guilt). The next day, seeing mother in a peer's company brought about ambivalence as well as some relief. The therapist remains receptive and reassuring, and with focus on the client indirectly conveying that she is important in her own right and is in charge of her own conduct. Her autonomy and initiative in introspection were anticipated throughout the expectation that change must come from within herself rather than her mother.

Sixth Contact

The therapist remains consistent and unperturbed with faith in selflessness and the eventual good of all. The message is that a good process (actions based on good principles) needs to be followed with patience even if there are some difficulties along the way. The basic assumption was that things would naturally work out in time. The mother-daughter conflict becomes a catalyst for better communication between them. Moreover, the involvement of others serves to disperse the mother's dependencies and the daughter's burdens. The client manages to emancipate from the mother-daughter relationship to a more mature adult-to-adult relationship with her mother. Stress and conflict are greatly reduced.

The therapist appears to be even more in the background now but without his support, the client would not have the required confidence and self-esteem, and might not continue with her efforts toward further resolution of the problems.

Seventh Contact

The therapist's discourses brought into the patient's awareness that the basic principles had been played out in her recent experiences. Her faith in the therapist and the wisdom of her culture's heritage gave her greater confidence. The discourses may not always coincide so well with individual experience but as one develops the habit of viewing unity, parallels over longer periods of time, become visible.

Eighth Contact

The unity of the basic human bond has been experienced across two generations. There is congenial equality and mutual respect between mother and daughter. The view of unity makes the notion of formal and rigid boundaries between "the mother's therapist" and "daughter's therapist" redundant. All can be helped by the same therapist in one small community because all are equal, belong together and, eventually are a part of the same Supreme Spirit. Separation is viewed as artificial and temporary.

Termination

Termination of therapy is unique. There is no such thing as a formal termination or formal re-initiation of contact. Instead, there is informal initiation of contact, and an ending based on mutual understanding. The "non-individualized" educational contact remains ongoing in the form of attendance at temple discourses and in obtaining blessings at the time of such attendance. The therapist does not belong to anyone other than God. Sharing him as a guide and leader is equivalent to many students sharing a teacher. Although the relationship with the priest in times of special need is one-on-one, confidential and personal, once the need is met it is possible to return to the original generalized relationship. This is possible due to the therapist's faith in his own spirituality and his or her detachment with all worldly relationships associated with the physical existence *(maya)*.

Conclusion

This system involves unconditional and unwavering trust in the therapist as long as his or her attitude and conduct are consistent with the spiritual philosophy. People can accept, and even take for granted, equal and fair treatment of all the individuals he helps. Further, it is understood that need of such help in humans will be recurrent and the therapist is appointed as a permanent guide, and helper in crisis situations, for one to access therapy or help immediately whenever the need occurs. There are no waiting lists, prior appointments, HMO prior authorization, and material payments for such services, hence services are offered based on human need, not on the ability to pay, nor on a formalized structure to meet the needs of the health-delivery system agencies. The system values flexibility and permits in the context of unity.

NOTES

1. Kulkarni S. D. (1995). *Dharma and vedic foundations: Bhishma's study of Indian history and culture, Vol. IX.* Bombay, India: Bhishma. pp. 1-77.

2. The word for deity in Sanskrit is *deva* or *deavata.* Often its inaccurate translation to represent the word "God," has caused misunderstandings. This gives the impression of polytheism while Hindu view is essentially monistic.

3. *Brahman* (not the same as the creator deity *Brahma*) is the Almighty, Supreme Spirit, or *Param-atman* or the one God and the cause for the total creation. The Sanskrit term "Sarva-lok-ik-natham" literally means the only one Lord of all universes.

4. In Sanskrit, *"atman"* means a soul in any being; *Param* means supreme; and *atman* (any soul) is the same as *Param-Atman* (the Supreme Soul). *Bhagavad Gita,* chapter II, verses 20-30.

5. Karma describes a definite relationship of actions (include thoughts and feelings) to outcomes. This spiritual cause and effect system is understood literally by some as karma being influential from one lifetime to future rebirths, and by others as consequences within one lifetime wherein each major change is a symbolic rebirth.

6. *Moksha* in Hinduism was conceptualized as the final merger with *Brahman* after many rebirths when the quality of individual karma enhanced to the highest level. In contrast, *Nirvana* is the Buddha's concept of liberation from all worldly involvements at the end of the only one lifetime.

7. Heaven is a rewarding shelter after death but there is no opposite place called "Hell." All the trouble, negatives, or suffering that occur on earth are symbolic "Hell" as a result of bad karma.

8. Good karma are positive actions that are individually role appropriate, and beneficial to society even when they are not connected to the desire to seek spiritual life or the Lord.

9. Bad karma are actions not beneficial to self, others, and society at large, even if connected with interest in spirituality and keenness for divine merger.

10. A *yogin* is an individual involved in the practice of yoga; his or her primary goal in life is attainment of spirituality.

11. Yoga as a process helps attain true spirituality along with the right attitude, dedication and efforts. It needs to be a constant (not occasional) requirement of spirituality, like we have regular necessary intake of food and air for physical life and exercise for health.

12. Eternal freedom is more a freedom of the soul (rather than the physical being and its activities), even though such freedom may include the physical aspect (e.g., reading is partially a physical activity but only in a secondary sense once an individ-

ual reads for understanding of the content). Sri Chinmoy (1973). *Commentary on the* Bhagavad Gita: *The song of the transcendent soul.* New York: Rudeep Steiner Publications. p. xvi.

13. "All-pervading" means uniformly and homogeneously present in every aspect of the creation.

14. "All-knowing" is a state of a general, automatic, intuitive awareness of all aspects of itself, without necessarily making an effort to supervise or keep track of all beings.

15. Suriyakumaran C. *Hinduism for Hindus and non Hindus (*1990). Sri Lanka. Department of Hindu Religion and Cultural Affairs.

16. Bhave, A.V. (1958). *Talks on the Gita.* Kashi, India: Akhil Bhartiya Seva Sangh Prakashan.

17. Vivekananda, Swami (1952). *Thoughts on the Gita.* Calcutta, India: Advaita ashram.

18. Chidbhavananda, S. (1996). *Sri Bhagavadgeeta.* Tirupparaitturai, India: Sri Ramakrishna Tapovanam.

19. Prabhupada, S. (1978). Bhagavad Gita *as it is.* Bombay, India: Bhaktivedanta Book Trust.

20. *Jiva* is a living being in any life form. This term is not limited to human beings. It is believed that God favors equally all animals, plant life, and what we see as nonliving materials.

21. Although self is the soul in an individual, Self is the Supreme Soul of which we all are exact, miniature representatives. The concept of Self-realization involves awareness of the "oneness" or unity of the two.

22. The so-called inert matter is only inert in appearance within our small units of time and due to the limited ability of our senses to perceive the latent and potential energy in it. Atomic research has shown that the same neutrons and protons are present in the inert materials as in the plant, animal and human cells.

23. Chinmayananda, S. (1980). *Discourses on Isvasya* Upanishad. Bombay, India: Central Chinmaya Mission Trust.

24. Chidbhavananda, *Sri Bhagavadgeeta,* pp. 60-61.

25. Gambhirnanda, S. (1954). *A short life of swami Vivekanada.* Calcutta, India: Sree Kali Press.

26. Chinmayananda, S. (1969). *Sreemad Bhagavad Geeta.* Chapters 12-18. Madras, Chinmaya Publications Trust.

27. *Patrika,* Newsletter of Hindu Society of Minnesota (Summer/fall 1998), pp. 2-3.

28. Tagore, R. (1966). *The religion of man: The Hilbert lectures of 1930.* Boston, MA: Beacon Press.

29. Chidbhavananda, *Sri Bhagavadgeeta,* pp. 60-61.

30. Chennakeshavan, S. (1974). *A critical study of Hinduism.* New York: Asia Publishing House. pp. 105-107.

31. Suriyakumaran, *Hinduism for Hindus and non Hindus,* pp. 5-7.

32. Ibid.

33. The word "attachment," in the *Bhagavad Gita* and Hindu philosophy writings, automatically includes the qualifications of "inappropriate and undue." If it is appropriate and due-attachment it is normal and therefore *dharma.* Then it is no lon-

ger called "attachment" but is a relationship. Divatia, H. J. (1970). *The art of life in the* Bhagavad-gita. Bombay, India: Bhartiya Vidya Bhavan. p. 69.

34. Gambhirnanda, S. (1954). *A short life of swami Vivekanada*. Calcutta, India: Sree Kali Press.

35. *OUM* is thought to be the first sound when the earth came into existence and also the sound of each revolution on its axis. A spiritual and religious symbol, O-U-M is worshipped at altars and is often placed on gold pendants to be used by Hindu devotees.

36. *Maya* is a Hinduism concept about life being an illusion. A misunderstanding of this idea led to the belief that the world is an illusion, and led many seekers to inaction because they left appropriate (spiritual) responsibilities of role function behind to become monks and lived in the Himalayas for years searching for "true spirituality" in order to counteract "*maya.*" The *Bhagavad Gita* states that such "inaction" is not only unnecessary but detrimental to human life, both social and personal. Instead, it is vital to create spiritual thoughts, feelings, attitudes, and outlook no matter what situation is faced by an individual.

37. Divatia, H.J. (1970). *The art of life in the* Bhagavadgita. Bombay, India: Bharatiya Vidya Bhavan. p. 69.

38. The *Bhagavadgita* sees the world as real enough but the subjective or personal meanings attached to various aspects of the world we perceive are illusory or *maya*. For instance, pessimism may make a person inactive and materialism may make a person neglect role function which includes relationships and spirituality at different stages of life. Therefore the strong beliefs in pessimism and the temporary satisfaction from materialism are illusions.

39. Dandekar, R. N. (1979). *Insights into Hinduism*. Delhi, India: Ajanta Publications.

40. Maier, *Three theories of child development,* pp. 75-143.

41. Chinmayananda, Chapters 5-11.

42. Chinmayananda, Chapters 12-18.

43. Chinmayananda, Chapters 1-4.

44. Chinmayananada, S. (1978). *The art of man-making: Talks on the* Bhagavad Geeta. Bombay, India: Central Chinmaya Mission Trust.

45. Easwaran, E. (1988). *The end of sorrow: The* Bhagvadgita *for daily living*. Pataluma, India: Nilgiri Press.

46. Bilpodiwala, Noshir (1962). *A synopsis of Acharya Vinoba Bhave's "the steadfast intelligence."* Tanjore, India: Sarvodaya Prachuralaya. pp. 1-30.

47. Chennakeshavan, *A critical study of Hinduism,* pp. 105-107.

48. Vivekananda, *Thoughts on the Gita.*

49. Desire is different from need, it is undue want/temptation in absence of a need.

50. *Ratnagiri,* the robber, later became *St. Valmiki* and authored the epic *Mahabharata.*

51. Easwaran, E. (1988). *The end of sorrow: The* Bhagvadgita *for daily living*. Pataluma, India: Nilgiri Press.

52. Vivekananda, S. (1962). *My master.* Calcutta, India: Advaita Ashram.

53. Easwaran, *The end of sorrow.*

54. Vivekananda, *Thoughts on the Gita.*

55. Maslow, A.H. (1962). *Toward a psychology of being.* New York: D. van Nostrand Company.

56. Rambachan, A. (1999). *Gitanidarsana: Similies of the* Bhagavadgita. Delhi, India: Motilal Banarasidas Publishers Private Limited.

57. Krishna had to leave his foster parents and take over the responsibilities of his kingdom. His foster father *Nanda* was devastated with separation anxiety and depression due to his positive attachment with the foster son whom he had raised as his own. Krishna's spontaneous therapeutic discussion with his foster father addressed the pain arising from attachment. This attachment had been appropriate when Krishna was a child but the foster father's dependence on the same type of daily face-to-face contact was unusual. Further, *Nanda* experienced emotional crisis and inability to survive emotionally without Krishna's presence in his home in the role of his child. Due to Krishna's compassionate and gentle discourse, the foster father was able to modify his beliefs and cognitions about separation and his painful conflict. He was able to "let go" of the adult offspring's constant presence.

58. Rambachan, *Gitamritam,* pp. 1-75.

59. *Sudama* was a school friend of Krishna in childhood. All contact between them had ceased after their departure from the boarding school. In adulthood, *Sudama* and his family found themselves in extreme poverty. There was no other way but to ask for help from someone with better resources. Nagged by his wife and concerned about food for the children, a very unwilling *Sudama* finally broke down and went to get help from King Krishna. *Sudama* had had no concept of royal lifestyle, and, upon arrival at the palace, he was dazzled by the riches and even more hesitant and self-conscious. He was reported to Krishna by the palace guards as a "totally lost, perplexed poor man asking for the King!". Krishna set an example of honoring friendship by running out barefoot to receive him and treated him as a cherished, royal guest besides helping him financially.

60. A beautiful dancer, *Vasavadatta's* charms were irresistible to most men, including kings and politicians of many kingdoms. Known as the "beauty queen" she found The Buddha's lack of romantic interest in her as a surprise and a challenge. However, despite her efforts, the Buddha remained uninterested. Many years later when *Vasavadatta* was ordered out of the city due to contagious diseases, and lay alone dying, The Buddha came to her aid. When no one else would come near her, The Buddha visited her with a nurturing attitude, in an effort to soothe and nurse her in a time of distress. His compassion and help to her in her ugly suffering state at the risk of his own health helped *Vasavadatta* see him as a true saint. This experience awakened spirituality in the dancer and she was able to rise above the "egoistic" identification she had with her appearance.

61. The salt law, imposed by the British rulers in India, was a very heavy tax payable to the British government by all companies manufacturing salt in India. Mahatma Gandhi opposed this law as unfair and unreasonable for the hard working and poor manufacturers especially because the tax collect was not being used for the public benefit. The nonviolent protestors were firm on their stand and were beaten by the British police until they either fainted or died.

62. Mahatma Gandhi was a political leader instrumental in helping to obtain India's freedom from the British rule in 1948 A.D. He was a follower of the *Bhagavad Gita* and was also given the title of "Maha-atma" (the great soul or the saintly soul) by the British rulers for his totally nonviolent self-assertion movement against the British government.

63. Vivekananda, *Thoughts on the Gita.*

64. Goble, F.G. (1970). *The psychology of Abraham Maslow: The third force.* New York: Pocket Books, Inc.

65. Kulkarni S. D. (1995). *Dharma and Vedic Foundations: Bhishma's study of Indian history and culture,* Vol. IX. Bombay, India: Bhishma. pp. 1-77.

66. Easwaran, *The end of sorrow.*

67. Vivekananda, S. (1963). *Work and its secret.* Calcutta, India: Advaita Ashram.

68. Existential anxiety is a term from Existentialism. It is anxiety specifically about own state of nonexistence. This is different from fear of death or sorrow for leaving the world or loved ones. It is purely anxiety only about the personal state of "not being."

69. *Diagnostic and Statistical Manual of Mental Disorders* (Fourth edition). American Psychiatric Association. pp. 393-438.

70. Saradananda, S. (1955). *Thus spake Sri Ramkrishna.* Madras, India: Sri Ramkrishna Math.

71. "Spirituality isn't opposed to rationality; it is the larger framework that reason fits into, one piece among many." For more details see Chopra D. (1998). *365 Days of Wisdom and Healing.* New York: Workman Publishing.

72. Thomas H. and Thomas D.L. (1988). In R.R. Divakar, and Ramkrishna (Eds.) *Living biographies of great religious leaders.* Bombay, India: Bhartiya Vidya Bhavan.

73. Ibid.

74. Zoroaster, an ancient prophet, lived in Northeast Iran in 1200 B.C. The religion Zoroastrianism, named after him, is followed by some in India. Bowker, *The Oxford dictionary of world religions.*

75. Bhave, A.V. (1958). *Talks on the Gita.* Kashi, India. Akhil Bhartiya Seva Sangh Prakashan.

76. Vivekananda, *Thoughts on the Gita.*

77. Saint Guru Nanak corrected a priest who was pressing a little boy to stop services to a hurt animal and go to attend the temple worship. The priest was gently made aware by Guru Nanak that the boy was already on the right spiritual track and the priest's pressure was disruptive of the boy's spiritual progress. The neglect of ritual worship was acceptable because the service to the ailing was a superior "worship."

78. Vivekananda, *My master.*

79. Vivekananda, *Thoughts on the Gita.*

80. Rychlak J.F. (1981). *Introduction to personality and psychotherapy.* Boston, MA: Houghton Mifflin Company. pp. 571-574.

81. Maslow, *Toward a psychology of being.*

82. Liebert, M. and Spiegler, D. (1982). *Personality: Strategies and issues.* Homewood, IL: The Dorsey Press. pp. 343-364.

83. Maslow, *Toward a psychology of being.*

84. Goyandaka, J.D. (1978). Bhagavad Gita *or the song divine.* Gorakhpur, India: The Gita Press.

85. Pereira, J. (1976). *Hindu theology: A reader.* New York: Doubleday and Company.

86. Gilliland, B., James R., and Bowman J. (1989). *Theories and strategies in counseling and psychotherapy.* Englewood Cliffs, NJ: Prentice-Hall Inc. pp. 90-110.

87. Ibid., pp. 111-154.

88. Rychlak, *Introduction to personality and psychotherapy,* pp. 577-616.

89. Gilliland, James, and Bowman. *Theories and strategies in counseling and psychotherapy,* pp. 66-89.

90. Rogers, C. (1961). *On becoming a person.* Boston, MA: Houghton Mifflin Company.

91. Sharma, P. (1979). *Hindu religion and ethics.* New Delhi, India: Asian Publication Services.

92. Maier, *Three theories of child development,* pp. 12-74.

Chapter 2

A Buddhist Psychology

Scott Kamilar

INTRODUCTION

Although Buddhism is usually classified as a religion, it is not based on faith in a Creator God. Buddhists are encouraged to follow the example of the Buddha, who resolved not to accept or believe in anything that he had not discovered for himself.[1] At the same time, Buddhism provides a path for spiritual awakening. For this reason, it can be called a nontheistic religion.

The Dalai Lama suggests that not only can Buddhism be considered a religion, but also a science of the mind, a philosophy, and a form of psychotherapy.[2] It is a science of the mind in that for 2,600 years Buddhists have studied their minds through meditation and developed an extremely sophisticated psychology. Buddhism can be considered a philosophy because it offers a fundamental view of reality (ontology), an epistemology, and a system of ethics. Finally, Buddhism can be considered to be a form of psychotherapy because it offers a theory of human distress and a method for alleviating suffering and promoting psychological growth. The Buddhist monk Punnaji wrote,

> Of course, the Buddhists of . . . Buddhist countries don't look upon Buddhism as a psychotherapy. It is mainly understood as a form of religion. Of course, those scholars who study the teaching of the Buddha . . . tend to regard the teaching as a philosophy. Now as I see it these two ways of thinking . . . can be seen as two extremes. . . . Avoiding these two extremes, I would like to take the Middle Path, which is to treat the teaching of the Buddha as a form of psychotherapy. . . . I would say that if Buddhism is introduced into the modern world as a psychotherapy, the message of the Buddha will be correctly understood.[3]

Buddha is a Sanskrit word meaning "the awakened or enlightened one." The founder of Buddhism, a prince named Siddhārtha Gautama, was born in India about 600 B.C. After living in the luxury and security of his father's palace for his first twenty-nine years, Siddhārtha began to feel his life was meaningless and was not satisfied with a life of material comforts. He set off into the world to seek an understanding of the nature of human life. Giving up all his wealth and possessions, he became a student of Hindu teachers who taught him a variety of yogic practices. Siddhārtha adhered to an ascetic discipline of extreme self-denial for several years. He scorched himself in fires and related to the energy of tantra by practicing a variety of visualization exercises.[4]

At first he felt exhilarated by his accrual of new and exotic experiences. He also felt pride in his mastery of difficult and fascinating techniques. However, these feelings eventually faded and he was left with the gnawing realization that he still had not found the awakened state of being he was searching for.

The time came to bid farewell to his teachers and to set out to discover the truth on his own.[5] After extensive travels, Siddhārtha stopped under a pipal tree on the bank of the Nairanjana river. There he remained for several years sitting on a large stone, eating and drinking very little. Finally he realized that leading an ascetic life and punishing himself did not result in enlightenment, so he went off to beg for some food. A wealthy woman gave him some boiled milk with honey in it. It tasted delicious and boosted his energy, allowing him to make great progress in his meditation practice. He then decided that sitting on a stone was too painful. A farmer gave him some kusa grass to use as a cushion, so that he could sit in comfort while meditating. Siddhārtha had discovered that trying to achieve enlightenment by force and privation would not work. He gave up all hope of achieving anything at all and decided, instead, to just sit comfortably. That night he realized the Awakened State of mind and became the Buddha.

Buddha then began to walk throughout India, and for nearly forty years he shared his wisdom in an effort to relieve the suffering of those he encountered. Three centuries after his death, his teachings were put into writing in the *Pali Cannon,* also known as the Tripitaka, "the three baskets." The first, the *Vinayapitaka,* is concerned with discipline. It spells out the practicalities of how to live one's life in a conscious way. The second "basket," the *Sutrapitaka,* includes the sermons of the Buddha and deals with meditation and various ways of training the mind.[6] The third "basket," the *Abhidharma,* is based on analysis of the data of experience. It is concerned with the workings of the mind and the states of human consciousness.

Since the time of Buddha, three main styles of Buddhism have developed: individualistic *(Hinayana),* universal *(Mahayana),* and apocalyptic *(Vajrayana)* styles. From approximately 500 B.C.E. to 0 C.E. the monastic or individualistic style was dominant.[7] Monastic Buddhism spread outside India to Sri Lanka, central Asia, Iran, and west Asia. Presently, Sri Lanka is the bastion of the monastic style. This style emphasizes the Hinayana path ("common or lesser vehicle"), which is also called *Theravadin* or the "Way of the Elders."

From 0 to 500 C.E. the universal or messianic style of Buddhism developed. This style, also called the Mahayana path ("greater vehicle"), extended the reach of Buddhism to central Asia and China. This style later spread to Japan and Korea in the form of Zen Buddhism.

From approximately 500 C.E. to 1000 C.E. the apocalyptic style of Buddhism developed and spread through the Buddhist world. This style is also called Vajrayana ("diamond or indestructible vehicle"). Vajrayana practices are described in a series of texts known as *tantras*. Only in Tibetan Buddhism is this style preserved in integration with the two previous styles.

The Hinayana path emphasizes renunciation, meditation, and the concept of impermanence. The goal is to attain liberation for oneself. When integrated with the other two paths, the logic of the Hinayana path is that before one can be of any use to others it is necessary to develop a clear state of mind.

The Mahayana path involves achieving liberation for the sake of others. The traveler on this path, a bodhisattva, vows to put off his or her own liberation so that he or she may work to relieve all other beings of suffering. The path of the bodhisattva is to develop *bodhichitta,* awakened heart.

According to Pema Chodron, an American Buddhist nun,

> *Bodhichitta* has three qualities: (1) it is soft and gentle, which is compassion; (2) at the same time, it is clear and sharp, which is called *prajna;* and (3) it is open. This last quality of *bodhichitta* is called *shunyata* and is also known as emptiness. Emptiness sounds cold. However, *bodhichitta* isn't cold at all, because there's a heart quality—the warmth of compassion—that pervades space and the clarity.[8]

What Vajrayana adds to the Hinayana and Mahayana paths is a description of enlightenment. Hinayana describes enlightenment as the rejection of *samsara* (endless suffering resulting from the definition of self as separate from the universe). Mahayana describes enlightenment as the separate coexistence of *samsara* and nirvana (freedom from *samsara*). In Vajrayana, enlightenment is the union of *samsara* and nirvana in pure, luminous awareness. Vajrayana utilizes visualizations, *mantras* (special formulas of syllables that use the spiritual power of sound vibration), and *mudras* (symbolic gestures that awaken spiritual receptivity and awareness).[9] There is also an emphasis on the guru. Through the power of his or her enlightened awareness, a guru can introduce the student to the nature of his or her own mind in a direct mind-to-mind transmission.

Chogyam Trungpa, a Tibetan Buddhist meditation master, described the path along the three *yanas* in this way:

We must begin our practice by walking the narrow path of simplicity, the [H]inayana path, before we can walk upon the open highway of compassionate action, the [M]ahayana path. And only after our high-way journey is well on its way need we concern ourselves about how to dance in the fields—the [V]ajrayana or tantric teachings.[10]

PERSONALITY THEORY

This discussion of personality theory consists of (a) personality structure in terms of karma and the emergence of the illusory ego in five stages *(skandhas)*, (b) personality dynamics in terms of the six realms of the Wheel of Samsara, (c) personality development through six psychological states, and (d) individual differences expressed in five personality styles *(buddha families)*.

Personality Structure

Maddi (1972) defines personality as "a stable set of characteristics and tendencies that determine those commonalities and differences in the psychological behavior (thoughts, feelings, and actions) of people that have continuity in time and that may or may not be easily understood in terms of the social and biological pressures of the immediate situation alone."[11] The concept in Buddhism that most closely fits this definition is karma.

Karma and the Illusion of a Stable Personality

In Buddhist psychology past actions are thought to create predispositions, tendencies, and attitudes to which we resort in relating to the present. Actions that grow out of this narrow, distorted view of the present, in turn, sow the seeds for future predispositions, tendencies, and attitudes.[12] However, karma differs from Maddi's definition of personality in that at any moment one can return to the "open-ended quality of the present." "If we do so, seeds of peace, joy, and happiness will be planted in us, and they will become strong. . . . Wherever we are, any time, we have the capacity to enjoy the sunshine, the presence of each other, the wonder of our breathing."[13] Thus, the "stability" of personality is, in Buddhism, an illusion.

The illusion of a stable personality results from the speediness of a confused mind. Just as a motion picture creates an illusion of continuous movement by projecting a series of still images fast enough so that the gaps between frames are not seen, so a confused mind creates the illusion of a continuous and solid identity out of a series of individual feelings, perceptions, and thoughts. This illusion of a solid and continuous identity is called "ego."

Ego Emerges in Five Stages

Buddhist psychology describes ego as emerging from open space in a sequence of five major stages and then fading back into spacious openness, just as clouds emerge from and then disappear back into the sky. The five stages, known as *skandhas,* reoccur from moment to moment. *Skandha* literally means "heap." It is a collection or pile of a lot of little details and aspects of psychological inclinations of different types. Ego is constructed of many particles rather than being one solid and continuous thing.[14] It emerges through five major stages of form, feeling, perception-impulse, conceptualization, and consciousness.

Form. The first *skandha* of form, emerges with the birth of ignorance, the beginning of a duality between self and other. Ignorance, in this context, refers to the ignoring of the basic ground of open awareness and the construction of an illusory separate self.

Feeling. The next stage in the development of ego is the *skandha* of feeling. At this point the world is an It, separate from me, so there is a tendency to ask whether the territory out there is hostile, friendly, or neutral. We reach out and feel the qualities of "other" in order to reassure ourselves that we exist. "If I can feel that out there, then I must be here."[15]

Perception-impulse. The third *skandha,* perception-impulse, is the stage in which the information transmitted during the *skandha* of feeling becomes the basis for making judgments and reacting with either passion, aggression, or ignorance. Passion in this sense is a strategy of seducing, pursuing, and possessing objects of desire. Aggression is a strategy of pushing away and rejecting threatening situations. Ignorance is a strategy of being indifferent to something or avoiding it. Known as the Three Poisons, these strategies are the basic ways in which we respond impulsively to perceptions of the outside world.

Conceptualization. Concept, the fourth *skandha,* is the next step in the process of protecting one's ignorance and armoring the self. At this stage we utilize intellect to name and categorize things and events. Elaborate schemes of interpretation, rationalization, and belief are used to appropriate more and more territory for ego.[16] In the *abhidharma,* fifty-one general types of mind/body patterns are described. The six types of egocentric patterns are ignorance, passion, anger, pride, doubt, and dogmatism. The four types of neutral patterns are slothfulness, intellectual speculation, remorse, and knowing. There are eleven patterns associated with "goodness" in that they are expressions of basic intelligence or buddha nature. Among these are surrendering or faith, awareness, discipline, equanimity, absence of passion, absence of anger, absence of ignorance, humility or shyness, a tendency of nonviolence, a tendency of energy or effort, or bravery.[17] These patterns are appropriated by ego in its pursuit of "spiritual materialism" which, according to Chogyam Trungpa, is when we "deceive ourselves into thinking we are developing spiritually when instead we are strengthening our egocentricity through spiritual techniques."[18]

Consciousness. In the final stage of ego's development, the fifth *skandha* of consciousness, all the previous *skandhas* flow together into the stream of consciousness. At this point there is an ongoing process of thinking and feeling, an inner dialogue that Trungpa calls "subconscious gossip." The cloudy mind of the fifth *skandha* contains a bank of collected memories including ashamed thoughts, irrelevant thoughts, and various other thoughts that have been hidden and suppressed. The maintenance of a dualistic separation between self and other has become highly efficient because the cloudy mind immediately supplies thoughts from its memory bank to fill in the naturally occurring gaps in the stream of consciousness.

Upon attaining the final stage of ego development, the chain of karma is complete. The predispositions, tendencies, and attitudes that might be called "personality" are constantly being reborn moment-to-moment in the form of the five *skandhas* and the primordial state of spacious openness is effectively ignored and forgotten.

Personality Dynamics: Six Realms

The Wheel of Life (Wheel of Samsara) is depicted in Buddhist art in circular form and is set into "the yawning jaws of Yama, the lord of death."[19] Depicted on the Wheel of Life are the six realms: the realm of the gods, the realm of the jealous gods, the human realm, the animal realm, the realm of the hungry ghosts, and the hell realm. Depicted in the center of the Wheel of Life are the three forces that drive us repeatedly through the same vicious feedback loops. These forces are greed represented by a red cock, hatred represented by a green snake, and delusion represented by a black hog. Each is biting the tail of its neighbor to indicate the circular nature of their interconnection. The basic motivating forces for all egocentric behavior are the greedy pursuit of pleasure, the hate-filled campaign to eradicate pain, and the deluded retreat into ignorance. At the most fundamental level these patterns are all designed to cocoon and promote the self.

Each time we are presented with an object of desire we feel an impulse to possess that object, whether it is a tasty morsel of food, a great job, an attractive member of the opposite sex, or a shiny new car. The project of acquiring this object can then propel us forward into action, during which all existential anxieties are ignored. Once the object is acquired, we can then begin to look around for the next object of desire. One's whole life can become a project of acquiring more money, better toys, tastier food, and sexier partners.

Underlying this whole project, however, will be a gnawing and, at times, stabbing pain. This is the painful recognition that no matter how much we manage to acquire, the pleasure of acquisition is short-lived and in the meantime we all grow older, get sick, and eventually die. We can hate what we perceive to be the sources of pain in our lives, our enemies, our spouses, or friends when they confront us about our habitually selfish patterns, our unruly emotions, our less than perfect bodies. We can aggressively seek to destroy what we perceive to be the sources of pain by killing or defeating our enemies, leaving our spouse or friend, pursuing the power of positive thinking, going on a diet, or getting plastic surgery. However, the underlying pain will always return. No matter how much we delude ourselves or push away the painful truth it will sneak up on us in those moments of satiation, disappointment, and boredom.

Personality Development: Six Psychological States

The six realms depicted on the Wheel of Life can be considered to be forms of existence through which sentient beings cycle from birth to rebirth. Karma dictates that harming others results in reincarnation in the hell realm, the pursuit of desire results in rebirth in the animal realm, while compassionate acts of generosity result in reincarnation in a more comfortable human or god realm.

On a psychological level, however, the realms of existence can be considered to be psychological states through which we may cycle in the course of a day or over a lifetime. Usually, a person's psychology is primarily located in one realm.[20] This realm is actually one of confusion, a dream world in which we can entertain and distract ourselves from our ultimate fear that we may not exist, that our carefully constructed ego is merely a "heap" of habitual patterns and delusions.

Blissful State

The god realm is described by Epstein as a peak experience in which ego boundaries are dissolved in an orgasmic experience of pleasure.[21] The infant at the breast, the lover absorbed in romantic bliss, the meditator experiencing inspiring visions and seemingly profound mental states, all could be considered experiences of the god realm. Obviously, all these experiences are temporary and eventually produce psychological rebirth in a lower and less pleasurable realm. Sooner or later, the breast is withdrawn, the romance fades, or the state of meditative absorption is interrupted by the demands of reality. Even people who have managed to amass great fortunes, develop wonderful relationships, and construct fascinating lives, must eventually face loss and death. Any resident of the god realm will come to have his or her blissful state shaken and faith in the continuity of the blissful state is also lost. Doubts and fears begin to creep their way into one's consciousness. This is the birth of the jealous god realm.

State of Distrust

The realm of the jealous gods is pictorially depicted by a fruit-laden "wishing-tree" that is fought over by the residents of this realm. The dominant characteristic of this psychological state is paranoia. Its mentality is extremely intelligent: it looks at situations from all angles. There is a constant striving to attain something higher and greater. Life situations are regarded as games, in the sense that there is always an opponent to be outwitted and defeated. The residents of this realm are preoccupied with comparison. They are perpetually striving to be number one, to have more, to accomplish more, and to enjoy more.

Pursuit of an Ideal

The only path off the Wheel of Life and into Buddhahood is in the human realm. Human birth is considered a precious opportunity to awaken, to realize one's true nature, and thereby, to stop producing unnecessary suffering for oneself and others. The essence of this realm is striving to achieve some high ideal. The psychological state characterizing the human realm is fascination with what one lacks. When a resident of the human realm hears of someone who possesses remarkable qualities, a strong identification with that person develops. In this realm, you criticize and condemn people who do not meet your standards and you reject things and experiences that are not exactly compatible with your style. You are "stuck in a huge traffic jam of discursive thought . . . there is a constant churning out of ideas, plans, hallucinations and dreams."[22]

State of Instinctual Gratification and Ignorance

The animal realm is characterized by ignorance. The essence of the animal style is the gratification of instinctual desires. This is an extremely serious, stubborn, and humorless way of relating to the world, and is traditionally symbolized by the pig. "The pig does not look to the right or left but just sniffs along, consuming whatever comes in front of its nose; it goes on and on, without any sense of discrimination—a very sincere pig."[23] The animal style is impervious to feedback from others. In this realm there is no possibility for enlightenment because there is no way of surrendering or opening up to the world. Instead there is a continual, self-justifying round of activity.

Acquisitive State

The hungry ghost realm is characterized by a sense of poverty and a preoccupation with acquiring and consuming. This realm is traditionally represented "by a hungry ghost who has a tiny mouth, the size of a needle, a thin neck and throat, skinny arms and legs and a gigantic stomach."[24] His strawlike neck and tiny mouth can never allow enough food to pass through them so that his tremendous belly can be filled and his desperate hunger satisfied. Food can represent any object of desire—money, sex, unconditional love, or power.

Even spiritual seekers can find themselves in the hungry ghost realm if they apply a poverty mentality to their search for a higher state of consciousness. When a spiritual breakthrough or insight occurs there is a natural tendency to cling to it. Over time this experience begins to fade and the search for new and more powerful experiences can grow more and more desperate. There are many spiritual hungry ghosts who go from teacher to teacher and accumulate experiences from a variety of traditions without ever satisfying their craving for enlightenment.

State of Aggression

The hell realm is symbolized in Tibetan paintings by beings boiling in hot oil, being torn from limb to limb by wild animals, and suffering a variety of other tortures. This realm is pervaded by aggression, which is symbolized by the sky and earth radiating red fire. There is no space to breathe. In this realm, you discover that the more you try to destroy your enemies, the stronger they become. The only way out of this realm is to observe one's feelings of anger and hatred clearly. This is symbolically represented by the Boddhisattva of Compassion holding a mirror.

Individual Differences: Five Personality Styles

Although the Hinayana and Mahayana versions of Buddhism present a psychology and a path that can apply to any human being interested in progressing spiritually, in tantric Buddhism individual differences are appreciated more fully. These differences dictate the "precise therapy" each person requires to progress on the tantric path.[25] Thus, in tantra we find that there are five principles of buddha nature, known as the five buddha families. These buddha families are: *vajra, ratna, padma, karma,* and *buddha.* A person could identify primarily with only one of these styles, all of them, or partially with several. Each family is associated with both a style of neurosis (not defined in the western psychological way but rather used to indicate a state of confusion) and a style of sanity.

Logical Style (Vajra)

The *vajra* buddha family is symbolized by the *vajra* scepter, or *dorje* in Tibetan.[26] *Vajra* is literally translated as "diamond," but in this context it conveys additional qualities associated with a diamond such as sharpness, crystallization, and indestructibility. The *vajra* scepter has five prongs representing piercing and cutting through the five emotions: aggression, pride, passion, jealousy, and ignorance. *Vajra* is thought to precisely correct any neurotic distortion of reality. A person in the *vajra* family is intellectually very sharp, logical, and analytical.

The neurotic aspect of *vajra* is associated with intellectual fixation and anger. When we become attached to an insight or fixated on a particular logic we can become rigid and unyielding. When our perspective or point of view is challenged we can react with anger or aggression.

Vajra can also be represented by the element of water. The defensiveness and aggression of the neurotic aspect of *vajra* is symbolized by cloudy, turbulent water. The sharpness, precision, and clarity of *vajra* wisdom is represented by the clear, calm water of a reflecting pool. For this reason, *vajra* wisdom is traditionally referred to as Mirrorlike Wisdom.

Expansive Style (Ratna)

The next buddha family is called *ratna,* which means "jewel," "gem," or "precious stone." *Ratna* is associated with a sense of richness and wealth of all kinds. There is also a tendency toward expansion, enrichment, and plentifulness. When this tendency is neurotic it manifests in ostentatious self-indulgence. Moreover there can be a need to maintain one's pride by adopting defense mechanisms—building an impenetrable fortress.

The neurotic pride of *ratna* can be transmuted into the Wisdom of Equanimity. The anxiety of having to maintain and fortify one's pride dissolves. Because there is a feeling of richness and wealth it is possible to extend oneself personally and spiritually. There is a corresponding sense of expansion and openness.

Ratna is associated with the earth and with fertility. It is similar to a rotting log that grows all kinds of mushrooms and plants and allows animals to nest in it. *Ratna* can be a lazy settling down and making oneself comfortable, inviting other people to come in and rest as well.

Passionate Style (Padma)

The next buddha family is *padma,* which means "lotus flower." The lotus grows and blooms in the mud remains still, pure and clean, virginal and clear. *Padma* neurosis is connected with passion and a desire to possess. A person suffering this kind of neurosis would be consumed by desire and determined to seduce the world. Such a person might relate to the people in his or her life as a slick salesperson or hustler.

When the neurotic passion of *padma* is transmuted it becomes Discriminating Awareness Wisdom. Instead of passion and seductiveness there is intense interest and curiosity about the world and other people. Because other people are seen with precise awareness and appreciated as unique individuals, genuine communication can take place.

Padma is associated with the element of fire. In its neurotic aspect, the fire of desire consumes and destroys everything in its path. When transmuted, it becomes the warmth of compassion.

Padma is connected with an appreciation of the visual qualities of objects, the colors and patterns of surfaces rather than the solidity of being. As a result, a person in the *padma* family would be more involved with art rather than science or practicality.

Active Style (Karma)

The fourth buddha family is *karma,* which literally means "action" or "activity." *Karma* is the energy of efficiency. In its neurotic aspect, there is a fear that you will never achieve any of your goals so there is a tendency to be speedy, pragmatic, and functional at all times. Anything that does not fit your scheme or agenda is ignored or destroyed. At the same time, the accomplishments of other people are irritating and there is a fear of being surpassed. The emotion associated with the neurotic aspect of *karma* is jealousy or envy. *Karma* is connected with the element of wind. The wind never blows in all directions at once, but blows in only one direction at a time. This is the one-way view of jealousy and envy that picks out one little virtue in another person and blows it out of proportion.

The enlightened aspect of *karma* is the Wisdom of All-Accomplishing Action. The emotion of jealousy or envy falls away, but the qualities of energy, fulfillment of action, and openness remain. One's actions are appropriate because they are no longer based on fear and envy. One sees the possibilities inherent in situations and automatically takes the appropriate course. The active aspect of wind is retained so that everything in one's path is touched.

Meditative Style (Buddha)

The fifth family is *buddha* and is associated with the element of space. As such, it is the "basic ground" or foundation that makes it possible for the other families or principles to function. The *buddha* family has a sedate, solid quality. A person in this family is highly meditative. The neurotic manifestation of the *buddha* family is a quality of being "spaced out" rather than spacious. A slothful, senseless quality is brought to all the other emotions. A person with *buddha* neurosis cannot be bothered by the mundane details of existence such as doing laundry or washing the dishes. Ignoring one's environment is much easier. Similarly, communicating with others is too much effort. Even when another person treats you badly or invades your territory you ignore them, perhaps rationalizing that it is really nothing when compared with the vastness of infinite space and time.

When the ignoring quality of *buddha* neurosis is transmuted into wisdom, it becomes the Wisdom of All-Encompassing Space. This wisdom contains great energy and intelligence and activates the other four wisdoms. It is vast and spacious, similar to the sky.

It is necessary to understand the five *buddha* families before embarking on the tantric path. Once we understand our unique qualities we can use them as stepping stones on the path of self-transmutation. Each individual belongs to certain *buddha* families and can develop awareness of their neurotic aspects so that their intrinsic enlightened aspects can be uncovered.[27]

THEORY OF DISTRESS

Four Noble Truths

When the Buddha became enlightened he first thought that teaching others would be impossible because no one could possibly understand what he had learned. When he finally decided that he would go out and teach, his first teachings were on the four noble truths, which outline the origin of suffering and how suffering can be alleviated.

Reality of Suffering

The first noble truth is the truth of suffering: life inevitably involves pain. There is the pain of birth, the pain of sickness, the pain of aging, and the pain of death. No matter how hard one tries to hold onto pleasure and avoid discomfort, pleasure is fleeting and discomfort cannot be avoided.

Origin of Suffering

The second noble truth is about the origin of suffering. Although pain is unavoidable, we increase our suffering unnecessarily each time we defend against it. Trungpa calls this unnecessary layer of self-created pain "negative negativity" or "double negativity."

> We would like to pretend that these "evil" and "foul-smelling" aspects of ourselves and our world are not really there, or that they should not be there. . . . so negative negativity is usually self-justifying, self-contained. It allows nothing to pierce its protective shell—a self-righteous way of trying to pretend that things are what we would like them to be instead of what they are.[28]

Psychotherapists often encounter very clear examples of double negativity. Panic attacks are usually caused when a person begins to get anxious about being anxious. The first sign of anxiety then becomes a signal to mobilize a defense against anxiety, which triggers more anxiety until a full blown panic attack results. Similarly, chronic insomnia can result from overreacting to occasional and entirely normal episodes of insomnia. As soon as difficulty falling asleep is labeled a problem, an unnecessary layer of anxiety exacerbates the difficulty. One last example of double negativity is the avoidance of normal grief, which unnecessarily prolongs and complicates the grieving process.

In all of these examples, a part of the self sits in judgment of another part, which it sees as alien and problematic. It is this split between what is identified with and what is pushed aside that is what Buddhist psychology defines as ego. Ego is, "the activity of identifying with the objects of consciousness (i.e., thoughts, feelings, perceptions) and grasping anything that maintains this identity."[29] When we desperately hold onto an identity, the world is split into an I and an It.

In the process of defending ourselves from pain, we also attack those people in our lives who hurt us, even when their intentions are benevolent. There is a natural tendency to push away or even strike out against those people who hurt us or reflect back to us our inadequacies. When this happens it is not unusual for those we have pushed away to return, now bearing a grudge and seeking vengeance. This vicious interpersonal circle can also be considered to be double negativity.

Cessation of Suffering

Although the first noble truth of suffering can sound extremely pessimistic and gloomy, good news is contained in the third noble truth about the cessation of suffering. Although we cannot stop ourselves from aging, becoming sick, dying, or experiencing losses, we can eliminate the unnecessary layer of suffering resulting from double negativity by, "letting go of holding on to ourselves . . . not resisting, not grasping, not getting caught in hope and fear, in good and in bad, but actually living completely."[30] In *Zen Mind, Beginner's Mind,* Shunryu Suzuki states that

> mind includes everything; when you think something comes from outside, it means only that something appears in your mind. Nothing outside yourself can cause any trouble. You yourself make the waves in our mind. If you leave your mind as it is, it will become calm. This mind is called big mind.[31]

Letting go of the hold we have on ourselves or big mind are different ways of describing egolessness.

It is important to note that egolessness does not mean entirely eliminating the Freudian ego. Egolessness is not a state of being completely driven by libidinal impulses so that one is unable to function effectively in society.

Another common misconception is that Buddhism promotes a state of egolessness in which one becomes completely passive and unfeeling or numb. This idea is exactly the antithesis of the goal of Buddhist psychology. In Richard Baker's introduction to *Zen Mind, Beginner's Mind,* the Zen master Shunryu Suzuki is described as existing,

> freely in the fullness of his whole being. The flow of his consciousness is not the fixed repetitive patterns of our usual self-centered consciousness, but rather arises spontaneously and naturally from the actual circumstances of the present. The results of this in terms of the quality of his life are extraordinary-buoyancy, vigor, straightforwardness, simplicity, humility, serenity, joyousness, uncanny perspicacity and unfathomable compassion.[32]

Clearly, egolessness is not a state of passive, numb inability to function.

End of Suffering Via the Middle Way

Although the third truth tells us that the cessation of suffering is possible by letting go of the grasping, dualistic tendencies, it is not clear how this can be accomplished. The fourth noble truth provides the path to the cessation of suffering, known as the "middle way." In the Buddha's first twenty-nine years of life he lived a life of pleasure and self-indulgence. After realizing that such a life could not lead to enlightenment he embarked on an ascetic path of self-denial and pain. Only when he avoided these two extremes could he attain liberation. The fourth noble truth describes a middle way known as the eightfold path (see pp. 240-245).

Although the four noble truths are the foundation of all styles and schools of Buddhism, Vajrayana goes further in its exploration of suffering and freedom from suffering. In tantric wisdom, *samsara* and *nirvana* are seen as inextricably linked. Whereas, in Mahayana there is an emphasis on *shunyata,* which means emptiness, as an alternative to *samsara.* Vajrayana teachings emphasize the transmuting of samsaric energy into nirvana.[33] Anger, sadness, fear, and pain all contain tremendous energy and intelligence. The goal of the Buddhist path is not to empty oneself of all negative emotion; rather, the goal is to learn to dance with the energies of these emotions. Only then can a truly indestructible state of awareness be realized. Chogyam Trungpa once wrote: "Hold the sadness and pain of samsara in your heart and at the same time the power and vision of the Great Eastern Sun. Then the warrior can make a proper cup of tea."[34] We are all born with a brain and a nervous system capable of producing a wide spectrum of feelings. Only when we embrace this fact of our existence can we be fully human.

THEORY OF THERAPY

Purpose of Psychotherapy

The Buddhist path is a vehicle for achieving self-knowledge and the alleviation of suffering. Consequently, it can be considered psychotherapeutic. Buddhism has influenced an increasing number of psychotherapists who have developed ways of integrating Buddhist psychology and meditation into their work as therapists. In the following sections, discussions of Buddhist "therapy" will refer to both those intrinsic aspects of the Buddhist path that can be considered psychotherapeutic and those systems, developed in the West, that explicitly integrate Buddhism and psychotherapy.

Growth-Oriented Therapy: Beyond Ego

The various approaches to psychotherapy can be categorized as being either problem solving or growth oriented. Problem-solving therapy tends to be short-term and directed toward resolving defined symptoms and dilemmas. Growth-oriented therapy tends to be long-term and directed toward self-exploration and psychological development. Buddhist therapy clearly goes beyond the narrow limits of problem solving and is definitely oriented toward the long-term process of self-exploration and development. As such it is a growth-oriented therapy. The symptoms and dilemmas presented to the Buddhist therapist are not seen as problems to be solved, but rather are seen as precious opportunities for developing greater awareness and self-acceptance. What Pema Chodron says about people who start on the Buddhist path can also apply to people seeking therapy:

> [T]hey often think that somehow they're going to improve, which is a sort of subtle aggression against who they really are. It's a bit like saying, "If I jog, I'll be a much better person." "If I could only get a nicer house, I'd be a better person." "If I could meditate and calm down, I'd be a better person."[35]

Instead of viewing self-improvement as the goal, Buddhist therapy focuses on developing loving-kindness toward ourselves *(maitri).* We are encouraged to befriend ourselves because by doing so we can discover that we already have everything we need to be a fully functional, joyful human being.

On the Buddhist path, the way we befriend ourselves is through meditation. Over time, the meditator begins to recognize his or her ways of maintaining a solid and stable identity. Gradually less time is spent in mindless activity and more time is spent in a state of egoless awareness. As a result, self-loathing and the project of self-improvement is given up.

The purpose of Buddhist psychotherapy, then, can be seen as the growth of awareness and the development of a less ego-based way of being. As stated in the third noble truth, such growth results in the cessation of unnecessary self-created suffering.

Principles of Psychotherapy

Whether working with oneself within the context of the Buddhist path or working with others in Buddhist psychotherapy, there are a number of principles that can provide guidance and inspiration. These principles include acceptance, adopting a right view, focusing on the here and now, rejection of mind-body dualism, appreciation of environmental factors, emphasis on basic sanity, and a description of the stages of healing.

Acceptance

A basic principle of Buddhist psychology is that each of us has "buddha nature" or "basic sanity." All neurosis contains wisdom. The Buddhist therapist must accept the client's neurotic patterns so that the wisdom within them can become apparent to the client.

To illustrate what accepting neurotic patterns really means, let us examine the method Buddhist psychology gives us for relating to emotions. When sitting in meditation we are instructed to feel the texture of feelings and then let them go. The same painful emotion may come up again and again, but each time the practice is the same, "touch and let go." When we attend to an emotion in this way, the story line or idea that feeds it begins to fall away leaving us with pure energy. For example, with anger, it is important

> to see it clearly with precision and honesty, and also to see it with gentleness. That means not judging yourself as a bad person, but also not bolstering yourself up by saying, "It's good that I'm this way. . . . other people are terrible, and I'm right to be so angry at them all the time." [36]

Accepting painful emotions clearly means not falling into the trap of either repressing or fighting them. For this reason, Buddhist therapy would not include the use of affirmations and "positive thinking."

> Affirmations are like screaming that you're okay in order to overcome this whispering that you're not. That's a big contrast to actually uncovering the whisper, realizing that it's passing memory, and moving closer to all those fears and all those edgy feelings that maybe you're not okay. [37]

The method of using positive thinking to overcome painful emotions reinforces our estrangement from ourselves. It is actually a subtle form of double-negativity. Instead of simply feeling fear, we give ourselves the message that fear is irrational. Feelings of fear then become opportunities to feel shame about how irrational we really are.

Accepting painful emotions also means not falling into the trap of acting them out. When we act out our emotions we are not fully experiencing them. In the case of anger,

> some of us may prefer to go into our room, lock the door, and punch a pillow. We call this "getting in touch with our anger." But I don't think this is getting in touch with our anger at all. In fact, I don't think it is even getting in touch with our pillow. If we are really in touch with the pillow, we know what a pillow is and we won't hit it.[38]

This does not mean that when hurt by another person we should passively accept their destructive behavior. Once the anger has been experienced and the story line fallen away, we are left with energy that can be channeled into skillful self-protection and assertiveness. If a situation calls for the assertive expression of anger, it is done with awareness and compassion. Therapists who advise their clients to express anger without an appreciation of these subtleties often reinforce destructive patterns and cause damage to their relationships.

In order to communicate an attitude of acceptance, it is also important that Buddhist therapy does not overemphasize the use of techniques. Techniques are usually used to eliminate symptoms and solve problems. If one technique does not work, another is tried until the symptom or problem is eliminated. The client is given the message: "there is something wrong with you and we will fix it."

One technique that is particularly incongruent with the principle of acceptance is Michael White's externalization of the symptom. Although it may temporarily feel good to see symptoms as external to one's self, in the long run this will reinforce the egoistic tendency to split off unwanted aspects of identity. In fact, it is often the case that the tendency to externalize symptoms is what exacerbated them to the point where therapy is needed.

Adopt a Right View

Adopting a right view is one of the aspects of the eightfold path outlined by Buddha. The wrong view is to see a situation through the filter of categories and concepts. Such a view screens out important details and fixes our way of relating to the situation. The right view, therefore, is nonconceptual.[39]

This does not mean that we erase from our minds all categories and concepts. Our ability to categorize and conceptualize grows out of our basic intelligence and helps us to function skillfully in the world. Instead, right view means not becoming attached to our categories and concepts. Although maps are useful they are not the territory; nor is thought identical with experience.

In a therapeutic situation, right view would mean not becoming attached to diagnostic categories and concepts. Skillful therapists realize the pitfalls involved in seeing clients as "borderline personality disorders" or "major depressions." Although such diagnoses can usefully inform one's behavior as a therapist, it is vital that the full complexity of each individual client is appreciated, and not screened out by imposed categories.

Focus on the Here and Now

Part of maintaining the right view is to not be caught up in memories and echoes from past experiences.

> Strictly speaking, there is no connection between I myself yesterday and I myself in this moment; there is no connection whatsoever. Dogen-zenji said, "Charcoal does not become ashes." Ashes are ashes; they do not belong to charcoal. They have their own past and future.[40]

By maintaining the focus on the here and now, Buddhist therapy avoids the trap of reinforcing the tendency to replay and become stuck in past experiences. Although it may be necessary to give clients a chance to tell their stories, this should be done with a present orientation.

> It is not purely a matter of retelling stories in order to reconnect to the past, but rather it is a question of seeing that the present situation has several levels: the basic ground, which could be in the past; the actual manifestation, which is happening now; and where the present is about to go. . . . Once you begin to approach a person's experience in that way, it comes alive.[41]

Affirm Body-Mind Unity

Western psychology was developed upon the foundation of mind-body dualism. For example radical behaviorism was based on the idea that the mind is a "black box" that can never be known objectively. For this reason behaviorists limited their focus of inquiry to observable behavior which, in their view, could be objectively measured and quantified. Cognitive behaviorists began to peak into the black box. However, they still operated from the premise that mind and body are separate entities. Cognitive-behavioral therapists therefore talk about how thoughts, which are mental phenomena, create feelings, which are anchored in the body.

In contrast, Buddhist psychology does not speak of the physical as opposed to the mental, but instead speaks of a body-mind unity, or simply, "body-mind."[42] Consequently, Buddhist therapy must attend to both thoughts and "bodily" sensations. A therapy that is too focused on "cognitions" and words can easily wander away from the experience of the present. Buddhist meditation uses mindfulness of the "bodily" sensations of breathing as an anchor to what is happening right here and right now. Rather than directing clients to attend to their "irrational" thoughts and assigning the project of replacing them with more rational and adaptive thoughts, as in cognitive therapy, the Buddhist practice is to simply acknowledge thoughts, whether "adaptive" or not, and then to let them go and return to one's awareness of the breath. Buddhist therapy is experiential and holistic.

Appreciate the Environment

The entirety of Buddhist psychology is based on the premise that the egoistic separation of self from other is an illusion. Therefore, a Buddhist therapy would not limit its focus to the individual. Instead, there would be an appreciation of the environment or context within which the client is embedded. The implications of this idea are far-reaching.

The first implication to be drawn from the Buddhist refusal to draw a sharp boundary separating people from their environment, is that the details of the therapeutic space will impact the therapy. Edward Podvoll, founder of the Department of Contemplative Psychotherapy at the Naropa Institute, states that, "mind and environment are in a continuous and subtle, even unconscious, interaction. When we enter a new environment there is an impact—the colors, the lighting, the space, the furnishings, the textures, the smells, the whole setup."[43] This means that the office or room in which therapy is conducted should be as clean, uncluttered, comfortable, and attractively decorated as possible. Similarly, the Buddhist therapist will realize the importance of his or her grooming and casual dress in creating a welcoming environment. Alan Watts pointed out that the beatniks of the fifties mistakenly concluded that Buddhist philosophy, with its concepts of "nonjudging" and stories of Zen monks behaving in outrageous and spontaneous ways, gives one license to live a completely undisciplined life with total disregard for conventional ideas such as cleanliness, neatness, and the importance of caring for one's appearance and material possessions.[44]

Another implication to be drawn from the Buddhist appreciation for the interaction between environment and mind is that the client's home and work environments should be within the scope of therapy. "Getting people to pay attention to details of sweeping the floor or putting away the dishes can help them bring body and mind together. This helps the mind to slow down and can be a big relief. It is an invitation to be mindful and grounded."[45]

Edward Podvoll extended this idea to the treatment of psychosis. The Windhorse Project, which he founded, treats psychosis by sending therapists trained in meditation and Buddhist psychology into the homes of their clients or bringing the clients into a therapeutic home. Assisting the client in cleaning and caring for the household environment becomes an essential part of the therapy.[46]

When considering the way a client's mind and environment interact, it is vital to understand the family context. Gregory Bateson, whose work provided a foundation for the development of family therapy, acknowledged the influence of Buddhist psychology on his thinking. Affirming a cybernetic epistemology, he stated that it is an epistemological error to think that a person's behavior can be entirely explained without looking at context.[47] Attempts to treat individuals without appreciating the importance of the family context will prove inadequate or even harmful. Buddhist psychotherapy is contextual.

Emphasize Sanity

An approach to psychotherapy that over-emphasizes psychopathology and ignores health can be inefficient or even harmful. Rather than focus on psychopathology, the Buddhist therapist looks for the sanity that accompanies all neurosis. Most clients have lost sight of their "basic sanity." Often symptoms and problems are maintained or exacerbated by the client's desperate attempts to eradicate them.

By focusing on neurosis and ignoring sanity, the therapist inadvertently reinforces this destructive pattern. For this reason, it is necessary for the Buddhist therapist to practice meditation so that the signs of one's own wakefulness and sanity become familiar. Having come to recognize these signs in oneself, it then is possible to recognize them in one's clients. This enables the therapist to gently direct the client's attention toward already existing experiences of wakefulness.

Six signs of sanity. Podvoll describes six signs of sanity that he learned to recognize from clinical experience.[48] The first is repulsion, which he defines as "fundamental estrangement and a feeling of nausea about one's way of living." In Alcoholics Anonymous this is called "hitting bottom." In order to become disgusted with one's endless cycle of self-destructive and habitual patterns of behavior, it is necessary to have a moment of clarity in which there is a recognition that there could be something different. This can only happen if there has been some past experience of something different. This could be an experience with a grandparent, teacher, or coach. In addition, it could be a period in one's life in which a state of health was maintained. If the therapist becomes curious about this past experience of health, the client can begin to reconnect with his or her history of sanity.

The second sign of sanity is a longing to transcend the sense of self. It is not unusual for a client to say, "I don't know who I am." An "identity crisis" is an opportunity for one to begin to see the unstable and fabricated nature of identity. Frequently, the result is a turning toward the spiritual dimension in one's life.

Repulsion and longing to transcend one's constricting identity often lead to a desire for simplicity and discipline, the third sign of sanity. If the therapist becomes curious about the details of past experiences with discipline, the client's understanding of and relationship to discipline will become apparent. Often experiences with discipline produce insight into how mind and body can come together. Athletics, playing a musical instrument, or cooking all require mindfulness and increase appreciation for the sensory world.

The fourth sign of sanity is longing for compassionate action. Frequently a client with intense self-hatred still demonstrates great compassion for other people or animals. Often a client in the midst of suffering and despair shows concern for the well-being of the therapist. One of the curative factors of group therapy is the opportunity to help others.[49]

The fifth sign of sanity is a sense of clarity and complete presence. Frequently, such moments occur during a psychotherapeutic encounter. When the therapeutic environment has the qualities of wakefulness, crispness, and simplicity, clients can observe the shifts in their state of mind. Moments of clarity are highlighted within the context of disciplines that synchronize body and mind. During an experience of rock climbing there is a state of focused attention and precision of movement. I have heard Vietnam veterans talk about how they never felt more alive than during the war when all of their senses were sharpened and they lived completely in the moment.

Finally, when investigating the client's history of sanity, the therapist should look for signs of courage. Clients who have survived traumatic and terrifying events always have a history of great bravery in the face of intense fear. Because seeking psychotherapy still is considered by many to be an admission of weakness and failure, the very act of entering a therapeutic relationship takes courage. Beyond that, the therapeutic process of uncovering and experiencing painful emotions is a courageous act. The therapist demonstrates courage in the determination to be authentic and present in the face of the client's intense pain and at times challenging behaviors. The experience of psychotherapy can be seen as an opportunity for heroic courage in both client and therapist.

Describe the Stages of Healing

As mentioned previously, the three *yanas* can be looked at as stages on the Buddhist path. Although we may aspire to go out into the world and help others, until we help ourselves we will only continue polluting the world and inadvertently harming those we seek to help. Therefore we must begin on the Hinayana path of "taming the mind" through meditation practice.

The meditation practice emphasized at this stage is called *shamatha,* which literally means development of peace.[50] This practice is also called "mindfulness," which means one is fully present to whatever one is doing. When doing sitting practice, we are present with our breath; when doing walking meditation, we are present with the process and sensations of each step. The Buddha is said to have taught a village woman how to be mindful while drawing water from a well. He instructed her to be precisely aware of the movement of her hands and arms as she drew up the water.[51] Similarly, we can practice mindfulness when drinking tea, arranging flowers, or even when washing the dishes. Thich Nhat Hanh says, "If I am incapable of washing dishes joyfully, if I want to finish them quickly so I can go and have dessert, I will be equally incapable of enjoying my dessert. . . . I must confess it takes me longer to do the dishes, but I live fully in every moment, and I am happy."[52] Mindfulness practice is especially important in our fast-paced, achievement-oriented society that breeds the mindless pursuit of material success.

Through mindfulness practice we begin to become familiar with our habitual patterns of thinking, feeling, and behaving. *Shamatha* slows down our minds so that we can see that there are naturally occurring gaps in our thought streams. We come to realize that our thought process is not problematic; we do not need the paranoid insurance policy of ego to keep us on the straight and narrow. As a result, we begin to relax with our thoughts and emotions and bodily sensations with whatever occurs in our practice.[53] This is the beginning of *vipashyana.*

Vipashyana is a sanskrit term that means insight, or clear seeing. As the precision of mindfulness naturally develops into the gentleness and spaciousness of *vipashyana,* we begin to notice the atmosphere around our practice. This is called awareness. Instead of focusing attention upon details, we bring awareness to the overall pattern. At this point we have attained the first spiritual level of the bodhisattva, the first *bhumi.*[54]

Ten spiritual levels (bhumis). The word bodhisattva means he who is brave enough to walk on the path of the awakened ones. The bodhisattva path consists of ten *bhumis,* or spiritual levels. Each *bhumi* is accompanied by a *paramita. Paramita* means arriving at the other side or shore. The bodhisattva goes beyond the river of *samsara,* the river of confusion.

The joyfulness of the first *bhumi* is accompanied by generosity, the first *paramita.* The transcendental generosity of this first stage does not arise out of pious or religious motives. There is no expectation of getting anything in return. There is also no connotation of looking down on someone lower or less fortunate, thinking that you are in a superior position and can save them. Instead, the generosity of the bodhisattva arises from having discovered one's own basic sanity and the resulting sense of richness. There is now something to offer one's fellow sentient beings. Because there is a sense of fundamental richness, rather than fundamental poverty, it is possible to delight in generosity.

The second *bhumi* is called the "spotless" *bhumi*. It is associated with the *shila paramita* of morality or discipline. The morality and discipline of the bodhisattva is not forced and painful. Instead it is based on making friends with yourself, loving yourself. There is no need to control yourself so as to avoid temptations and follow the rules, no need to apply detergent to your natural condition.[55] Because the bodhisattva has practiced *shamatha-vipashyana* and developed insight and awareness, it feels natural to follow appropriate patterns of conduct.

One type of discipline known as the "gathering of virtue" involves relating properly to physical things. The bodhisattva does not relate to a cup of tea by knocking it over. With mindfulness and awareness it is possible to pick up the cup, sip from it, and put it down properly, without frivolousness. There is no need to waste energy on unnecessary or anxiety driven pursuits. When ego-based activity is eliminated, activity becomes deliberate, precise and sane.[56]

The *paramita* associated with the third *bhumi* is patience. The conventional notion of patience is to wait and hold your temper, repressing your restlessness. In contrast, because the bodhisattva is free from expectations and the compulsive concern with time, it is possible to just sit patiently without "waiting" for something else to happen. Although the bodhisattva's action has a sense of timelessness, this does not mean that everything is done so slowly that inefficiency results. In fact, because the bodhisattva's action is direct, persevering it is extremely efficient. Finally, the *paramita* of patience does not mean passive enduring of pain, allowing someone to torture you. The bodhisattva is not afraid to subjugate what needs to be subjugated, to destroy what needs to be destroyed, and to welcome that which needs to be welcomed.

The fourth *bhumi* is connected with the *paramita* of energy or taking delight in working with everyday situations. Because one's whole life has been opened by generosity, activated by discipline, and strengthened by patience, one arrives at the stage of joyous energy. The bodhisattva does not work hard out of a sense of obligation. At this stage it is possible to see the tremendous opportunities inherent in situations and derive inspiration from one's creative potentials. We can take delight in what is and then work with it.

The *paramita* associated with the fifth *bhumi* is *dhyana,* which literally means "awareness." In the Chinese tradition it is called *ch'an* and it is called Zen in the Japanese tradition. All these words refer to a state of total involvement, awareness without a watcher. In common parlance, "awareness" means egocentric watching, which is quite complicated. We watch ourselves and judge how we are doing, at all times keeping in mind the goal and fearing loss of control. In contrast, *dhyana* or Zen, is awareness without a watcher. "As long as we are alive, we are always doing something. But as long as you think, 'I am doing this,' or 'I have to do this,' or 'I must attain something special,' you are actually not doing anything."[57]

The sixth *bhumi* is associated with the *paramita* of *prajna*, which means "super knowledge," accurate and complete knowledge. "*Prajna* is traditionally symbolized by a sharp, two-edged sword that cuts through all confusion."[58] It is two-edged because it cuts through any dualistic tendency to separate "that" and "this." *Prajna* cuts through subtle attitudes of self-righteousness or piety and allows the bodhisattva to sail through situations without having to self-monitor.

The *paramita* of *upaya* or "skillful means" is connected with the seventh *bhumi*. At the more advanced stages of the bodhisattva path, progress becomes more and more subtle. In the first six *bhumis* there is still a faint undercurrent of spiritual materialism, which is an ego-centered version of spirituality in which spiritual techniques inadvertently strengthen egocentricity. In the seventh *bhumi,* spiritual materialism is completely left behind. The bodhisattva's actions then become completely uninhibited and perfectly skillful.

The *paramita* of the eighth *bhumi* is *pranidhana,* which literally means "wishful thinking" or "best wishes," but really refers to a vision of how future developments might occur. The present is seen as pregnant with possibilities for the future.

The ninth *bhumi* is connected with the *paramita* of power. Power in this context is a further expression of the confidence of skillful means.

Enlightened power leads into the tenth *bhumi, dharmamegha* or dharma cloud, which involves the development of the *paramita* of wisdom.

> Wisdom, is non-identification with the teaching, non-identification with the path, non-identification with the technique. The bodhisattva doesn't identify with the path any longer because he has become the path. He is the path. He has worked on himself, trod on himself, until he has become the path and the chariot as well as the occupant of the chariot, all at the same time.[59]

At the tenth and last stage of the bodhisattva path, the experience of *shunyata,* or emptiness, falls away, exposing the luminous nature of form, the vivid, precise, colorful aspect of things. This is the beginning of Vajrayana, or *tantra,* which is connected with working with energy. Because the mind has been tamed in the Hinayana path, and trained in the Mahayana path, energy can be stimulated in the Vajrayana path without becoming intoxicating. According to the Buddhist scriptures, a person who has not prepared adequately for tantra can become intoxicated with energy, similar to a drunken elephant who runs wild without considering where he is going.

PRACTICE OF THERAPY

This section begins with an outline of how the eightfold path and meditation can be applied to the practice of therapy. The remainder of the section consists of a discussion of the role and behavior of the Buddhist therapist and suggestions for applying Buddhist therapy to couples, family, and group therapy.

Eightfold Path

The fourth noble truth outlines a way to achieve the cessation of suffering known as the eightfold path. This path can apply to one who is formally pursuing Buddhism as a spiritual discipline, to a client in Buddhist therapy, and to the Buddhist therapist as well. The eightfold path consists of the right view, intention, speech, morality, livelihood, effort, mindfulness, and absorption.

Right view. The first aspect of the eightfold path is "right view." In order to understand right view and the other aspects of the eightfold path, it is important to understand what Buddha meant by "right." He did not mean right in the sense of not morally wrong. Instead the term "right" is used to mean "complete." The right view is a view that is free from conceptualization and prejudice and therefore completely accurate. Whenever we view situations through the filter of preconceived categories and beliefs we screen out important information and distort reality. Most clients in psychotherapy suffer needlessly from rigid negative self-concepts and inaccurate assumptions about other people. For this reason almost every school of psychotherapy focuses on helping clients drop their rigid and maladaptive concepts. In Buddhist therapy, the therapist also adopts a nonconceptual view of the client. As mentioned previously, therapists who treat "borderlines" or "depressives" lose the ability to have a genuine encounter with their clients.

Right intention. The second aspect of the eightfold path is "right intention." Ordinary intention is based on preconceptions and prejudices. Right intention, springs from right view. It is inclined only toward what is. Right intention is neither wishful thinking nor catastrophizing. Clients usually base their behavior on the intention to defend themselves from pain or the intention to pursue pleasure. As seen in the discussion of double negativity, the result is unnecessary pain and suffering. Therapists who intend to rescue their clients from pain can inadvertently reinforce their clients' symptomatic patterns.

Right speech. The third aspect of the eightfold path is "right speech," meaning speech which is true and direct. For clients this might involve learning to assertively express their thoughts and feelings rather than being passive-aggressive or manipulative. For therapists practicing right speech might involve the cultivation of authenticity and congruence.

Right morality. The fourth aspect of the eightfold path is "right morality" or "right discipline." In ordinary or samsaric discipline we give up conveniences and comforts in order to make ourselves "better." As the Buddha found, this only perpetuates the dualism of ego. The good and disciplined part of me attempts to defeat the selfish or evil part of me making the self into a battleground. As Jungian psychologists have demonstrated, the "shadow" never disappears; it only goes underground where it continues to influence our thoughts, feelings and behavior. People who come into therapy frequently have been taught to deny their own needs and never allow themselves to feel pride in their accomplishments. In contrast, right discipline is nondualistic and grows out of our "basic goodness." As we grow in mindfulness and awareness we experience a natural impulse to simplify our lives and to treat others with respect. For example, clients in therapy often discover that the mindless pursuit of money and material possessions has caused them to miss out on the simple pleasures of life. As a result, therapy commonly leads to the deliberate adoption of a less extravagant lifestyle.

Right livelihood. The fifth aspect is "right livelihood." This means that we do not resent the fact that we have to spend time on the job in order to afford food, clothing, and shelter. Neither do we need to be embarrassed by dealing with money. Work is seen as a natural fact of life. Furthermore, because we spend such a large portion of our lives in the workplace, work becomes an opportunity for spiritual practice. By practicing mindfulness and exercising compassion in relationships with customers and co-workers, time on the job becomes an integral part of the spiritual path. Clients often present with work-related conflicts and problems. For Buddhist therapists, work is an especially good opportunity for spiritual practice because the practice of psychotherapy demands awareness and compassion and inevitably exposes one's unresolved issues. Also, because people often become therapists for altruistic reasons, therapists tend to fall into the trap of being embarrassed by having to deal with money and payments. By seeing one's work as right livelihood, this problem is avoided.

Right effort. The next point of the eightfold path is "right effort." This is the same principle as in the *paramita* of energy. Effort need not be drudging and without humor. There is a story of how the Buddha once gave meditation instruction to a famous sitar player.

> The musician asked, "Should I control my mind or should I completely let go?" The Buddha answered, "Since you are a great musician, tell me how you would tune the strings of your instrument." The musician said, "I would make them not too tight and not too loose."

"Likewise," said the Buddha, "in your meditation practice you should not impose anything too forcefully on your mind, nor should you let it wander."[60]

Meditation and therapy both need the spaciousness of effort, noneffort, effort, noneffort. Some clients pursue therapy and self-help so seriously and intensely that it becomes necessary for the therapist to suggest that they take time off from the project of self-improvement and simply enjoy living life without an agenda. Therapists who work too hard and lack a sense of humor are subject to burnout.

Right mindfulness. "Right mindfulness," the seventh aspect, is environmental or panoramic. Awareness extends beyond the object of attention to the entire context. Typically when we run into a problem our vision "zooms in" on the problem and we see little else. Therapy helps clients to step back and see a more complete picture. Therapists who practice right mindfulness focus not only on the client and the client's context but also on their own posture, breath, and feelings. This heightens their ability to work with countertransference.

Right absorption. The final aspect of the eightfold path is "right absorption," which means being thoroughly and fully involved in a nondualistic way. Right absorption in sitting meditation means that the technique and you are one. Right absorption in a therapy context occurs in moments of intensity when the interaction between therapist and client flows. In such moments the separation between client and therapist disappears.

Meditation

Concentration versus Mindfulness

All meditation practices fit into one of two broad categories, concentration and mindfulness. *Shamatha-vipashyana* is a mindfulness practice, as is *zazen,* the sitting practice used in Zen Buddhism.

Concentration practices are based on focusing the mind on a particular point in order to control the mind and focus attention. The object of attention can be a visual image, a mantra, a chant, or a prayer. Electroencephalogram (EEG) studies of yoga meditation revealed that there was no response in the yogi's brain to external stimuli during meditation.[61] In effect, concentration practices produce a state of relaxation by shutting out all distracting or anxiety arousing perceptions and thoughts.

Most schools of Buddhism do not recommend concentration practices for those starting out on the spiritual journey because they can inadvertently be ego-reinforcing. The ability to "control" the mind and block out all distractions could easily be seen as a weapon in ego's arsenal used to promote ego's agenda of self-aggrandizement.[62]

Mindfulness practices are characterized by an expansion of the field of attention. Although the technique varies slightly among the Buddhist traditions, the basic idea is the same in every Buddhist mindfulness practice. Awareness of breath is used as an anchor to the present moment. Although relaxation can and often does develop during the course of mindfulness meditation, this is not the goal. Instead of focusing concentration and awareness by shutting out distractions, mindfulness practice opens up and expands awareness.

EEG studies of Zen meditators confirm that mindfulness meditation differs dramatically from concentration meditation. Not only did the brains of Zen masters respond to external stimuli, but they also did not show the habituation that ordinarily would result from exposure to a repetitive stimulus. Normal subjects, when exposed to a click repeated every fifteen seconds, show a decrease in the response of the brain's electrical activity after the third or fourth click. Zen masters sitting in meditation for five minutes responded to the last click in exactly the same way as they did to the first.[63] "Zen mind" is truly "beginner's mind" in this sense. Every experience is fresh and unfiltered by learned concepts and judgments.

Instructions in Shamatha-Vipashyana *Meditation*

The following technique for *shamatha-vipashyana* meditation was taught by Chogyam Trungpa, a Tibetan Buddhist meditation master who spent many years in America teaching Buddhist practices in forms that were tailored to his American students. Other Buddhist traditions may differ slightly in the details of the technique.

Although *shamatha-vipashyana* is traditionally practiced sitting cross-legged on a cushion, it can also be done while sitting in a chair with both feet on the floor. First, relax and take a comfortable posture, upright but not rigid. The head, shoulders, and spine are vertically aligned, but without tension. This posture expresses wakefulness.[64] Next, rest your hands comfortably on your thighs, palms down. Keep your eyes open, and direct your gaze slightly downward. Avoid staring at one point with a sharp focus, and gently take in the immediate environment.

Attend to your breath for a few exhalations. Feel the physical breath going out and dissolving into space, not just a mental picture of the breath. It is not necessary to block out awareness of sounds, visual stimuli, or other perceptions. Only about 25 percent of the awareness is on the breath so that a sense of relaxation and being fully present can develop.

> But being with one's breath is only part of the technique. These thoughts that run through our minds continually are the other part. . . . The instruction is that when you realize you've been thinking you label it "thinking." When your mind wanders off, you say to yourself,

"thinking." Whether your thoughts are violent or passionate or full of ignorance and denial; whether your thoughts are worried or fearful, whether your thoughts are spiritual thoughts, pleasing thoughts of how well you're doing, comforting thoughts, uplifting thoughts, whatever they are, without judgment or harshness simply label it all "thinking," and do that with honesty and gentleness.[65]

It is very important that labeling is not done in a harsh or scolding tone. The labeling of thoughts is an opportunity to develop a sense of friendliness and compassion for yourself. When labeling thoughts is done in a self-critical way, meditation becomes an egoistic project to build a better and holier "me."

Integrating Meditation into Psychotherapy

A number of Buddhist psychotherapists have taught their clients meditation as a part of the therapy process. Jon Kabat-Zinn has developed a structured program of yoga, relaxation exercises and mindfulness training, which he offers to people suffering from physical and or psychological pain.[66] David Brazier, author of *Zen Therapy,* states that "in suitable cases" *zazen* can be taught to clients as an "antidote to stress" and a "powerful aid in breaking habits."[67] Mark Epstein believes that meditation can aid both therapist and patient by teaching them how to stay in the present.[68]

Although there are clients who are interested in meditation and capable of pursuing the discipline of a formal sitting practice, many clients lack such motivation, or they are so overwhelmed with anxiety or depression that a regular meditation practice is impossible. Nonetheless, it is still possible to utilize mindfulness within therapy sessions with these clients. Brazier states that, "The therapist whose inner calm is well established remains minutely attentive, but does not react in the predictable manner. When this happens, therapy is rather like a meditation for two."[69] Similarly, according to Jack Kornfield, "the best of modern therapy is much like a process of shared meditation, where therapist and client sit together, learning to pay close attention to those aspects and dimensions of the self that the client may be unable to touch on his or her own."[70]

Aspects of mindfulness-awareness meditation can be brought into the therapy in concrete ways. When therapists ask their clients to pay attention to each breath and the bodily sensations associated with feelings of anxiety or anger, they are having clients practice the first foundation of mindfulness, known as mindfulness of body. The common therapeutic technique of asking clients to record incidences of symptomatology during the week between sessions, is a way of bringing mindfulness to what is usually mindless behavior. So-called "paradoxical techniques" of asking clients to voluntarily produce or exaggerate symptoms can similarly be seen as exercises in making conscious behaviors which are normally unconscious.

Just as mindfulness practices can facilitate the practice of psychotherapy, so can psychotherapy be a useful or even necessary part of the Westerner's spiritual journey. Buddhist psychology does not have a theory of psycho pathology. In the Eastern cultures where Buddhism developed, it is assumed that a person has a capacity for empathy, relaxation of outer ego boundaries, emotional attunement and receptivity, and a sense of belonging.[71] When the Dalai Lama met with a group of Western therapists he was incredulous at the notion of "low self-esteem" that was described to him. When he asked each Westerner if they suffered from this and, "they all nodded yes, he just shook his head in disbelief."[72] In 1993, Kornfield found that at least half of the students at a three-month retreat were unable to meditate because so much unresolved grief, fear, and unfinished developmental business emerged.[73] Because many Westerners do not start on the Buddhist path with a positive sense of self, meditation and psychotherapy often need to be combined.

A common trap Westerners fall into is the use of meditation to avoid having to deal with life's challenges. Notions like nonattachment, emptiness, egolessness, and renunciation can become rationales for passivity, social withdrawal, avoidance of conflict, and suppression of painful feelings. For such people, psychotherapy can help them gain the courage to confront life head-on. Uncomfortable and painful feelings and relationships can then become opportunities to practice "meditation in action."

Tonglen *and* Lojong *Meditation Practice*

Although *shamatha-vipashyana* is a way to "tame" the mind and can be thought of as a Hinayana discipline leading to individual liberation, in Mahayana practice we begin to "train" the mind. *Lojong* is a Tibetan word meaning training the mind.[74] The seven points of mind training were developed by the Indian Buddhist teacher Atisa, who transmitted this body of wisdom to his Tibetan disciple. In the twelfth century C.E., *The Root Text of the Seven Points of Training the Mind* was written. This text summarized the practical application of mahayana Buddhism in a list of fifty-nine slogans. The seventh slogan in this list describes the meditation practice associated with mind training *(tonglen)*. *Tonglen* is Tibetan for sending and taking. In Sanskrit this practice is called *maitri bhavana,* meaning warmth or friendliness meditation.

Lojong practice is based on the idea that we can make friends with what we reject and see as "bad" in ourselves and other people, while learning to be generous with what we cherish and see as "good."[75] Through this practice we discover *bodhichitta,* or awakened heart.

The basic message of the lojong teachings is that if it's painful, you can learn to hold your seat and move closer to that pain. Reverse the usual pattern, which is to split, to escape . . . if it's painful, you become willing not just to endure it, but also to let it awaken your heart and soften you. . . . The lojong teachings encourage us, if we enjoy what we are experiencing, to think of other people and wish for them to feel that. Share the wealth . . . Be generous with your insights and delights. Instead of fearing that they're going to slip away and holding onto them, share them.[76]

This practice is not based on the traditional moralistic notion that we must strive with all our might to eradicate evil and promote good in ourselves and others. Because *lojong* practice rests on the foundation of mindfulness and awareness, the practice of compassion is natural and spontaneous. Having tamed our own minds and made friends with ourselves, we begin to look around and see others suffering from mindlessness and ignorance. We can share our wealth with them because we can afford to. We can take in their pain because we know it is not solid and overwhelming. As Shakespeare said, "The quality of mercy is not strained, it falleth as the gentle rain from heaven." The traditional Buddhist metaphor for compassion is the sun, which shines naturally on everyone equally.[77]

The practice of *tonglen* begins with briefly resting your mind in a state of openness. In the second stage, you imagine breathing in darkness, heaviness, and heat, and breathing out brightness, lightness, and cool. The experience of neurotic suffering typically feels dark, heavy, and stifling. On the other hand when we experience a gap in our neurotic struggles there is a sense of lightness and bright, fresh openness, clear and cool as an alpine stream. We work with these textures until they have become synchronized. The heavy, dark heat of neurosis is coming in and the light, bright, coolness of openness is going out on the medium of the breath.

> The third stage is working with a specific heartfelt object of suffering. You breathe in the pain of a specific person or animal that you wish to help. You breathe out to that person spaciousness or kindness or a good meal or a cup of coffee—whatever you feel would lighten their load. You can do this for anyone: the homeless mother that you pass on the street, your suicidal uncle, or yourself and the pain you are feeling at that very moment.[78]

The fourth stage extends your compassion and wish to relieve the suffering of an individual to all beings who are suffering in the same way, to all those who are homeless or suicidal or in pain as you are.

Postmeditation *lojong* practice consists of memorizing the slogans so that they can arise spontaneously in the course of your everyday life. By letting the slogans permeate your whole being, everyday life becomes the path of awakening and compassion. One slogan, which expresses the spirit of *lojong* is, "Gain and victory to others, loss and defeat to myself." This slogan does not suggest that you become a self-denying masochist. What it does mean is that you can open your heart and mind and really experience defeat.

> You feel too short, you have indigestion, you're too fat and too stupid. You say to yourself, "Nobody loves me, I'm always left out. I have no teeth, my hair's getting gray, I have blotchy skin, my nose runs." That all comes under the category of defeat, the defeat of ego. We're always not wanting to be who we are. However, we can never connect with our fundamental wealth as long as we are buying into this advertisement hype that we have to be someone else, that we have to smell different or have to look different.[79]

Because we have already discovered impermanence and basic goodness through the practice of *shamatha-vipashyana,* experiencing the defeat of ego does not lead to chronic depression. Similarly, sharing victories with others does not lead to excessive self-denial. Other examples of slogans that can be worked with in the course of ordinary living are, "Don't be jealous" or "Be grateful to everyone."

Although the *lojong* teachings and the practice of *tonglen* can be wonderful techniques for advancing on the Buddhist path, they obviously would not be taught to the majority of clients in psychotherapy. They can, however, be extremely useful to therapists, who often need a way to work with "difficult" clients in a compassionate way. Moreover, a therapist who is steeped in these teachings would be much less influenced by our culture's emphasis on individuality and hedonism at the expense of altruism and generosity. This is compatible with recent trends in the field of psychotherapy toward a renewed appreciation for morality[80] and forgiveness, and away from the former emphasis on self-fulfillment and the perpetrator/victim dynamic. Buddhist psychotherapists will nurture compassion in their clients and, when appropriate, move clients through anger and rage to the healing that comes with forgiveness and empathy.

Koans

Koan is a Japanese word meaning "test." It refers to a problem not subject to logical solution, which is given by the Zen master to a student. The most commonly cited koan is: "What is the sound of one hand clapping?"

Alan Watts states that the koan is actually a concealed form of a question the student has asked the master, "How can I attain liberation?"[81] The koan asks the question, "Who asks the question? Who wants to be liberated?" The student cannot respond with a verbal, pre-planned answer. As a result the student is put into a double-bind that cannot be solved by the logic of ego. There is a Zen analogy that says this is "like being a fish with an iron ball stuck in one's jaws. The fish can neither swallow it nor spit it out."[82] Ultimately, after much effort and struggle, the student gives up and surrenders.

As in the first step in the Alcoholics Anonymous program, the acknowledgment of powerlessness has a paradoxical effect. When the alcoholic admits powerlessness over alcohol, recovery begins. When the Zen student surrenders, it becomes possible to present the master with his or her true and spontaneous self as the answer to the koan. An example of a completely spontaneous response to a koan occurred when the master presented his staff and asked, "If you say it is a staff, you affirm; if you do not call it a staff, you negate. Apart from negation and affirmation, what would you call it?"[83] A monk took the staff away from the master, broke it in two and threw the pieces on the ground.

David Brazier conceptualizes the life problems people present within therapy as koans:

> The mental construction of a self-centered universe inevitably generates contradictions. These crystallize as koans, life tests, which may drive a person to seek therapy. The client wants the therapist to remove the source of the discomfort. The koan, however, represents an opportunity for bringing matters to a head, and the Zen therapist is likely to approach it with this in mind.[84]

By encouraging clients to hold their feelings and problems in awareness, Buddhist therapists allow an opportunity for wisdom to emerge from confusion. Examples of koans in common life include: "Who am I?" (usually asked during important developmental transitions); "Can I love?" (often asked when experiencing difficulties with intimate relationships); "What makes me happy?" (often asked when experiencing depression or boredom); and, "How can I control my mind and/or body?" (asked when the central issue is anxiety).

Therapist's Behavior

In Western psychotherapy, Rogers' core conditions of empathy, positive regard, and congruence are acknowledged to be necessary for a person to have a therapeutic effect on clients. However, little or no training is offered for the development of these qualities in psychotherapists. In contrast, Buddhism describes in great detail the process of developing one's potential for therapeutic impact. The bodhisattva path can be considered a training program for the development of the ideal therapist.[85] Bodhisattvas dedicate their lives to developing the wisdom and compassion necessary for helping others.

Because the Buddhist therapist utilizes mindfulness and awareness to remain focused in the present moment and to maintain equanimity, the client's feelings and behavior are seen clearly and reflected back without being colored or distorted by the therapist's personal agenda. By serving as a mirror, a Buddhist therapist gives clients an opportunity to become aware of their own behavior.

There are times, however, when simple mirroring is not sufficient for helping a person grow. The history of Buddhism is replete with stories of masters who behaved in outrageous ways to wake their students. Tilopa demonstrated "crazy wisdom" when he transmitted enlightenment to Naropa by removing his sandal and slapping him in the face.[86] From a conventional viewpoint this is bizarre and cruel behavior. However, because Tilopa knew that Naropa had erected a barrier that could only be penetrated by a sudden jolt, this tactic was actually very precise, skillful, and compassionate.

In the conventional way of thinking, compassion is equated with kindness, warmth, and gentleness. In the Buddhist scriptures this kind of compassion is called "grandmother's love."[87] In contrast, a person who has developed skillful means exercises "ruthless compassion." In Zen stories, "teachers complimented their students by criticism, blows even. When they praised, it usually meant belittling. This was the custom. They had a deep concern for their pupils, but showed it in presence not words."[88] An extreme example is the Zen story of Gutei.

> [Gutei] raised his finger whenever he was asked a question about Zen. A boy attendant began to imitate him in this way. When anyone asked the boy what his master preached about, the boy would raise his finger. Gutei heard about the boy's mischief. He seized him and cut off his finger. The boy cried and ran away. Gutei called and stopped him. When the boy turned his head to Gutei, Gutei raised his own finger. In that instant the boy was enlightened.[89]

Although finger amputation will obviously not be in the Buddhist therapist's repertoire of interventions, cutting through a client's confusion and neurosis will be relevant. When need be, the Buddhist therapist can operate with a sharp scalpel.

Applications to Couples, Family, and Group Therapy

As stated previously, Buddhist psychotherapy is environmental in that individuals are understood to be embedded in context. The idea of a clear boundary between self and other is an illusion. For this reason Buddhist psychotherapists appreciate the importance of working with the family and relationship contexts.

Couples Therapy

John Welwood, in his books *Journey of the Heart*[90] and *Love and Awakening,*[91] outlines how an intimate relationship can be a path for spiritual development. He integrates systemic ideas from marriage and family therapy with the Buddhist emphasis on awareness, awakened heart, and skillful means.

Marital partners are seen as bringing family-of-origin wounds and patterns into their relationship. Therapists who counsel couples often observe how each partner has come to carry the projections and split off parts of the other. Couples therapy then, becomes an opportunity for each partner to reclaim their wholeness by reintegrating the split-off parts and bringing awareness and compassion to the relationship. Because a committed intimate relationship brings to the surface all of the ways in which we continue to cling to our well-learned neurotic patterns, it is one of the richest opportunities we have for self-discovery and transformation.

This approach rejects the behavioral idea of couples therapy as a process of negotiating a "quid pro quo." Such an approach makes an intimate relationship into a business deal and inevitably debases the sacred aspect of marriage. In Japan, a form of therapy called Naikan, developed in the 1950s by a Buddhist, involves completely letting go of the common Western notion that relationships are an opportunity to get one's "needs met." Instead, Naikan involves intense examination of one's past life in relation to others.[92]

Clients are asked to consider three questions about each relationship, beginning with their own mother and father, then onto other significant relationships, and finally examining even casual relationships. The questions are: (1) "What did this person do for you?" (2) "What did you do in return?" and (3) "What trouble and worries did you cause them?"

The point of these questions is to develop a deep sense of gratitude for all of the ways in which we have been nurtured and cared for so that we can awaken the desire to give of ourselves to others. The underlying assumption is that a relationship in which each partner is focused on how their needs can be gratified by the other will inevitably be conflictual and unfulfilling.

A Buddhist approach to couples therapy incorporates these ideas by emphasizing the spiritual nature of a committed relationship, utilizing the couple's approach to spirituality whether Buddhist, Judeo-Christian, Native American, or one of the countless other traditions. Within this context it is possible to shift the couple from blame to forgiveness, selfishness to selflessness, and victimhood to responsibility.

Family Therapy

Just as a committed intimate relationship can be a sacred path for awakening the heart, so can parenting. Every parent knows how a child's innocence and vulnerability can powerfully cut through one's armor and crack open one's heart. Every parent also can appreciate how a child's zen-like spontaneity and beginner's mind can inspire them to reclaim their own playfulness and wonder. Furthermore, many parents have had the experience of suddenly realizing that they were repeating the words of their father or mother, the words they had smugly known would never come from their lips! Children, then, can be our most powerful teachers.

In *Everyday Blessings,* Myla and Jon Kabat-Zinn describe how "mindful parenting" can nurture the growth of both parents and children. Parenting

> calls us to recreate our world every day, to meet it freshly in every moment. Such a calling is in actuality nothing less than a rigorous spiritual discipline—a quest to realize our truest, deepest nature as a human being. The very fact that we are a parent is continually asking us to find and express what is most nourishing, most loving, most wise and caring in ourselves, to be as much as we can, our best selves.[93]

A Buddhist approach to family therapy appeals to the parents' natural love and innate tendency to make sacrifices for the sake of their children. As in couples therapy, the spirituality of the family is included in the process. Rather than motivating parents through guilt, a Buddhist therapist uncovers the primordial parental instinct for nurturance and empathy. At the same time, children are given a safe place in which to express their true nature, which always includes an idealization of their parents and a poignant eagerness to please. The Buddhist therapist, having cultivated the skillful means of communication, is well-prepared to teach effective and respectful communication to families.

When doing family-of-origin work with adults, a Buddhist therapist would not deliberately or inadvertently reinforce a client's tendency to blame a parent or both parents for his or her current problems and pain. Although there are times when anger needs to be brought to the surface before it can be worked with mindfully, it is never helpful for a therapist to promote the vilification of a client's parents or to foster unnecessary conflict or distance between an adult client and that client's parents.

Of course, in cases where parents are abusive, clients are assisted in drawing appropriate boundaries. However, even in such cases, the Buddhist therapist respects the need we all have to understand and honor our ancestors for whatever they managed to provide for us, despite the imperfections and limitations imposed by their own neurotic and ego-based patterns. The empathy and unlimited compassion of the bodhisattva therapist will pervade work with even the most horrendous cases of abuse.

Group Therapy

Irvin Yalom's *The Theory and Practice of Group Psychotherapy* includes altruism as one of the therapeutic factors in group therapy. He points out that "many patients are immersed in a morbid self-absorption which takes the form of obsessive introspection or a teeth-gritting effort to 'actualize' oneself. But self-actualization can never be attained via deliberate, self-conscious pursuit."[94] This idea is certainly consistent with the Buddhist idea that ego is the cause of unnecessary suffering and bodhisattvas vow to put off their own liberation in order to work to relieve all other beings of suffering.

Group therapy, as described by Yalom, is compatible with Buddhism in another respect. The "here and now" focus recommended by Yalom is exactly the approach taken by the Buddhist therapist. Group therapy, more so than individual therapy, provides an opportunity to become mindful of neurotic ego-based patterns. The group is a social microcosm that inevitably evokes the patterns of thinking, feeling, and behaving that have been problematic for the client in life outside the group. The variety of personalities and the presence of peers as well as the authority figure of the therapist, makes group therapy a laboratory for the study of one's habitual patterns and the learning of new patterns.

EVALUATION

Buddhist Theories of Personality and Psychotherapy

Buddhist psychology was not developed to describe either personality structure, its development, or its dynamics. Neither was it developed as an approach to psychotherapy, as practiced in the West. Buddhist psychology was developed over 2,600 years from the experiences of meditators intent on discovering truth, and alleviating their own suffering and the suffering of others. As a result, the emphasis in Buddhism is on describing the mind, the cause of suffering, and the way to attain liberation or enlightenment. As a theory of mind and suffering, Buddhism is unsurpassed by anything Western psychology has to offer; however, as a theory of personality and psychotherapy, it is incomplete and limited.

Western psychologists are just beginning to investigate how Buddhism can contribute to Western theories of personality and psychotherapy. Because the goal of the Buddhist path is far beyond the goals of traditional Western therapies, it can be considered to pick up where Western psychotherapy leaves off. Freud's statement that even the best therapy can only return us to a state of "common unhappiness"[95] would be considered extremely pessimistic and limited from the perspective of Buddhism.

Research

Because Buddhist psychology is only beginning to be integrated into the practice of psychotherapy, there is no outcome research on Buddhist psychotherapy. However, there have been more than 1,500 studies published that demonstrate a variety of psychological, physiological, and therapeutic effects of meditation.[96] Examples are provided here in all three areas.

Numerous psychological effects of meditation have been found. Studies have shown enhancement of creativity, perceptual sensitivity, empathy, lucid dreaming, self-actualization, self-control, and marital satisfaction. An interesting study of Rorschach Test responses of Buddhist meditators found that subjects who had reached the initial stage of enlightenment still had normal conflicts around issues such as dependency, sexuality, and aggression, but they demonstrated little defensiveness or reactivity to these conflicts. Meditators at more advanced stages of enlightenment showed no evidence of drive or psychological conflicts.

Of the physiological effects of meditation, one of the clearest is the reduction of heart rate, and with regular practice, a decrease in blood pressure. For this reason, meditation can be an effective treatment for high blood pressure. Other physiological effects include a shift in blood chemistry, modification of hormone levels, decreased lactate levels (sometimes regarded as a measure of relaxation), and reduction of cholesterol levels. The EEG slows and alpha waves (eight to thirteen cycles per second) may appear in meditation. The slowing is greater in more advanced practitioners and theta patterns (four to seven cycles per second) may appear, consistent with deep relaxation. Brain waves also show increasing synchronization or coherence between different cortical areas.[97]

Meditation has been found therapeutic for a variety of psychological, psychosomatic, and social disorders. Psychological disorders in which therapeutic effects have been found include anxiety, phobias, posttraumatic stress, muscle tension, insomnia, and mild depression. Regular, long-term meditation has been found to reduce legal and illegal drug use and, in prisoners, anxiety, aggression and recidivism are reduced. Psychosomatic disorders responsive to meditation are high blood pressure and cholesterol levels, asthma, migraine, and chronic pain.

Although there is no clear evidence that meditation is more effective for clinical disorders than other self-regulation strategies such as relaxation training, biofeedback, or self-hypnosis, meditators often report that their practice is more meaningful, more enjoyable, and easier to continue over time than other approaches. In addition, meditation is reported to foster an interest in self-exploration.

Deane Shapiro calls for future research to find the active components of meditation and discover whether these components can be profitably combined with other self-regulation strategies.[98] He also suggests the development of a subject profile of those for whom meditation is likely to be an effective clinical intervention. Finally, he recommends that researchers study meditation phenomenologically.

An additional direction for future research is suggested by Roger Walsh, who calls for studies of, "advanced practitioners and their transpersonal goals such as enhanced concentration, ethics, love, compassion, generosity, wisdom, and service."[99]

POINTS OF DIALOGUE

Dialogues with Other Religions

Judaism

There are many Jews who are exploring Buddhism and other meditative paths. This has raised concern within the Jewish community that the future of Judaism could be jeopardized by a widespread conversion of Jews to Buddhism and other Eastern religions. In part, to address this concern, in October, 1990, a meeting took place in Dharamsala, India, between the Dalai Lama and a group of Jewish delegates.

From the Dalai Lama's point of view, this meeting provided him with an opportunity to ask about "the secret of Jewish spiritual survival in exile."[100] The Jewish people had survived the destruction of the Temple and thousands of years of persecution, culminating in the Nazi genocide. The Dalai Lama, as the spiritual leader of the Tibetan people, wanted to learn how Tibetan Buddhism could survive the Chinese army occupation in 1950 and the subsequent murder of 1.2 million Tibetans, and the systematic pillaging and razing of more than 6,000 Buddhist monasteries.

In the course of this meeting, described in *The Jew in the Lotus,* many similarities were found between the two traditions, particularly between the Buddhist *tantra* and the Jewish *kabala.* In fact, it is possible that some of these similarities are the result of past contact between Judaism and Buddhism in Alexandria, Egypt, in the first century.[101]

Both religions encourage the cultivation of "right intention" and the importance of bringing awareness to everyday life through mindfulness in Buddhism and prayer and ritual in Judaism. The name the kabalists used for God is *ain sof,* sometimes translated as "nothing," a term reminiscent of the Buddhist idea of *shunyata.* As in Buddhism, spiritual leaders in Judaism are considered "geologists of the soul" who can tell you where to dig for the soul's treasures but "the digging you have to do yourself."[102]

The Dalai Lama learned about Jewish strategies for survival such as the democratization of religious education and the practice of the home rituals of keeping kosher and making blessings over bread and wine. Jews who explore Buddhism often find that meditation experiences help them to see Jewish prayer and ritual as a powerful and profound spiritual path. Sylvia Boorstein, in *That's Funny, You Don't Look Buddhist,* describes how "Practicing mindfulness I felt peaceful and happy. Feeling peaceful and happy caused me to say blessings. . . . My meditation experiences, especially those that presented themselves in terms of Scripture imagery, reminded me to read Scripture again."[103]

Christianity

A very rich and lively dialogue has grown between Buddhism and Christianity. The Naropa Institute, a contemplative college in Boulder, Colorado, sponsors an annual conference devoted to this topic. Thomas Merton, a Catholic monk who pioneered this dialogue, illustrated the influence of Buddhism on his thinking when he said,

> The contemplative is not one who directs a magic spiritual intuition upon other objects, but one who, being perfectly unified in himself and recollected in the center of his humility, enters into contact with reality by an immediacy that forgets the division between subject and object.[104]

Forgetting the division between subject and object is one of the primary goals of the Buddhist path.

Anthony deMello, a Jesuit priest, drew parallels between Buddhist thought and the insights of two prominent Christian mystics, St. Teresa of Ávila and Meister Eckhart. When deMello says, "Suffering exists in 'me,' so when you identify 'I' with 'me,' suffering begins,"[105] he is echoing the second noble truth. The influence of Buddhism is also evident in his statement,

> There is far too much God talk; the world is sick of it. There is too little awareness, too little love, too little happiness, but let's not use those words either. There's too little dropping of illusions, dropping of errors, dropping of attachments and cruelty, too little awareness. . . . Religion is supposed to be about a lack of awareness, of waking up.[106]

The Dalai Lama said, "I believe it is possible to progress along a spiritual path and reconcile Christianity with Buddhism."[107] He also expressed the belief that Buddhists could learn from the example of Christian monks and nuns who "have taken on great responsibilities in the realms of education and health care—they really do serve humanity, all over the world."[108] At the same time, "Christian followers could in turn learn certain techniques for developing love, compassion, one-pointed concentration, and for improving altruism, from their Tibetan counterparts."[109]

Hinduism

As noted previously, the Buddha spent a significant portion of his life studying with Hindu teachers. Some Buddhist concentration exercises, and Buddhist ideas of reincarnation and karma, have their roots in Hinduism and yoga. For this reason, Buddhism can be seen to have developed out of a dialogue with Hinduism. Continuing dialogue between Buddhists and Hindus can only enrich both traditions.

Taoism

When Buddhism was brought from India to China it was mixed with the native Taoism. The result was *Ch'an,* which spread to Japan, where it became known as Zen. The most subtle principle of Taoism is *wu-wei,* which literally means "non-doing." A more meaningful translation is "to act without forcing-to move in accordance with the flow of nature's course which is signified by the word Tao."[110] The *Tao te Ching* states:

> Being favored and disgraced both bring fearful anticipation. Honor and misfortune are the normal conditions of the self. What is meant by fearful anticipation? Being favored puts one in a vulnerable position. It's a surprise to receive a favor; but fear of losing it leads to anguish. What is meant by normal conditions of honor and misfortune? I bring about my own misfortune because of my own self-interest. If I have no self, how could it have misfortune? Therefore, he who understands the cultivation of selflessness can be entrusted with the world.[111]

From this it is clear that Buddhism, with its idea that ego is the cause of unnecessary suffering, is in harmony with Taoism.

Native American Spirituality

In 1984 the Tibetan Buddhist Chogyam Trungpa met with Gerald Red Elk, an Ogala Sioux shaman-chief. Gerald Red Elk had expressed a desire to meet a Tibetan lama, "because we understand the heart of what they are. We call anybody in that state of mind a 'common man of the earth' because they live the laws of the earth, they understand, and we could communicate without talking."[112] After meeting and talking together for about forty minutes, Trungpa said, "I think we can work together. It is very magical."[113] When he gave Gerald a copy of his book *Shambala: The Sacred Path of the Warrior,* Gerald exclaimed, "The sacred path of the warrior, this is what we believe in. The honor is there. The honor is there." Later Trungpa commented, "He understood the whole book just from the cover," while Gerald said, "We understood each other completely without needing to say anything."

As Gerald Red Elk walked away after he and Trungpa had embraced, a torrential downpour flooded the valley. The night before, Gerald had had a dream of rain and lightening during the meeting, which he took to be the god's approval of the meeting.

Dialogues with Other Theories of Personality and Psychotherapy

It has been noted previously that Buddhism can provide a training method for the development of the Rogerian core conditions that constitute a therapeutic relationship, which facilitates the client's self-exploration and self-actualization. There are many other potential benefits from a dialogue between Buddhism and Western theories of personality and psychotherapy. In this section, Buddhism is placed in dialogue with the following Western theories: psychoanalysis, Bateson's cybernetic epistemology, Ericksonian hypnosis and therapy, narrative therapy and constructionism, and cognitive-behavioral therapy.

Psychoanalysis

In 1960 Erich Fromm, D. T. Suzuki, and Richard DeMartino wrote *Zen Buddhism and Psychoanalysis*. This book marked the beginning of the dialogue between psychoanalyis and Buddhism. Fromm noted that this dialogue could be fruitful for both traditions because they shared a common goal, "insight into one's nature, the achievement of freedom, happiness and love, liberation of energy, salvation from being insane or crippled."[114]

Both Zen and psychoanalysis adhere to the principle that knowledge leads to transformation. Freud and Zen recognize the limitations of the conventional rationalistic mode of thinking which, in the Western world, is highly valued. Freud used free association to break through the conscious thought system, while Zen uses koans and meditation.[115]

In 1995 Mark Epstein wrote *Thoughts Without a Thinker,* in which he extended the dialogue between Buddhism and psychoanalysis. Epstein goes as far as to contend that Buddha may have been the original psychoanalyst, in that he used the same mode of analytic inquiry as Freud.[116] The observing ego, which engages in free association, is strengthened through the practice of meditation. Epstein describes how a psychoanalyst he knew, who had been through five years of psychoanalysis, attended a meditation retreat where he felt he understood for the first time what it meant to free-associate.[117]

The period between 1960 and 1995 saw the development of self-psychology and object relations theory, and Epstein was able to include this material in his discussion of Buddhism and psychoanalysis. He notes the question of the self is common to Buddhism and contemporary psychoanalysis. However, although psychotherapy can identify the problem of the restless and insecure self, "bring it out, point out some of the childhood deficiencies that contributed to its development, and help diminish the ways in which erotic and aggressive strivings become intertwined with the search for a satisfying feeling of self,"[118] it is unable to deliver freedom from narcissistic craving.

One additional way in which Buddhism and contemporary psychoanalysis overlap is that they both offer methods for creating what Winnicott called a "holding environment" for rage and other uncomfortable thoughts, feelings, and sensations. In psychoanalysis, the holding environment is created by the analyst while in Buddhism, meditation creates an internal holding environment.

Bateson's Cybernetic Epistemology

Gregory Bateson was an anthropologist who studied communication in cultures, the families of schizophrenics, and animals. He developed what he called a cybernetic epistemology in order to correct what he considered to be fundamental errors in Western or occidental thinking. The field of systemic family therapy grew out of his notion that in order to understand human behavior and communication it is always necessary to broaden the focus from the individual to the context or system within which the individual is embedded.

In his article "The Cybernetics of 'Self': A Theory of Alcoholism," Bateson proposed that the power of Alcoholics Anonymous in treating alcoholism resides in its "first step," the acknowledgment of one's powerlessness and inability to control one's drinking. This step is designed to eliminate alcoholic "pride," the tendency of alcoholics to stubbornly cling to the conviction that they are strong enough to control their drinking, as if drinking is something outside of the self.

Bateson saw alcoholic "pride" as a natural outgrowth of the more widespread occidental view that the "self" is transcendent in that it can unilaterally control that which is non-self (the body, ego-alien unconscious processes, and objects in the environment). As opposed to the occidental view, Bateson proposed that the self is immanent in the totality of consciousness and unconscious mentation, and it is, "not bounded by the skin but includes all external pathways along which information can travel."[119] This view is consistent with the Buddhist idea that the ego is a fiction, and with the second noble truth that it is ego which creates unnecessary suffering.

Buddhism provides a corrective to Bateson's cybernetic epistemology. Bateson had a tendency toward a "systemic fatalism" in his overemphasis of the limits of conscious purpose. For example, he criticized the deliberate use of pesticides to achieve the narrow conscious purpose of increasing crop yields while inadvertently disrupting the ecosystem, but refused to consciously intervene in the ecosystem of his mouth through visits to a dentist, which resulted in his teeth rotting.[120]

Buddhism takes a more reasonable and balanced view that although a bodhisattva may not have attained perfect wisdom, it is still important to take action in the world. Cybernetic epistemology and the field of family therapy can also help Buddhists learn how to relieve suffering more effectively in family and social systems, an activity which has historically been underemphasized in the Buddhist tradition.

Ericksonian Hypnosis and Therapy

As with Bateson, Milton Erickson considered purposive consciousness to be extremely limited:

> Consciousness, programmed by the typical attitudes and beliefs of modern rationalistic man, is grievously limited. It has been estimated that, at best most people do not utilize more than ten percent of their mental capacity. . . . Patients have problems because their conscious programming has too severely limited their capacities. The solution is to help them break through the limitations of their conscious attitudes to free their unconscious potential for problem solving.[121]

From a Buddhist perspective, consciousness programmed by the typical attitudes and beliefs of modern rationalistic man is ego-based consciousness.

Erickson used hypnosis and trance to bypass the habitual patterns of the conscious mind in order to tap into the potential of the unconscious mind, which he considered to be a vast reservoir of learning and creativity. Earnest Rossi, Erickson's closest collaborator in his later years, initiated a dialogue with Buddhism when he wrote:

> Trance is a state of awareness wherein the normal organizing and structuring function of left-hemispheric consciousness or the ego is minimal. In this less organized state, awareness can maintain its receptive function and sometimes its observer function as well. I wonder if this is similar to the state of "no-mind" which the Zen Buddhists strive for.[122]

Buddhist psychology would respond that no-mind is a state of pure awareness in which there is no subject-object dualism and consequently no "observer function." In this way it differs from the trance state. No-mind is similar to trance, however, in that both states minimize the normal organizing function of the ego.

Both Ericksonian and Buddhist conceptions of mind are also similar in their recognition of the fact that ordinary awareness contains gaps. In *Hypnotic Realities,* Erickson and Rossi state:

> the apparent continuity of consciousness that exists in everyday normal awareness is in fact a precarious illusion that is only made possible by the associative connections that exist between related bits of conversation, task orientation, and so on. We have all experienced the instant amnesias that occur when we go too far on some tangent so we "lose the thread of thought" or "forget just what we were going to do."[123]

The *abhidharma* considers these naturally occurring gaps to be glimpses of no-mind or egolessness.

Once we have understood the similarities between Buddhist and Ericksonian conceptions of mind, it becomes clear that it is not coincidental that Erickson utilized many of the same teaching and change-inducing techniques as have innumerable Buddhist masters. Techniques such as the utilization of confusion, surprise, paradox, and metaphorical communication are all effective because they disengage or bypass the conscious mind (ego). As a result, the wisdom of the unconscious becomes manifest and change ensues.

Although Ericksonian and Buddhist conceptions of mind are similar in some respects, there are important ways in which they differ. While developing his legendary skills as a hypnotist, Erickson found it efficacious to talk to subjects about the conscious and unconscious minds as if they were independent entities. This Ericksonian bifurcation of the mind into the conscious and unconscious is deficient in two respects. First, unnecessary confusion is created when Erickson and Rossi use phrases such as "habitual conscious patterns" or "conscious programming." From a Buddhist perspective habitual or programmed patterns of behavior are unconscious. Rather than use the concepts of conscious and unconscious mind, Buddhism uses the concepts of ego and egolessness (or pure awareness).

Second, the Ericksonian conception of mind overemphasizes the limitations of the conscious mind and the wisdom of the unconscious. Erickson and Rossi's writings could easily give the impression that the conscious mind is a dangerous enemy. The implication is that to realize one's potential, one must plunge headlong into a life of complete spontaneity and mindless abandon. Again from a Buddhist perspective, what is lacking in the Ericksonian model of mind is the concept of pure awareness or no-mind. It is this nondualistic awareness that frees us from mindless habitual patterns, regardless of whether they are considered conscious or unconscious.

Dialogue between Ericksonian therapists and Buddhism could give Buddhist change agents innovative techniques for liberating people from suffering unnecessarily in self-defeating habitual patterns.

Narrative Therapy and Constructionism

The field of psychotherapy has seen a proliferation of approaches framed within a postmodern and social constructionist orientation. Social constructionism and narrative therapy share with Buddhism the idea that a fixed self or identity is an illusion developed through social conditioning. Both narrative therapy and the Buddhist path involve becoming aware of the narratives that guide our thinking and behavior. Such awareness allows us to "deconstruct" the stories we tell ourselves, which perpetuates psychological symptoms.

In constructionist and narrative approaches, once a symptom-perpetuating story has been deconstructed it becomes possible to write a new story, one which will liberate the individual from symptomatic patterns. This is an important point of divergence from Buddhism, which takes the more radical approach of letting go of all stories and narratives. From the standpoint of Buddhist psychology, all stories unnecessarily restrict our view of reality and reinforce the dualism of ego.

A second important difference between Buddhism and post-modern narrative approaches is that they take different positions with respect to hierarchical relationships. Postmodern narrative approaches attempt to be nonhierarchical in order to ensure that an oppressive hierarchy between therapist and client does not develop. In contrast, Buddhism does not assume that hierarchy inevitably leads to oppression. While there is a recognition that on the absolute level student and teacher are not separated by a hierarchical dualism, on the relative, practical level there is a recognition that an enlightened or "natural hierarchy" can be useful.

For example, in a family it is important for parents to comfortably exercise their benevolent authority by maintaining a clear and respectful hierarchy with their children.

> Leadership is natural in a good human society. People who practice the warrior's disciplines together—the disciplines of mindfulness and awareness, gentleness and fearlessness . . . know who their leaders are. A leader with authentic presence raises people up—encourages them to follow the path of warriorship so that they can surpass that leader.[124]

Similarly a teacher or therapist with authentic presence is not afraid to take his or her place in a natural hierarchy with students or clients. Through the practice of skillful means, the teacher or therapist can powerfully utilize this hierarchy in helping students and clients to discover their own wisdom.

Cognitive-Behavioral Therapy

Cognitive-behavioral therapy emphasizes symptom elimination, goal-setting, and other particular techniques. While these emphases would seem to be antithetical to Buddhist therapy, there has actually been a fruitful dialogue between the two approaches. One important way in which they overlap is in cultivating awareness of habitual patterns of thinking and behaving. The first step in behavioral therapy is frequently self-observation of symptomatic behaviors or feelings. The client is asked to record antecedents of the symptom, rate the severity of the symptom, and record cognitions that are associated with the symptom. Although the intent is to use this data to develop strategies for behavior management, it is often the case that the very act of self-observation produces symptom reduction. From a Buddhist point of view this makes perfect sense.

Furthermore, cognitive therapy can be facilitated by having the client practice mindfulness-awareness meditation. For many clients the substitution of healthy rational beliefs and self-statements for irrational and unhealthy beliefs and self-statements is impossible because they are not aware of feelings and associated cognitions, and they have great difficulty developing such awareness. The practice of meditation is particularly effective for developing the habit of awareness.

By encouraging the development of nonevaluative awareness, meditation also sidesteps a frequently encountered obstacle to change in cognitive therapy. This obstacle develops when the client applies a judgmental attitude to the process of observing thoughts. Such an attitude produces what was earlier described as double negativity. When the neurotic style of ego permeates the process of self-observation, the result can only be further confusion and suffering. Only the unconditioned awareness of egolessness can transform confusion into wisdom.

Deane Shapiro has elaborated a system for integrating Buddhist psychology and behaviorism in his book *Precision Nirvana.*[125] More recently, Marsha Linehan has developed an approach to working with borderline clients, which also brings Buddhism to behaviorism. This approach, called Dialectical Behavioral Therapy,

> goes a step further than standard cognitive-behavioral therapy in emphasizing the necessity of teaching clients to fully accept themselves and their world as they are in the moment. The acceptance advocated is quite radical—it is not acceptance in order to create change. The focus on acceptance in DBT is an integration of Eastern psychological

and spiritual practices (primarily Zen practice) in Western approaches to treatment.[126]

CASE STUDY*

For purposes of case formulation, it is assumed that the client selected for analysis throughout this text is a practicing Buddhist. Following discussion of her presenting problem, five therapeutic strategies will be presented, each derived from a Buddhist perspective.

Presenting Problem

The presenting problem of depression and guilt related to the client's relationship with her mother can be understood within the framework of the four noble truths. The first noble truth recognizes that life inevitably brings the pain of sickness and aging. We all must face sickness and aging in ourselves and those we love. When the client struggles with her relationship with her demented mother she is faced with this truth.

According to the second noble truth, we create unnecessary pain for ourselves and others by avoiding and fighting the truth of suffering. Ego is the tendency for one part of the self to sit in judgment of another part, which it sees as problematic. The client creates unnecessary pain for herself when she engages in "double negativity" by avoiding the painful memories of her childhood, thereby perpetuating neurotic patterns of self-blame. Her anxiety and guilt are generated by attitudes and habitual patterns that support the bureaucracy of her ego.

For example, in order to maintain her position as a "dutiful daughter" she must attack herself when she realizes that she sometimes wishes that her mother would die. Her social and family conditioning tells her that a good daughter could never wish for her mother's death. Her egoistic attachment to her self-concept therefore requires that she flagellate herself.

Buddhist Interventions

A Buddhist approach to therapy with this client might include an emphasis on the use of "touch and go" in relating to emotions, attention to her history of sanity, a discussion of "right morality," a recommendation that she

---

*The case selected is the analysis of a forty-two-year-old, married, employed, Caucasian woman suffering from a major depressive episode. Madill and Barkham (1997). From "Discourse analysis of a theme in one successful case of brief psychodynamic-interpersonal psychotherapy," *Journal of Counseling Psychology, 44* (2), 232-244.

practice tonglen, and attention to her environment, particularly the role of her husband in the presenting problem.

Touch and Go

When a Buddhist therapist works with a Buddhist client the therapy is based on the belief that painful memories and emotions should be approached with mindfulness. In this case, the client would be encouraged to respond with mindfulness to painful memories, thoughts, and feelings. For example, rather than fight or repress childhood memories, the memories and associated feelings could be labeled "thinking," and then the attention could be gently brought back to the here and now. She would "touch" and feel the texture of negative emotions such as guilt or anxiety and then "let go" of them, repeatedly if necessary. One expected result would be a form of desensitization or extinction.

History of Sanity

The Buddhist therapist would listen carefully for "signs of sanity." In the transcript excerpts there are several examples of the client manifesting basic sanity. The first sign of sanity, estrangement from one's way of living, is evident when the client admits that her mother would be much better off in a nursing home and then asks herself "so why the guilt? Why must I feel so damn guilty?"[127] A Buddhist therapist would emphasize to the client that her dissatisfaction with her pervasive and overwhelming guilt is a reflection of basic sanity and a desire for psychological health.

The fourth sign of sanity, longing for compassionate action, is obviously evident in the client's great desire to attend to her mother's needs. In fact, it is the client's desire to act compassionately that has led her to ignore her own needs. A Buddhist therapist would acknowledge the client's compassion, while questioning the skillfulness of her chosen course of action. The discussion of "right morality" that follows will clarify how this aspect of the eightfold path could be made relevant to the client.

The fifth sign of sanity is a sense of clarity, which is evident when the client said "something inside me does tell me that I don't have any reason to be guilty."[128] A Buddhist therapist would view this statement as reflective of her unconditioned "original mind" and would nurture its expression.

The last sign of sanity manifested by the client is courage. Despite being emotionally abused by her mother as a child, the client devoted herself to her mother's care in a way that could be seen as heroic. There are many adult children in similar circumstances who choose to cut themselves off from parents who abused them in childhood.

Right Morality

Right morality is nondualistic in the sense that is not based on a struggle between good and evil. Buddhism views people as having inherent wisdom and goodness, which emerges with the growth of mindfulness and awareness. As one drops the conditioning of ego and experiences harmony and peace, skillful and compassionate action follows.

In the case in question, the client knows that her mother would be better off in an adult care facility. She also knows that caring for her mother at home is overwhelming and has contributed to her own depression. The client's choice to care for her mother at home grows out of her conditioned concept of what a "good daughter" should do for her mother. A Buddhist therapist would point this out, thereby reframing her actions as neurotic or misguided rather than moral.

Tonglen

As a practicing Buddhist, it is assumed that the client would be receptive to *shamatha-vipashyana* meditation. This practice would help her relate to her emotions and thoughts with clarity and precision. A Buddhist therapist could inquire further about whether she also practices *tonglen*. Suggestions could be made for utilizing this practice in her relationship with her mother. It is possible that the client's unworkable attempt to be the sole caregiver to her mother was the only way she knew to exercise her compassion. The practice of *tonglen* would provide her with a means for exercising compassion which is not self-destructive and unskillful. Whenever she felt her mother's pain she could take it in, while sending out comfort and peace to her mother and all other beings who are sick and suffering. When feeling guilt the client could practice *tonglen* by taking it in while sending herself love and understanding.

Environment

Because Buddhist therapists see separation of self from other as an egoistic illusion, they inquire about the client's environment. Particularly the social context is an extremely important part of all presenting problems. For this reason, it would be helpful to explore the part the client's husband plays in her relationship with her mother. How does he get along with her mother? What is his opinion about placing her in a care facility and how strongly does he express it? Similarly, what is the client's larger family-of-origin context? Does she have siblings and if so what role do they play in her mother's care? Assuming her father is deceased, what was her relationship to him? What would he tell her to do if he were still alive? Finally, it would be important to examine the cultural context. Is the client aware of the messages sent to women in our culture regarding their roles as caregivers? By raising these questions and teaching meditation, Buddhist psychotherapy could be an effective intervention for this woman suffering with depression.

NOTES

1. Trungpa, C. (1969). *Meditation in action*. Boulder, CO: Shambhala, p. 12.
2. Dalai Lama XIV (1996). *Beyond dogma*. Berkeley, CA: North Atlantic Press, p. 100.
3. Brazier, D. (1995). *Zen therapy*. New York: John Wiley and Sons, p. 20.
4. Trungpa, C. (1976). *The myth of freedom*. Berkeley, CA: Shambhala, p. 57.
5. Trungpa, *Meditation in action,* p. 12.
6. Clifford, T. (1984). *Tibetan Buddhist medicine and psychiatry*. York Beach, ME: Samuel Weiser, p. 24.
7. Thurman, R. A. F. (1995). *Essential Tibetan Buddhism*. San Francisco, CA: HarperCollins, p. 16.
8. Chodron, P. (1994). *Start where you are*. Boston, MA: Shambhala, p. 11.
9. Clifford, *Tibetan Buddhist medicine and psychiatry,* p. 31.
10. Trungpa, C. (1976). *The myth of freedom*. Berkeley, CA: Shambhala, p. 4.
11. Maddi, S. R. (1972). *Personality theories: A comparative analysis*. Homewood, IL: The Dorsey Press, p. 9.
12. Trungpa, C. (1980). Becoming a full human being. *Naropa Institute Journal of Psychology,* 1 (1), 4-20.
13. Hanh, T. C. (1991). *Peace is every step*. New York: Bantam Books, p. 78.
14. Trungpa, C. (1975). *Glimpses of abhidharma*. Boulder, CO: Prajna Press, p. 15.
15. Trungpa, C. (1973). *Cutting through spiritual materialism*. Berkeley, CA: Shambhala, p. 126.
16. Welwood, J. and Wilber, K. (1979). On ego strength and egolessness. In J. Welwood (Ed.). *The meeting of the ways*. New York: Schocken Books, p. 107.
17. Trungpa, C. (1975). *Glimpses of abhidharma*. Boulder, CO: Prajna Press, p. 41.
18. Trungpa, *Cutting through spiritual materialism,* p. 3.
19. Epstein, M. (1995). *Thoughts without a thinker*. New York: Basic Books, p. 15.
20. Trungpa, *The myth of freedom,* p. 24.
21. Epstein, *Thoughts without a thinker,* p. 31.
22. Trungpa, *The myth of freedom,* p. 31.
23. Ibid., p. 35.
24. Ibid., p. 36.
25. Thurman, R. A. F. (1995). *Essential Tibetan Buddhism*. San Francisco, CA: HarperCollins, p. 25.
26. Trungpa, C. (1981). *Journey without goal*. Boulder, CO: Prajna Press, p. 79.
27. Ibid., p. 85.
28. Trungpa, *The myth of freedom,* p. 73.
29. Welwood, J. and Wilber, K. (1979). On ego strength and egolessness. In J. Welwood (Ed.). *The meeting of the ways*. New York: Schocken Books, p. 104.

30. Chodron, P. (1991). *The wisdom of no escape*. Boston, MA: Shambhala, pp. 41-42.

31. Suzuki, S. (1970). *Zen mind, beginner's mind*. Tokyo, Japan: Weatherhill, p. 35.

32. Baker, R. (1970). Introduction. In Suzuki, S. *Zen mind, beginner's mind*. Tokyo, Japan: Weatherhill, p. 18.

33. Trungpa, *Cutting through spiritual materialism*, p. 221.

34. Chodron, *The wisdom of no escape*, p. 76.

35. Ibid., pp. 3-4.

36. Ibid., p. 15.

37. Chodron, *Start where you are*, p. 19.

38. Hanh, T. C. (1991). *Peace is every step*. New York: Bantam Books, p. 59.

39. Trungpa, *The myth of freedom*, pp. 93-94.

40. Suzuki, *Zen mind, beginner's mind*, p. 105.

41. Trungpa, C. (1983). Becoming a full human being. In J. Welwood (Ed.), *Awakening the heart*. Boston, MA: New Science Library, p. 128.

42. Guenther, H. (1963). *The life and teaching of Naropa*. Oxford, England: Oxford University Press, p. 148.

43. Podvoll, E. (1990). *The seduction of madness*. New York: HarperCollins, p. 238.

44. Watts, A. (1960). *This is it*. New York: Vintage Books, pp. 79-110.

45. Wegela, K. (1996). *How to be a help instead of a nuisance*. Boston, MA: Shambhala, pp. 178-179.

46. Podvoll, E. (1990). *The seduction of madness*. New York: HarperCollins, pp. 223-226.

47. Bateson, G. (1972). *Steps to an ecology of mind*. New York: Ballantine Books, p. 319.

48. Podvoll, E. (1983). Uncovering a patient's history of sanity. In J. Welwood (Ed.). *Awakening the heart*. Boston, MA: New Science Library, p. 185.

49. Yalom, I. (1985). *The theory and practice of group psychotherapy*. New York: Basic Books, pp. 13-15.

50. Hayward, J. (1984). *Perceiving ordinary magic*. Boston, MA: New Science Library, p. 261.

51. Trungpa, *Cutting through spiritual materialism*, p. 157.

52. Hanh, T. N. (1991). *Peace is every step*. New York: Bantam Books, pp. 26-27.

53. Tendzin, O. (1982). *Buddha in the palm of your hand*. Boulder, CO: Shambhala, p. 38.

54. Trungpa, *Cutting through spiritual materialism*, p. 168.

55. Trungpa, *The myth of freedom*, p. 111.

56. Ibid., pp. 112-113.

57. Suzuki, *Zen mind, beginner's mind*, p. 47.

58. Trungpa, *Cutting through spiritual materialism*, p. 177.

59. Trungpa, *The myth of freedom*, p. 123.

60. Trungpa, *Cutting through spiritual materialism*, p. 10.

61. Naranjo, C. and Ornstein, R. (1971). *On the psychology of meditation*. New York: The Viking Press, p. 241.

62. Trungpa, *Cutting through spiritual materialism,* pp. 154-155.

63. Naranjo, C. and Ornstein, R. (1971). *On the psychology of meditation.* New York: The Viking Press, p. 242.

64. Tendzin, O. (1982). *Buddha in the palm of your hand.* Boulder, CO: Shambhala, p. 33.

65. Chodron, *Start where you are,* p. 6.

66. Kabat-Zinn, J. (1990). *Full catastrophe living: Using the wisdom of your body and mind to face pain, stress, and illness.* New York: Dell, pp. 1-14.

67. Brazier, D. (1995). *Zen therapy.* New York: John Wiley and Sons, p. 55.

68. Epstein, M. (1995). *Thoughts without a thinker.* New York: Basic Books, p. 184.

69. Brazier, *Zen therapy,* p. 61.

70. Kornfield, J. (1993). *A path with heart.* New York: Bantam Books, p. 245.

71. Epstein, *Thoughts without a thinker,* p. 177.

72. Ibid.

73. Kornfield, *A path with heart,* p. 246.

74. Trungpa, C. (1993). *Training the mind.* Boston, MA: Shambhala, p. 3.

75. Chodron, *Start where you are.* Boston, pp. 6-7.

76. Ibid., p. 7.

77. Quoted lines are from *The Merchant of Venice,* Act IV, Scene i. Lief, J. (1993). Editor's foreword. In C. Trungpa. Training the mind. Boston, MA: Shambhala, p. xxi.

78. Chodron, *Start where you are,* pp. 38-39.

79. Ibid., p. 9.

80. Doherty, W. (1995). *Soul searching.* New York: Basic Books.

81. Watts, A. (1961). *Psychotherapy east and west.* New York: Ballantine Books, p. 152.

82. Brazier, *Zen therapy,* p. 249.

83. Suzuki, D. T. (1960). Lectures on Zen Buddhism. In E. Fromm, D. T. Suzuki, and R. DeMartino. *Zen Buddhism and psychoanalysis.* New York: Harper Colophon Books, p. 44.

84. Brazier, *Zen therapy,* p. 105.

85. Ibid., p. 14.

86. Trungpa, *Cutting through spiritual materialism,* p. 221.

87. Ibid., p. 210.

88. Ekai, (1934) The gateless gate. In P. Reps (Compiler). *Zen flesh, Zen bones.* New York: Anchor Books, p. 85.

89. Ibid., pp. 92-93.

90. Welwood, J. (1991). *Journey of the heart.* New York: HarperPerennial.

91. Welwood, J. (1996). *Love and awakening.* New York: HarperCollins.

92. Brazier, *Zen therapy,* p. 131.

93. Kabat-Zinn, M. and Kabat-Zinn, J. (1997). *Everyday blessings.* New York: Hyperion, p. 15.

94. Yalom, *The theory and practice of group psychotherapy,* pp. 14-15.

95. Epstein, *Thoughts without a thinker,* p. 161.

96. Walsh, R. (1996). Meditation research: The state of the art. In B. Scotton, A. Chinen, and J. Battista (Eds.). *Textbook of transpersonal psychiatry and psychology.* New York: Basic Books, p. 167.

97. Ibid., pp. 169-170.

98. Shapiro, D. (1980). *Meditation.* New York: Aldine Publishing Company, p. 160.

99. Walsh, Meditation research: The state of the art, p. 175.

100. Kamenetz, R. (1994). *The Jew in the lotus.* New York: HarperSanFrancisco, p. 2.

101. Ibid., pp. 273-274.

102. Ibid., pp. 125-126.

103. Boorstein, S. (1997). *That's funny, you don't look Buddhist.* New York: HarperSanFrancisco, p. 143.

104. Hayward, J. (1984). *Perceiving ordinary magic.* Boston, MA: New Science Library, pp. 259-260.

105. deMello, A. (1990). *Awareness.* New York: Doubleday, p. 50.

106. Ibid., p. 162.

107. Dalai Lama XIV (1996). *Beyond dogma.* Berkeley, CA: North Atlantic Press, p. 155.

108. Ibid., p. 101.

109. Ibid., p. 91.

110. Watts, A. (1973). Foreword. In A. Chung-liang Huang, *Embrace tiger, return to mountain.* Moab, UT: Real People Press, p. 2.

111. Chung-liang Huang, A. (1973). *Embrace tiger, return to mountain.* Moab, UT: Real People Press, p. 172.

112. Hayward, J. (1995). *Sacred world.* New York: Bantam Books, p. 223.

113. Ibid., p. 224.

114. Fromm, E. (1960). Psychoanalysis and Zen Buddhism. In E. Fromm, D.T. Suzuki, and R. Demartino. *Zen Buddhism and psychoanalysis.* New York: Harper Colophon Books, p. 122.

115. Epstein, *Thoughts without a thinker,* p. 9.

116. Ibid., p. 135.

117. Ibid., p. 6.

118. Ibid., p. 101.

119. Bateson, G. (1971). The cybernetics of "self": A theory of alcoholism. *Psychiatry, 34* (1), 1-18. In Bateson, G. (1972). *Steps to an ecology of mind.* New York: Ballantine Books, p. 319.

120. Bateson, M. C. (1984). *With a daughter's eye.* New York: HarperPerennial, p. 219.

121. Erickson, M., Rossi, E., and Rossi, S. (1976). *Hypnotic realities.* New York: Irvington, pp. 17-18.

122. Erickson, M. and Rossi, E. (1981). *Experiencing hypnosis.* New York: Irvington, p. 90.

123. Erickson, Rossi, and Rossi, *Hypnotic realities,* p. 299.

124. Hayward, J. (1995). *Sacred world.* New York: Bantam Books, p. 239.

125. Shapiro, D. (1978). *Precision nirvana.* Englewood Cliffs, NJ: Prentice-Hall, Inc.

126. Linehan, M. (1993). *Skills training manual for treating borderline personality disorder.* New York: The Guilford Press, pp. 5-6.

127. Madill and Barkham (1997). Discourse analysis of a theme in one successful case of brief psychodynamic-interpersonal psychotherapy. *Journal of Counseling Psychology, 44* (2), 232-244 (extract 8, session 5, lines 8-9).

128. Ibid., extract 9, session 5, lines 1-2.

Chapter 3

Taoism and Psychology

Lynne Hagen

INTRODUCTION

Tao is the source of the ten thousand things.
It is the treasure of the good man, and the refuge of the bad . . .
Why does everyone like the Tao at first?
Isn't it because you find what you seek and are forgiven when you sin?
Therefore this is the greatest treasure of the universe.[1]

The Tao is the underlying force that fosters existence, growth, and flexibility. It encourages us to open our hearts and minds. It teaches us that life is ever-changing, and to be respectful of all that exists. Followers of the Tao find guidance, wisdom, comfort, compassion, and unconditional acceptance. As we experience the gentle manner of the Tao, we gain understanding of the rhythms and interconnections among all within the universe.

The Tao

The Tao is not considered the creator of the universe. It is all things; but it is not the law of all things.[2] According to the Tao, if things are allowed to follow their own pattern or direction, they will harmonize with others not because of any imposed rule, but by mutual cooperation and innate interdependence. The universe is a symbiosis of all that exists. When a particular part of the universe is analyzed, classified, and compartmentalized, conflict arises and the larger pattern and meaning within the universe is lost. Nature's way is that larger animals feed upon smaller animals. If the life of the mouse is analyzed, one could become angry at the cat that eats the mouse, yet this occurrence is simply part of the larger biological cycle of life in the universe. It simply happens because of itself, without being pushed or pulled.[3] Each act creates another and another according to the principle of mutual arising *(hsiang sheng).*[4]

As we become conscious, we begin to conceptualize how the universe works. The human concept of causality is our feeble attempt to connect identified stages of events so that these events can be described with words. When we do this, however, the full meaning of the event is lost. Each event is the universe itself. No event is separate, and each always affects the way of the universe.[5]

The Tao is not a personal God, but it can be intuitively known.[6] In Western thinking, it is sometimes helpful to view the Tao as a type of all-encompassing energy. It cannot be grasped or touched, but we know intuitively that it is all around us. The Tao is the source of all things conscious and unconscious. It is the basis of all being and cannot be named, but we give it a name in an effort to make sense of it.[7]

Naming is one way we acknowledge the existence of Tao, but the way to perceive the Tao is by observing the patterns and processes in nature and through meditation, which allows our minds to become quiet and aware of what is, without putting it into words. Words judge events, and when judgment occurs the Tao is effaced.[8] The Tao must be experienced and apprehended, not merely labeled or conceptualized with words.

Knowledge

Didactic learning can increase knowledge especially when it is combined with experiential and Socratic learning imbued with paradox to stimulate thought and understanding of self, others, and nature. Book knowledge can be intimidating. In addition, scholastic knowledge can be difficult to understand when it is not holistic and does not match the experience of ordinary people.

Western philosophy tends to divide and compartmentalize people, objects, and concepts. Complex analyses can leave us feeling disorganized and vulnerable. Oftentimes, learning from books is valued rather than direct experience, and impressive words can keep us from comparing scholarship to actual experience. Words can cover up and distort life experiences, and they prevent us from facing what is occurring in our lives. Book learning is helpful in Taoism, but life must be experienced in order to gain a true understanding of it. Life must be brought into full awareness regardless if the knowledge that is uncovered is judged "right or wrong."[9] In Taoism appearances are not important. Appearances disguise the genuine self and get in the way of wisdom and happiness. When arrogance and complexity are cast off, the natural uncarved life is revealed. When this natural state is found, one can enjoy being quiet and living simply. This childlike state of being allows life to be spontaneous *(tzu-jan)* and fun.[10]

Intuition

Taoism is experiential and intuitive. As experiences are allowed into consciousness, we begin to know and trust our inner nature. When this occurs, we know intuitively what is right for us.[11] Taoism is an intuitive approach to life. We begin to understand that everything in nature has its own place. This does not mean we leave our life to fate; rather it emphasizes the need to simply recognize what is going on around us, what is there. Some have called this awareness "facing the facts," or facing our own limitations. Once limitations are recognized, they can be understood and managed, so that limitations can become strengths rather than unconsciously ignored problems that work against us. Intuitive awareness allows us to choose the path that leads straight from the heart and helps us remember that we are part of the eternal Tao.[12]

Intuition is a term that is not only difficult to define; it is a word that the scientific practitioner both desires and resists, since it is subjective and not readily observable. Consequently, intuition and "felt meanings" have been likened to mysticism, magic, and even voodoo.[13] To rely upon one's intuition means one has fervent confidence in the wisdom of one's feelings.[14] Intuition is a form of knowledge gained from experience rather than solely from scientific study. Consequently, intuition is private, personal, and subjective.[15] Conclusions are reached without explanation of how or why they occurred.[16]

Despite psychology's desire to be an objective science, clinicians continue to devote considerable effort to developing their intuitive sense[17] and frequently claim they function intuitively.[18] Clinical intuition is sometimes cited as a hallmark of an experienced psychologist. Ironically, however, clinicians are reluctant to say they acted without knowing why they acted, because that suggests incompetence.[19] It seems more professional to use the term "clinical judgment."

In the Taoist sense, intuition arrives spontaneously and is believed to be a noncognitive process,[20] or a "gut" feeling.[21] Intuition is developed through experiential learning and formal education. It is not something that can be learned in textbooks, but arises through combined effects of experiential and formal learning. Intuition is developed by being open minded, fully present to experiences, and by affirming the validity in knowledge that cannot be objectified. Intuitive thinking is the Taoist person's way of cooperating with the course of the natural world. It is similar to the patterns found naturally in water and wood.[22] The intuitive individual is mindful of the natural rhythms of nature, knows and trusts one's inner self, and lives fully in the present.

Mindfulness

From the Taoist perspective the only way to truly enjoy life is to live mindfully, in the present moment.[23] *Taoist mindfulness is silent, nonverbal, nonconceptual, and nonintellectual.* Mindfulness is manifested in the extraordinary musician or athlete, who gives a masterful and "effortless" performance without any apparent, deliberate, or intentional step-by-step verbal instruction. Mindfulness is the ability to be in the present moment, to focus, and to be aware of the most basic and simplest of actions, such as breathing and walking.[24]

Mindfulness is not the Western psychological notion of bringing thoughts, feelings, behaviors, or self-talk into awareness. Being mindful allows one to be in the present moment and fully focused on the process of attaining a goal rather than the end result of the goal.[25] In the West, we are usually preoccupied with goals and future-oriented events. Westerners seem to believe that in order to be happy, they must engage in considerable planning, endure hardships, and sacrifice now to have a better future. But if attention is on the future, the opportunity for happiness in the present is missed. How can we find meaning and happiness while reliving the past or worrying about the future? If we do not enjoy the present, how will we enjoy the future when it becomes the present? Life cannot be fulfilling if we continually compare current experiences to the past or wishes for change in the future. Comfort, happiness, peace, and appreciation are not qualities to be attained in the future through struggle and hard work now; they can be found by immersing ourselves in the present moment.[26] Being precedes doing and thinking.

In the Taoist sense, being mindful is to be in the present moment and being fully focused on the activity rather than the goal.[27] As Csikszentmihalyi suggests, the best times in our lives are when we are so involved in an activity that nothing else matters and time seems to fly by. When we are absorbed in the present moment, we forget about the past, the future, and ourselves. Sometimes after we have achieved a goal following a particularly difficult struggle, we find that the process of reaching that goal was much more enjoyable that its actual attainment. The activity we are participating in becomes spontaneous and automatic, and we experience the intrinsic reward of feeling connected to the world.[28]

When one's thinking remains open, and untainted by both perceptions of the past and fantasies of the future, understanding of self and others is enhanced. Each moment can be experienced to its fullest, free from discrimination and premeditated ideas. Being mindful allows one to be immersed in the moment and to perceive clearly and accurately. The open mind allows acceptance and compassion toward all and recognizes that all are worthy of attention.[29] Acceptance is the natural response when all aspects of an individual are at peace.

Therapy from a Taoist perspective leads to greater consciousness. As present-mindedness, acceptance of the genuine self, and recognition of the ever-changing nature of life develops, compassion for one's self, others, and nature grow. Through this process, feelings of alienation are replaced with the strength and guidance that emanates from the awareness that all in nature, including humans, are interdependent. We are never truly alone, but always supported by all that surrounds us. As a result, our life purpose can become clearer and more meaningful.[30]

Taoism is described as "timeless Chinese wisdom" that is "medicine for the ills of the West. Yet, paradoxically, it must not be taken as medicine, an intellectually swallowed 'pill,' but allowed joyously to infuse our total being and so transform our individual lives and through them our society."[31]

The wisdom of the Tao is practical and fun-loving, with teachers that come in many forms (e.g., water, earth, heavenly, animal, human, botanical, circumstance, etc.).[32] These teachers help one to experience the Tao by letting go of opinions and philosophies, and become inquisitive, attentive, and unfamiliar with intellectualism. It is a state of sensing and experiencing in the present while letting go of the worries of the past and the future.[33] Taoism encourages living in the present moment. Regular practice of present-mindedness develops a relaxed way of thinking that is open to accomplishment without dwelling on past failures or future desires. Success naturally arises when one is mindfully involved in the achievement of a desired goal rather than worrying about potential positive or negative outcomes.[34]

Many journeys have a beginning and an ending. In Taoism, however, there is no final destination because change is ever constant and cyclical. Bodies grow and change as they progress through the life cycle, continually evolving physically, mentally, emotionally, and spiritually. Attitudes and beliefs shift as new skills are learned and ineffective or dissatisfying ones are revised or discarded. Through this process, what "can be" is redefined through the amplification of genuine strengths and the release of self-limiting, self-defeating thoughts. Taoism is a way of accepting and being comfortable with change, rather than wasting energy fighting against change.[35] To a Taoist, peace can be realized through mindfulness, letting go of self-defeating, negative thoughts, and recognizing and honoring the cycles of nature, including those within one's self.

Internal strength is nurtured through the study and application of Taoist teachings, and confidence grows as one learns to interact harmoniously with life's demands.[36] The essence of Taoism is compassionate cooperation rather than self-interest and competition.[37] Following the Tao develops a passion for a higher good beyond self-interest, and builds inner strength, integrity, and interdependence.[38] As we learn to unconditionally accept and care for all aspects of creation, we grain a sense of balance and connectedness in our lives, and realize that difficulties and pain appear when we isolate, separate, or set ourselves apart from others and from nature.[39] Taoism promotes unconditional acceptance and respect of all of nature through positive holistic attitudes.

The following text reviews the meaning of Taoism, Contemplative and Hsien Taoism, a brief historical overview including references to the Age of Perfect Virtue and the Great Separation story, Taoist sacred scriptures, and basic Taoist principles. The discussion of Taoism and psychology contained in this chapter is not meant to be a precise or a complete representation of Taoism, but hopefully captures the spirit of the Tao from a Western cultural perspective and how its principles may be applied to psychology and therapy.

Meaning of Taoism

> The Tao that can be told is not the eternal Tao.
> The name that can be named is not the eternal name.
> The nameless is the beginning of heaven and earth.
> The named is the mother of ten thousand things.[40]

The Tao is a neither a personal God, a divine ruler, nor the designer of the universe. Tao is absolute reality, energy of the universe, motherly, and the beginning and ending of all things.[41] The Tao was not created; rather it is a "primeval reality that well precedes gods and human beings."[42] There is no similarity between Taoism and Western ideas of good, what should and should not be obeyed, or what is divine law. In Taoist thought, laws and rules are developed only when people do not realize that they cannot stray from the underlying forces of nature.[43] Ultimately, one can only follow the Tao because all of nature, including humans, is part of the integral force of Tao. Even though we call this force, "Tao," it is recognized that "Tao" is only a label used to describe something that cannot be categorized or described by words.[44] The Tao only can be felt and intuited; it cannot be created, classified, or explained. The Tao "is," and those who feel or intuit the Tao, simply acknowledge and accept its presence. Water is often used as a teaching metaphor to aid understanding of the Tao and the reason why Watts refers to Taoism as The Watercourse Way.[45,46]

Taoism is based on the Chinese principle that if you cannot trust your intuitive self or "gut," you cannot trust others or nature. Ironically, inability to trust yourself limits your ability to know when you should not trust yourself, others, or nature. Without trust in others, the environment, and ourselves, we are stuck and powerless.[47] Taoism posits that all things in the universe are equal, interdependent, and work together as a unified whole to survive, grow, and flourish. In Western thinking, nature is separated and categorized by species, higher and lower forms of intelligence, diagnostic codes, stages of development, social status, etc. To follow the Tao requires courage, faith, and trust to set aside Western isolationist beliefs and linear logic and begin thinking and acting from the perspective of universal interconnections and interdependence.[48]

Contemplative Taoism

Contemplative Taoism is based upon the authoritative writings of three men: Lao-tzu, presumed author of the *Tao Te Ching*, written approximately 2,500 years ago;[49] Chuang-tzu, who, approximately 2,000 years ago, authored several works including *The Chuang Tzu* and founded a school of writers and philosophers; and the Yellow Emperor who ruled China 4,500 years ago and is credited with the development of Taoist meditative, alchemical, and healing principles and practices.[50]

Taoism is a spiritual path that is to be consciously followed in order to gain understanding, morality, compassion, and wisdom. It is a way of being and living.[51] Taoism does not promote intellectualism, but encourages living a simplified, natural way of life.[52] In Taoism, knowledge per se is not synonymous to either wisdom or virtue.[53] From the Taoist perspective, one knows him or her self through a variety of experiences that includes both formal and informal education. In addition, a highly developed intuitive sense is promoted to understand both oneself and others, and to maintain personal safety.[54] A Taoist values the freedom to work and play without outside regulation. Intellectuals often presume laws and regulations are necessary to control and manage human behavior when, in fact, they deprive individuals of their own power to develop the skills necessary for survival.[55]

Furthermore, since there is no proof of heaven or hell, contemplative Taoists do not believe it is realistic to believe in an afterlife, gods, ritual, or clerical authority. For similar reasons, Eastern beliefs in reincarnation are denied. Most important, Taoism values genuine personal exploration to achieve inner understanding.[56] Taoism is a spirituality that assists in the management of what is already known.

To follow the Tao is to observe nature (e.g., the flow of water) and its cycles (i.e., the order of the seasons). The Tao is impartial, impersonal, and the *rational* law of all things. It must be followed if humans want to live in peace. The early philosophers believed that a simple uncomplicated life surrounded by nature creates and sustains peace within one's self. The Taoist has an unimpassioned obedience to nature and trusts nature's commands. The mark of a wise person is the refusal to interfere with the natural course of things.[57]

Hsien Taoism

In contrast to the here and now emphasis of contemplative Taoism, Hsien Taoism is focused on a search for immortality and supernormal powers through ascetic and yogic practices that are believed to have arisen among

Taoists by the second and first centuries, B.C.E. The teachings of Hsien Taoism are nearly the opposite of the teachings of Lao-tzu and Chuang-tzu. Followers of Hsien Taoism are called Hsiens. Hsiens use special forms of breathing, diet, drugs, and exercise in an effort to become immortal.[58]

The focus of this chapter is not on Hsien Taoism, but on Contemplative Taoism where alienation and separateness is set aside and interdependence and cooperation among all humans and nature is paramount.

Historical Overview

Taoism developed in China in an effort to counterbalance the teachings of K'ung-Fu-tzu or Confucius. Confucianism was mainly interested in preserving social order within Chinese society. Its followers emphasized rigid conformity and an authoritarian attitude toward life. Some of its major principles are loyalty, duty, filial piety, social protocol and order, and day-to-day interpersonal conduct. It has contributed to the development of Chinese government, business, family relations, and reverence of ancestors. Taoism, on the other hand, places greater emphasis on an individual's relationship with the world and nature. Its contributions to society have largely been scientific, artistic, and spiritual. The difference between Taoism and Confucianism is partly in emotional tone. Confucianism tends to be patriarchal and strict, whereas Taoism is matriarchal, gentle, fun loving, and serene.[59]

During the fourth, fifth, and sixth centuries B.C.E., Chinese philosophers described a way of life that they called Taoism or "The Way." This ancient Way of being was introduced in China 500 years before Christ and has become the cultural basis of Taoism.[60] These philosophers were not the founders of Taoism, although they organized and communicated the tenets of Taoism. Taoism actually began long before these philosophies were born during what Chuang-tzu described as the Age of Perfect Virtue before the Great Separation.[61]

Age of Perfect Virtue

During the Age of Perfect Virtue, all of nature lived together in egalitarian harmony where none were separated or classified as better than or less than the other. All remained genuine to their true selves and lived simply and purely. All were accepting of one another despite their intellectual ability, achievement, or level of wisdom. During this age, all creatures loved, respected, and supported each other without laws and regulation.[62] Today, this way of life can be seen in American Indian, Buddhist, and Shinto beliefs. In China, it is passed along through Taoism.[63]

Great Separation Story

During the Age of Perfect Virtue, people lived in harmony with the earth and all of its creatures. All forms of life communicated telepathically and were considered equal. They harmoniously worked together, and learned from and cared for each other. As time went by, however, humans grew to believe that they were more important than other forms of life and began to act in ways that upset the cooperative harmony among life. The Great Separation occurred when humans separated themselves and placed themselves above nature. In an effort to help the humans realize the importance of cooperation, equality, and interdependence, nature exiled the humans from their paradise where they were cut off from food, social support, and peace. As a consequence of being cast out and alienated from nature, humans began experiencing isolation and loneliness. Thus began the frenetic quest to recover the happiness they had known. They tried to regain their lost happiness through the collection of things, but found it only brought them short-term contentment. In fact, this process brought even more distress into their lives, because they needed to continually search for more and more things to sustain peace and happiness. Eventually, humans learned that "things" were only a substitute for the belongingness, contentment, peace, and joy they had known before the Great Separation.[64]

Since humans could no longer communicate telepathically with other forms of life, they tried to understand their world through linear logic and began to categorize nature. Unfortunately, these techniques were limiting and did not capture the full understanding of the aspect of nature they were attempting to classify. Eventually, Taoist prophets (e.g., Lao-tzu) were born to teach humans the truth of what had nearly been forgotten. These prophets began teaching that peace and harmony with all of life is possible and that all life has wisdom and divine presence. Peace and harmony within one's self and within the world can be found, if one is able to set aside ego and is willing to cooperate with the natural laws of the universe.[65]

Following the Tao is living in harmony with nature. Ever since the Great Separation, the goal of Taoists has been to attain the state of Perfect Virtue by abandoning all that thwarts harmony in the universe.[66]

Sacred Scriptures

The essence of Taoism is contained in the *Tao Te Ching,* which remains a significant influence on Chinese thought and culture.[67] Over the last fifty years, Chinese, Japanese, and European scholars have agreed that even though the authorship of the *Tao Te Ching* has been attributed to Lao-tzu, it may be a collection of Taoist sayings compiled by various writers.[68]

Regardless of the authorship of the *Tao Te Ching,* it is believed to have originated in China during the fourth century B.C.E. The *Tao Te Ching* was written during the Warring State Period (475 to 221 B.C.E.) as guidance in surviving this very troubled time.[69] The *Tao Te Ching* is translated as a path, principle, or Way of being that leads from the heart. It is a compilation of verses that teaches about the Tao and how to live simply, practically, cooperatively, compassionately, and serenely without unreasonable ambition.[70]

The *I Ching* appears to have influenced Taoism some time after the *Tao Te Ching* was written. Both texts are similar in that they recognize the existence and interdependence of polar opposites. The *I Ching* also recognizes a higher internal wisdom that in psychological terms we call unconscious, inner-self, intuitive knowing, etc. This internal knowledge may be called upon through a method of random sorting of milfoil twigs or coins. The twigs or coins are thrown six times while the participant holds a serious question in his or her mind. Each throw results in a yin or yang, which eventually become a six-sided geometric design. The *I Ching* is then consulted for the meaning of the design. The meanings are oracular and ambiguous, but one may use the diagram and its predictions analogous to a Rorschach Ink Blot test or other projective psychological measure to project the unconscious onto a medium to increase understanding of unconscious thoughts, feelings, motives, etc. Throughout this process it is important to examine one's thoughts regardless of logic or morality, similar to free association in psychoanalysis.[71]

Principles of Taoism

The basic tenets of Taoism include: natural simplicity *(p'u);* spontaneity *(tzu-jan);* harmonious action *(wu wei)* and cyclical growth; virtue and personal power *(te);* and the *yin-yang* polarity.[72]

Natural Simplicity (P'u)

P'u refers to the beauty, grace, and power of all things in their natural, original, or simple state. Taoists value the strength, energy, and beauty of what they call the "uncarved block" or nature in its original state. When a natural state is tampered with, it is believed it loses some of its natural power and beauty.[73]

The wisdom of the uncarved block simply exists and cannot be accurately described with words. It is practical and focuses on common sense. *P'u* is uncovered when complexity is abandoned and the childlike, mysterious, and fun parts of life and one's true nature are uncovered. By developing the state of mind of the uncarved block, one becomes able to enjoy a life that is simple, ordinary, calm, and straightforward. One learns to work with the flow of life rather than against it and to act spontaneously.[74]

Taoism is holistic; the Tao does not separate nature or human beings into parts or categories, nor does it analyze characteristics in an effort to organize and understand human beings. Consistent with the principle of natural simplicity, the whole is valued more than composite parts. The whole is simpler than complex interactions among multiple parts. From the Taoist perspective, any attempt to categorize personality into discrete parts does not allow complete understanding of the individual in one's environment.

According to Taoism, human beings, animals, plants, earth, and sky are all intimately connected and share the same atmosphere, energy, and attitudes. Attempts at separation actually confuse thinking and the picture of the whole becomes lost in the analysis of the constituent parts. Compartmentalization leaves one feeling disorganized, vulnerable, and egocentric. [75]

Spontaneity (Tzu-jan)

The Tao is a name for spontaneity.[76] Actions and events harmonious with Tao are effortless, independent, and inexhaustible. If all things in nature are allowed to grow at their own pace and on their own volition,[77] harmony will arise. Mutual interdependence among things will unfold naturally, because all things are naturally interdependent. We need all elements in the universe as much as they need us. All things in nature are what they are because they are interconnected and interrelated. As Watts indicated, "the sun would not be light without eyes, nor would the universe 'exist' without consciousness. . . ."[78] We are what we are in relation to other people, things, and events. Therefore, individuals are never separate from community. We are never alone because we always exist in relation to someone or something.[79]

Since the Tao is free from any external necessity, it does not need to impose its rules upon the universe. When all things in nature are allowed to go their own way, harmony spontaneously arises effortlessly. The order of the natural world is not forced, and there are no laws that can command nature to behave in a certain way. Nature is not rigid and realizes everything has its own way of being. Mutual interdependence among all things will unfold. As Watts describes, our internal organs grow in cooperation with our outside growth.[80] Both differ in size, proportion, and appearance, but they cannot be separated.

The peace and order that arises spontaneously when we are in harmony with nature is called *li*. *Li* is not always easily recognized because of its multidimensional nature. It is most discernible in patterns in wood grains, the order found in moving water, clouds, frost crystals, etc. When the pattern and beauty are pointed out, the become recognizable to us even though we may not have the words to say why it is clear to us.[81]

Unfortunately, many people do not appreciate that order emerges spontaneously and naturally. They become frustrated, fearful, disgusted, or angry with that which appears to lack order. Rules and designs are adopted so that life appears predictable and consistent with their own expectations and plans, all guided by Western linear logic of cause and effect. Unwilling to accept that a natural order will arise spontaneously, they try to impose their own definitions of order upon nature. Taoist teachers often use water metaphors to gently encourage understanding.

The flow of water cannot be controlled, e.g., flood waters will find their own path. Similarly, a linear pattern cannot be forced upon either clouds or frost crystals, and yet they have order. Nature does not need to order and classify itself because it realizes that order and understanding spontaneously arise when one remains quietly attentive and open-minded to nonlinear logic. In Western culture, however, we prefer to separate and classify nature, including human nature, in an effort to increase order, understanding, and control.[82]

Harmonious Action (Wu Wei)

One of the paradoxes in Taoism is that "the Tao does nothing, but nothing is left undone."[83] This paradox affirms a way of being: action through inaction. *Wei* means forcing, interfering, deceiving, or going against the grain of natural order *(li)*. *Wu wei* is action without bureaucratic, competitive, aggressive, or self-serving effort. *Wu wei* is a way of being that comes from an internal sensitivity to the natural rhythms of the universe, similar to water flowing over or around rocks, logs, or islands in a stream. When we learn our own inner nature and the natural laws in action around us, we act with minimal effort by following the principles of the natural world.[84] In other words, we are in sync with nature, and therefore at one with Tao. We learn that the way to do is to be.

Wu wei is embodied in the allegory of the mighty oak and willow tree. When covered with heavy snow, the rigid oak branches crack under the weight of the snow. The willow branch, however, yields to the snow's weight lowering itself and allowing the snow to fall off. The willow is not flaccid, but flexible, resourceful, and resilient. It bends with the forces of nature and allows its branches to remain whole and unbroken.[85] Similar to the willow tree, human personality also benefits from being flexible in order to be resilient and to remain whole.

Wu wei is a way of being that produces *tzu-jan*. When life goes along effortlessly, there are no real accidents. Events may appear strange or uncomfortable at times, but they can be worked out, especially when they are allowed to be worked out by themselves. *Wu wei* is working with whatever happens instead of lamenting over what has happened in the past, or trying to make the present fit our vision of an ideal future. *Wu wei* is accepting whatever circumstance one encounters, and being sensitive to both the external circumstances and to our own internal wisdom. In this way, problems seem to solve themselves. The power of problems is neutralized because we remove the frustration, anxiety, and anger, which sustain or escalate them.[86]

Wu wei is not only a way of living, but also a form of intelligence. Through observation and experience, intuition and insight, knowledge of human and natural affairs became so engrained that one uses little physical, emotional, or mental energy in dealing with them. This intelligence combines conscious learning with intuitive knowledge of the body and nature.[87]

Wu wei is akin to the intelligence involved in putting together a jigsaw puzzle. One can take the time to enjoy the process of putting the puzzle together, considering each piece chosen as neither a good or bad choice, but simply a choice that either works toward completion or tells one to choose another piece. Alternatively, one can become frustrated when the puzzle is not completed by an imposed deadline, and waste time trying to figure out why certain pieces that should fit together do not. As a form of intelligence, *wu wei* does not try to find out why certain pieces fit in certain places; it does not place limitations on the person or activity; it just places them where they fit.

Wu wei is nonjudgmental and unconditional. Judgments are not attached to events, situations, or people. When life becomes difficult, Taoists allow themselves time and space to contemplate solutions to the presenting problem. Anxiety and frustration are likely to result with excessive deliberation. One who lives according to *wu wei* accepts reality without the need to know the how or why things work. No judgment is attached to solutions; results simply exist if one is open and willing to see them.[88]

When practicing *wu wei,* the conscious wisdom of the mind is combined with the unconscious knowledge of the body. The result is that one learns to act in a manner that produces the least resistance, yielding a quality of effort that is unforced, natural, and congruent. One applies intuitive and intellectual knowledge to work with the forces of nature so that the most fruitful response is realized moment to moment.[89]

To illustrate the principle of *wu wei,* Watts describes how, in judo, one steps aside when an adversary throws a blow.[90] Forward motion is used only when the opponent is off balance. The wise use of the opponent's energy *(chi)* will place him or her off balance, allowing the individual to remain safe. Taoism teaches us to act in harmony with the force or power of nature. By contrast, when we force change, we expend vital energy and go against the grain of spontaneous living. Consequently, we waste energy that could be used for things that can be accomplished. We must learn to trust others, ourselves, the rhythm and timing of the universe, and that it is ok to be fully and honestly human, imperfections and all *(jen).*[91]

To be fully human means accepting both achievement and disappointment. People who value only their virtues remain unaware of their dangerous shadows. As they live and arrange their world according to a set of unyielding and never deviating rules, they find themselves unable to compromise, and to accept the frailties found in themselves and the world. They are unable to trust human nature and to accept both the good and bad in all human beings. To trust in human nature is to accept the good and the bad of all of humankind, although it is extremely difficult to trust those who cannot admit they have imperfections.[92]

Any deliberate effort to cultivate doing without doing *(wu wei)* through directed study appears contradictory to the principle. Understanding *wu wei* is gained through intuitive awareness where one is able to experience it with body and soul, so to speak, often with a Taoist master guiding one in the principles and practices of meditation. Through meditation, both the *yin* and *yang* of life are encountered, problems are solved intuitively, and joy is found. Meditation is not intended for self-improvement, but to facilitate personal growth by separating one's self from forcefulness and letting life simply exist, letting life be, and flowing with nature's currents.[93]

Wu wei is not a conscious state or thought. *Wu wei* is a dream-like state of consciousness wherein one can experience thoughts and feelings without judgment, and freely let them go. This state of mind can be likened to a ball bouncing in a stream; it goes wherever the water takes it. It has been called flowing with the moment,[94] or "going with the flow." In this state, we become one with Tao and problems vanish. There is no notion of being separate from the Tao. Only when we sense we are different from the Tao does tension build.

When we stop fighting tension, accept it, and do not try to force it away, it eventually disappears. Understanding melts tension, anxiety, and loneliness. *To resist going with the flow creates stress, strain, and illness.* One cannot go with the Tao until one realizes there is no alternative and that all things are the Tao. There is no separateness; nothing exists apart from the Tao. We are all alike within the Tao.[95]

Releasing oneself to the Tao does not guarantee safety, profit, or happiness. If we follow the Tao specifically for that reason, however, it is nearly guaranteed that these things will not be found because that way of being is not the Way of Tao. Through realization that we are one with Tao, we embody its power. But, similar to Christian Grace, the power of the Tao is not something we achieve or possess.[96]

Virtue (Te)

"He who is filled with Virtue is like a newborn child."[97] *Te* is a special quality that comes from the inner nature of things. It is a unique attribute or spiritual strength, which one can possess without awareness. It is not a quality that is easily labeled, nor is it something that can be passed from one individual's heart to another.[98]

Te values sensitivity and modesty. Taoism emphasizes the might of the child, the female, that which is small, and the spirit of the valley rather than the mountain. These images connote *te*. Conversely, the West generally considers being sensitive, childlike, female, small, or low as negative traits that one needs to improve upon or to extinguish.[99] In the West worry and pessimism are thought to lead to illness, but to be sensitive to and accepting of the needs of the body, heart, and mind.[100]

Taoism affirms that as sensitivity develops, so do practical skills. Both traits and abilities develop interdependently. For example, as psychologists become more sensitive to their own inner experience and being, they often become more aware and sensitive to the psychological states and emotional distress of their clients. Greater awareness and recognition of client difficulties can allow psychologists to intervene more effectively. As one area increases learning, other areas grow and change as well. As individuals become more alert and aware of both their inner-self and their environment, they learn how to be more sensitive to their needs and the needs of others and the environment.

To be sensitive is to cooperate with the forces of nature. The virtuous person *(te)* is sensitive to, and respectful of his or her surroundings and works with the situations entered. As Hoff emphasizes, in full awareness the Taoist blends in with situations, lets go of excess ego, and becomes one with the situation.[101]

When we set aside our pride, uncover our genuine selves, and act based upon what our hearts truly tell us, we will find peace, contentment, self-acceptance, and love. By being honest and genuine with our universe and ourselves, we uncover our virtue *(te)*.[102] Sometimes this is called uncovering the child's mind inside of us. Taoist wisdom retains and respects the child's uncomplicated state of mind. A child's mind is not cluttered with ego (thoughts and feelings surrounding who and what we are and do) and abstractions. It is similar to the "beginner's mind" described in Zen Buddhism. When ego is eliminated, the energy of the Tao flows with clarity, creativity, directness, honesty, and liveliness.[103] The Tao promotes the ability to see clearly, act decisively and deliberately, and it provides the personal power/belief to make a difference in our personal lives and in our environment.

The Taoist "Way" is inexhaustible in its ability to be compassionate, supportive, and nurturing; but until we stop blaming others and ourselves for mistakes in life, we cannot truly accept the compassion of the Tao in our lives. Rather than blaming ourselves or others for the tribulations in life, the Taoist finds ways that naturally and harmoniously bring forth their true spirit.[104] *Te* produces self-acceptance by setting aside self-criticism and promoting respect of our internal cycles that, in turn, allow talent and creativity to be expressed. Transcendence of ego allows genuineness, authenticity, and congruency of thoughts, emotions, and behaviors. When one's self is accepted, compassion, patience, and acceptance of others naturally occur with light-hearted spirit.[105] When one follows the Tao, all of nature is respected.[106]

The power of te *means living in the present, accepting life's current circumstances and making the best of the situation.* The past is remembered, but not dwelt upon, and the future is not a steady focus of attention. Life is embraced through lightheartedness, love, and energy from the freedom of self-criticism. Life is approached with courage, jubilation, and amusement. Success occurs as a result of living mindfully in the present, creatively, and deliberately, with love and energy. The virtuous life is characterized by sensitivity, modesty, and acceptance of both oneself and situations in cooperation with natural cycles.[107]

Yin-Yang *Polarity*

The core of Chinese thinking is the dialectical principle of the *yin-yang* polarity, respecting and honoring the naturally occurring cycles in nature. Their Chinese ideograms represent the sunny and shady sides of a hill, and they symbolize contrasts such as masculine and feminine, firm and yielding, strong and weak, dark and light, rising and falling, earth and heaven, spicy and bland.[108] The key to life is balancing *yin* and *yang*. Both are part of the universe. *Yin* is necessary to have *yang* and *yang* is necessary to experience *yin*. They coexist and complement each other. According to the principle of *hsiang sheng,*[109] *yin* and *yang* arise mutually and they are inseparable. As Lao-tzu states:

> Under heaven all can see beauty as beauty
> only because there is ugliness.
> All can know good as good only because
> there is evil.[110]

There is a dualistic quality implied by the principles of *yin* and *yang*. This is not the form of dualism that asserts that the world is made up of only two elements (mind and matter), nor that the individual consists of a mind-body dualism. All polarities implied by *yin* and *yang* are complementary; they cooperate with one another analogous to the way strands of DNA from each gender work together to form a double helix. Without both strands of DNA, an individual would not exist.[111]

Another expression of the *yin-yang* principle is that both being and nonbeing are mutually generative and supportive. For Westerners, this can be a difficult concept to grasp since we usually believe that when there is nothing, we and perhaps the world will cease to exist, and that nothingness is not useful or purposeful.[112] Taoists, on the other hand, explain that something always comes from nothing, a void, or nonbeing that is creative and generative. For example, sound comes from silence and light from darkness.[113] Lao-tzu states:

> Thirty spokes share the wheel's hub;
> It is the center hole that makes it useful.
> Shape clay into a vessel;
> It is the space within that makes it useful.
> Cut doors and windows for a room;
> It is the holes which make it useful.
> Therefore profit comes from what is there;
> Usefulness from what is not there.[114]

All somethings and nothings are necessary components of existence. One cannot exist without the other. In order to know one, we need to know the other.

The *yin-yang* principle expresses the dynamic cycles of nature in addition to the polar quality of all that exists. These cycles have no beginning or end; they are everlasting. In Taoism there is no notion of original sin. There are only natural occurring cycles of birth and death, fortune and misfortune, peace and war, and so forth.[115] Taoism views individuals as one with the universe and/or inseparable from it.

Consequently, it is beneficial to work cooperatively with the natural rhythms of the universe (e.g., its seasons, principles of growth and decay, youth and maturity). Accepting the natural rhythms of the universe allows one to appreciate life and to live in peace and harmony. The Taoist personality is characterized by a sense of calmness, and an easygoing acceptance of self, others, and the world. This way of being is achieved without rigorous living by laws, rules, or commandments.[116] The calmness of the Taoist does not come from forcing oneself to be calm in all situations, but from a willingness to do what comes naturally in all circumstances. "By working with the situations life presents, the Taoist finds that life itself, when understood and utilized for what it is, is sweet,"[117] and that something that may initially appear negative can have value.[118]

PERSONALITY THEORY

In this section, a biopsychosocial paradigm of personality is presented, followed by discussion of suggested Taoist conceptions of personality structure, dynamics, individual differences, and personality development.

Biopsychosocial Paradigm

The biopsychosocial approach in clinical psychology emphasizes prevention and wellness, community work, and scientific research to facilitate and maintain physical and mental health.[119] This comprehensive approach states that health and disease occur as a consequence of interactions between biological factors (genetic and/or biochemical), psychological factors (personality, coping strategies, and behavioral attributes), and social factors (family, social support, trauma, etc.)[120] The biopsychosocial model suggests that numerous factors contribute to personality formation.

Taoist psychology is more comprehensive than the biopsychosocial approach of clinical psychology. Throughout history, native healers have said that health is the integrated balance between the mental, physical, emotional, and spiritual aspects of life. In Taoist psychology, human beings also must be looked upon as a whole system in which physical, emotional, social/environmental, and spiritual aspects are integrated. Any attempt to abstract information from the whole leaves understanding of the person fragmented and incomplete. Taoist psychology avoids the Western reductionist approach wherein mind, body, and spirit are analyzed as separate parts.[121]

Taoism is not an idealistic philosophy. The physical realm is affirmed. The human body is valued as a medium of the same kind of natural intelligence manifest in nature's ecosystems. The internal workings of the body must be watched with as much patience and respect as one observes a phenomenon in nature.[122] Taoist psychology adds, however, that the movements of the human spirit must be respected as well.

Personality Structure

Personality, according to Stone, is the individual, typical, and enduring manner each of us evolves for conveying our emotions, gestures, and behavior to those around us."[123] Personality, as all of the ten thousand things, arises from Tao. Personality is an amalgamation of genetics and life experiences. We are all that we experience physically, emotionally, consciously, and unconsciously.

Knowledge of the unconscious arises from intuitive knowing, uncovered through the art of meditation, or involvement in activities that allow reconnection with one's genuine self, for example praying, horseback riding, hiking, painting, playing music, or playing with children.[124] Taoist psychology attempts to assist humans in becoming more aware of themselves, others, and the environment they live in. Through this awareness, they develop their intuitive power, gain knowledge of their strengths and weaknesses, amplify their strengths by setting aside their weaknesses, work toward self-acceptance, and gain greater personal and interpersonal peace, all of which contribute to one's personality structure. However, in

Taoism, personality cannot be accurately categorized or differentiated because it is continually shifting and evolving. Personality structure is viewed more as a process than as a fixed substance or entity. Personality simply consists of whatever experiences have been encountered and the attributes one has been given by birth.

Personality Dynamics

As noted previously, the dialectical principle of *yin* and *yang* is the foundation of Taoist philosophy. The *yin-yang* principle explains how all of nature came into being and how nature continues to express itself.

> The Tao begot one.
> One begot two.
> Two begot three.
> And three begot the ten thousand things.
> The ten thousand things carry yin and embrace yang.
> They achieve harmony by combining these forces.[125]

Personality dynamics are explained in terms of both of the polarities of *yin* and *yang,* and the three levels of existence. The one represents the beginning of being; the two *yin* and *yang;* and the three refers to the three treasures *(chi, jing, shen)* or three levels of existence—physical, mental, spiritual.[126]

Chi *(Physical)*

The energy of all life is called *chi. Chi* is manifest in all that is in the universe, and all that is in the universe is a manifestation of *chi. Chi* is derived from the food we eat and the air we breathe. By caring for the body, one is caring for the most sacred gift of all—life itself.[127] This reverence for life is the reason that Taoists emphasize the importance of balanced breath, nutrition, and exercise.[128]

Jing *(Mental)*

Jing is the combination of *chi* from both parents that is received at conception. *Jing* provides us with our basic temperament, and accounts for our physical and personality characteristics.[129] The quality of *jing* from our parents also determines how well our body functions. *Jing* is finite and can be wasted or conserved. Those who are prone to illness can learn how to preserve and care for their *jing* to overcome personal adversity. Aging occurs as we use up our *jing.* Human beings can learn how to manage their *jing* to be the most helpful in consideration of their overall constitution.[130]

Shen *(Spiritual)*

Shen is the third treasure or level of existence.[131] *Shen* is spirit or consciousness. It refers to the human essence—that which makes us human and who we truly are. We are essentially spirit. *Shen* lives in our heart, and functions as the executive of the mind. Thinking, reasoning, and memory are all part of *shen*. *Shen* can be replenished.[132]

References to all three levels of existence suggest that Taoist psychology incorporates both a spiritual and a holistic perspective. Taoism encourages the study of wholeness and harmony through uncovering wisdom and knowledge of the genuine self and the conditioned self. This uncovering is accomplished through gentle encountering and confronting both biopsychosocial and spiritual obstacles within oneself and in one's relationships with people and nature.

Followers of Tao believe in the magnificence of the whole, not in the preeminence of individual parts. Taoism is concerned about interconnections with others, nature, and something larger than ourselves. From birth, we all have the innate desire to belong. As our wisdom grows, we learn that our purpose in life is not to remain separated, alienated, and isolated from the universe, but to realize our place within it, thereby uniting with Tao.

Individual Differences

Humans affect and are affected by everything in the universe: weather, human and animal behavior, health, and illness. When we are in balance with the universe and ourselves, we are happy, comfortable, and healthy. However, perfect balance is rarely achieved, so we need assistance from others in our environment to move toward it. As one gains greater understanding of how to gently correct our physical, emotional, social, and spiritual imbalances, and as one gains greater understanding and awareness of the natural cycles of one's self and the universe, reliance upon mental health practitioners is likely to decrease.

Personality could be differentiated based upon varying gradations of atonement with the Tao, but this distinction would not express the wholeness and uniqueness of an individual's experience. Individual differences occur as a consequence of spontaneity *(li)*, inherited patterns, and the variety of experiences organisms encounter throughout their lives. Just as each snowflake has its own unique design, so do individuals. The organization of physical organisms is far too complex to be understood by analyzing their component parts. As human beings, we have an irresistible temptation to find out how and why people and things work. We take things apart in order to find the answer to why behavior occurs, and proceed to explain how things work in words. Watts described this analytical proclivity by using the metaphor of learning how to perform a beautiful dance.[133] We learn the footsteps in a step-wise linear fashion, but somehow when the dance is performed in such a mechanical or sequential fashion, its beauty, fluidity, and rhythm is missing or lost. The same is true about descriptions of personality and its pathology. Specific attributes of disorders can be analyzed and categorized according to the terms contained in the DSM-IV,[134] but that does not provide understanding of a person's whole experience. To appreciate the uniqueness and individuality of organisms one must appreciate their whole. By viewing individuals analytically, the whole experience is lost.

Development of the Sage Personality

The goal of a Taoist is to become a person similar to the Sage, an emotionally and spiritually balanced individual who relates harmoniously with others and with nature. Chuang-tzu described the Sage as a free and easy traveler whose behavior appears purposeless.[135] There is enjoyment in the journey or process, rather than the actual destination. In a relaxed state of awareness, the Sage is in step as the environment shifts, allowing the Sage to respond to whatever life presents in a manner that is natural, creative, and spontaneous. One lives in the present moment, goes with the flow of life, and finds novel ways to make use of what is currently available. The Sage values self and all others as unique and integral components of nature. The Sage is resourceful, realizes potentialities, and imagines life not as it is, but as it could be. The Sage lives a full life in quiet cooperation and accepts all that he or she encounters.[136]

The eight primary characteristics of the Sage[137] are: humbleness, simplicity, genuineness, flexibility, adaptability, spontaneity, persistence, and acceptance.

Humbleness

The Sage is nonjudgmental, nondiscriminatory, and avoids using labels to describe others or make situations fit personal needs or desires. The Sage adapts to the changes that are constantly occurring rather than attempting to control surrounding events. Humbleness means having the ability to be a follower rather than a leader, and feeling comfortable doing so.[138]

Humbleness permits one to experience whatever occurs. If happiness is present, happiness is felt; if sorrow is present, the Sage grieves. The Sage is emotionally congruent with the environment and the moment. Once accepts oneself and others, realizing that everyone is an integral part of the great Tao.[139]

Simplicity

Simplicity means knowing when to go ahead and when to retreat. The Sage has the ability to simplify and clarify thoughts and perceptions.[140] The Sage avoids complexity and noise by seeking a quiet life, and knows intuitively when enough is enough. The Sage does not desire fame or fortune, and does not work to be noticed.[141] The Sage knows that all human beings are the same underneath their clothes and skin. All people share the same basic bodily structures and functions. It is a waste of energy to strive for advantage over equals.

The Sage lives according to personal experiences and not by that decreed by society. The Sage does not work to please others, enjoys spontaneity, and does not suppress or repress his or her internal states, especially humor. Being a true master of life, the Sage constantly seeks a moderate lifestyle by resisting the desire to acquire more and more things. Rather, he or she lets go of more and more until simplicity is reached.[142] The Sage finds enjoyment in living a simple, uncluttered, natural life, including simple clothing. The Sage does not need to rush about to meet deadlines because he or she knows the work will be completed when the natural rhythms within the self and the universe are in balance.[143]

Genuineness

Followers of Tao are open-minded and accepting of all of life. They believe in living honestly and genuinely, "innocence is inside us," and we need to go inside to find it.[144] Clear understanding is only possible when the uncarved block *(p'u)* is uncovered. The Sage realizes that when one is in touch with the natural, genuine self, one's direction is clear, goal-directed, and the best fit for him or her self.[145]

The Sage looks to the intuitive self for clear direction in living authentically. We are truly human when we allow our original nature to be expressed. The Sage is true to nature and character as the uncarved block *(p'u)*. The Sage is self-accepting, without pretense. The Sage is loyal to family, friends, and ideals, and is unafraid to act openly, honestly, and compassionately with others. The orchid, refined and impartial, symbolizes the character of the Sage.[146]

Flexibility

The flexible attitude required to achieve emotional and spiritual balance is symbolized by water. Water can remain still, yet it is open continuously to movement and change. In winter, a change in temperature changes water from flowing freely to slush and ice. In the spring, the temperature rises and changes water's constitution from apparent stillness to movement again.

Water does not refuse to become ice in the winter just as it does not refuse to become fluid in the spring. It changes with the rhythms in nature.[147]

Life involves continuous change. The human body is continually exchanging and replacing atoms through the breathing, digestive, and growth processes.[148] Even though the body looks the same, it is in a constant state of fluctuation. For example, the lining in our stomach is replaced every five days and every year the majority of the atoms in our body will be replaced with new ones.[149] Just as our bodies automatically adjust to physical change and growth, so too can we adjust to changes elsewhere in our lives, eventually becoming as flexible as the willow tree.

Flexibility involves being aware of the constant movement of Tao illustrated through the interdependence of *yin* and *yang*. Being open to movement does not mean flitting from one relationship, job, or situation to another or meaningless busyness. It does mean dynamic involvement in life and being ready, willing, and able to experience life as it occurs. The Sage's flexibility does not mean accepting what happens in life passively or fatalistically. Taoist flexibility is an intentional acceptance of the way things are, with an appreciation that life is always changing. As soon as one thing occurs, another will likely occur.[150]

The Sage realizes that his or her situation in life changes cyclically, just as water changes form with the seasons.[151] *Yin* and *yang* are not static. Sometimes *yang* appears greater than *yin,* and at other times *yin* appears greater than *yang.* Neither absolute *yin* nor absolute *yang* is right for a situation. The Sage is willing and able to blend both *yin* (internal knowing) and *yang* (learned skills, education) to create a dynamic balance between the two powers.[152] Behavior is guided by the innate instincts of *yin* and the learning we have accrued throughout life *(yang).*

Balancing *yin* and *yang* can be compared to walking on a tight rope. One combines instinctive knowledge of bodily balance and the skills learned from tight rope masters. As the tight rope is crossed, constant small adjustments are made depending upon one's internal feelings and assessment of the external situation. To refuse to adjust, or to refuse to be flexible, results in a potentially disastrous fall. Life is similar to a tight rope, and we need to make adjustments constantly in our thinking, feeling, and acting to account for whatever is occurring in our environment. To become a Sage, one must be dedicated to understand and accept internal cycles, and to learn how to integrate them skillfully with the cycles that occur in others and in the environment.[153]

Adaptability

The Sage is never too proud to adapt to changing circumstances or to adjust to new situations. To resist adaptation disrupts the flow of life, creates frustration and unhappiness, and depletes energy.

Adaptation involves reviewing problems from many perspectives in order to develop alternatives to achieve goals and maintain peace and contentment without depleting excessive energy. One chooses to let the obstacle exist and learns to go around it at times, and at other times finds it necessary to overcome the obstacles that thwart one's goals, perhaps through greater experience, education, or training.[154] The Sage knows that destiny must be obeyed, but that one's destiny is not absolutely predetermined. Life is constantly changing and we all are on a dynamic journey. What we do on our journey makes a difference. Today's decisions and actions will affect choices available to us in the future. The Sage is adaptable because he or she realizes that it is important to accept and understand limitations and to adjust responses in light of personal limitations and situational constraints.[155]

The Sage chooses to adapt because he or she trusts in Tao. With trust in Tao, life flows easily and naturally. The Sage views life as a river. He or she knows where the rocks are, where the current is swift, and watches for branches and debris that may impede progress. By studying nature, including human nature, we gain the experience and knowledge to navigate the river of life.[156] To become a Sage is to accept the flow of life. The Sage floats wherever the Tao takes him or her.

The Sage knows that every experience in life forms a path and that each person's path is unique to his or her life experiences. No one can walk the path of another. Regardless of the path one chooses to traverse in career or relationships, the Sage accepts the choice of self-determination. The Sage knows that only one path can be traveled at a time. He or she does not linger on "what ifs" when unhappiness occurs. Paths are formed one moment at a time, and can be especially fruitful when we are fully involved in our life and have been making deliberate decisions. The Sage knows it is very important to review life periodically throughout the aging process, to gain perspective of what remains unfulfilled in life. The Sage realizes that the better one knows oneself, the greater the likelihood that life goals will be fulfilled, and peace and contentment will be maintained.

Spontaneity

The Sage is open to all within Tao; hence, being spontaneous resides deep within the Sage's nature.[157] He or she recognizes that the basic desire of all things is to unite with Tao because listening to Tao can bring harmony and understanding. The only way to unite with Tao is through connecting with the true self or inner core. When this inner spirit *(shen)* is neglected, union with Tao is disrupted and unhappiness ensues. The path to becoming a Sage and connecting with the inner spirit and Tao is not easy and requires daily meditation and self-centering.[158] Becoming and being a Sage is not always fun and exciting. It is a way of being that develops from many uninteresting, dull moments spiced with occasional excitement.

Persistence

The Sage realizes that suffering is a natural part of life. Everyone experiences distressing events. Panic and fear interfere with the ability to think clearly, to face difficulties, and to act decisively. When difficulties are encountered, the Sage knows it is the time to be diligent and remain calm and clear-headed. Fortune and misfortune come and go, and the Sage realizes that in order to survive, one must adapt to the situation.[159] The Sage does not seek misfortune, but when it occurs, the lessons it brings are observed and valued.

The Sage is patient. When pain and suffering are experienced, the Sage has faith that health and joy will follow because all in Tao is balanced through the interaction of *yin* and *yang*. The Sage is ever hopeful and this hope gives strength to persevere despite pain and suffering. The Sage openly shares this belief in hope openly and freely with others, in a manner reminiscent of the Bodhisattva's concern for others in the Buddhist tradition.

The Sage accepts that all things are achieved through a series of small steps. Everything worthwhile takes time and effort. The Sage recognizes the need for goals and direction, especially during adversity. One must always have determination, patience, and a sense of direction. It is easy to ignore the spirit's intuition, to follow the confusion of society, and to do what is popular. The Sage makes a daily conscious choice to follow Tao.[160]

Acceptance

All of us are on a journey. We do not know what will happen to us tomorrow, but we have the wisdom of today. This wisdom includes accepting one's self, one's place in life's journey, and realization of how far one has to go. The Sage realizes that along life's journey good choices are made and, at other times, mistakes occur from which one can learn. Following Tao is the only possible action in life; but to follow Tao means taking risks.[161] To become a more fully functioning, genuine human being, one must become engaged and connected with life. The Sage does not fear error, but values the lessons learned from mistakes. If one does not like what happens, an alternate course of action is chosen. The Sage is nonjudgmental, compassionate, and accepting first of oneself in order to be nonjudgmental, compassionate, and accepting of others.

The following list summarizes the personality characteristics valued in Taoism and developed in the Sage personality.

- Genuine
- Meets obstacles and finds creative ways to manage them
- Enjoys life with all of its ups and downs
- Childlike curiosity
- Good sense of humor
- Subtle
- Happy
- Calm
- Strong intuitive and logical knowledge
- Balanced
- Present minded
- Compassionate toward self, others, nature
- Empty, clear mind
- Gentle
- Does not seek fame or fortune
- Does not set self apart from others

- Seeks simplicity
- Resourceful
- Flexible
- Adaptable
- Open minded
- Mindful of own natural rhythms and those around him or her
- Easygoing
- Knowledge of personal strengths and weaknesses
- Enjoys the journey
- Sees self as integral part of all nature
- Relatively free of anxiety
- Listens to voice within
- Contemplative
- Values experiential learning
- Humble

Stages of Personality Development

Taoism encourages childlike curiosity, flexibility, resilience, naturalness, simplicity, compassion, interconnectedness, and wisdom. These characteristics do not occur according to some prescribed time; rather, they can occur at any age.

From birth, humans encounter experiences that teach separateness and narcissism, which lead to inflexibility and judgmentalness of others and ourselves. Therefore, a prerequisite of the fully functioning personality is to be nonjudgmental and compassionate toward all things, learning to benefit from positive and negative experiences, and to remain open to possibility and change.[162] The goal of a Taoist is to achieve clarity of heart and mind through introspection.[163]

Taoism respects wisdom in both the young and the old.[164] There are many stories of how the secrets of life have been uncovered by children. Discovering these secrets helps to maintain a youthful appearance, life perspective, and energy. Sages of all ages are known for their youthful attitude, appearance, and energy as a result of a quiet inner-life that is relatively free of anxiety.[165]

As children, we are aware of and enjoy our surroundings. We are also quite helpless and need nurturing from parents. As adolescence is approached, we still need care and nurturing from our parents, but we experiment with independence. Adulthood is characterized by wisdom and maturity to care for others.[166]

Personality development does not end with attainment of adulthood. To realize the wisdom of the Tao, one must become once again a child at heart and one who has emptied the mind of clutter to allow the great wisdom of the Tao to enter.[167] One cannot become a Sage until all distinctions between the self and nature have disappeared, that is, until one is united with Tao. After uniting with Tao, knowing is intuitive and immediate.[168]

According to Chuang-tzu, the Sage knows that it does not make sense to say one is separate from the environment, because we are all part of nature or Tao. The Sage's awareness is not limited by the idea of being a separate self. One's sense of self is lost in the ubiquitous Tao.[169] Nevertheless, the Sage realizes the potential in the self and others, and sees self, others, and nature not as they are, but as they could be. With an accepting attitude toward all of nature, the Sage is able to see with open-mindedness, which allows one to witness and appreciate miracles in ordinary situations.[170] As the Sage embraces life, attuned to the everlasting flow of life, he or she knows that resisting the Tao would create conflict.

In summary, the characteristics of the Sage personality are freedom from preoccupation with self; receptivity; respect for action through nonaction; spontaneity; acceptance of self and others; and nonattachment to things, emotions, or thinking. The Sage is resourceful, virtuous, and easygoing.[171]

THEORY OF DISTRESS

From the Taoist perspective, distress results when humans are disconnected from themselves, other human beings, nature, and the universe that supports them. In contrast to Western medicine, symptoms are not explained by linear cause and effect logic.

Internal and external imbalances create disharmony and disease. Internal imbalances may consist of poor nutrition, weak constitution, overwork, stress, drug or alcohol use, and/or unbalanced emotions. When *chi* is depleted, the client may experience symptoms such as a very soft voice, slow movement, lethargy, shallow breathing, or exhibit a pale complexion. On the other hand, excessive *chi* can result in extreme energy that may be reflected in a red face, loud voice, forceful movements, headaches, and heavy breathing.[172]

Many of us inside and outside of the public arena, are not connected to our internal core or self, and consequently, are out of step with our natural surroundings and ourselves.[173] Towler suggests we all need a therapeutic system that nurtures the whole person: physical, psychological, social, and spiritual aspects of a person and one's environment. No one lives in isolation. We are all interconnected with nature, the universe, and with other people. In order to recover from illness and to maintain health, we need to become sensitive to the body, the mind, the self, the heart, and all that surrounds us.[174]

The Taoist theory of human suffering can be summarized in several principles. Similar to the First Noble Truth of Buddhism, Taoism affirms as a fundamental principle that suffering is a natural part of life. We may not like it, but there is no life without suffering. Once we acknowledge the things we do not like, we can choose whether we want to change, accept, or use them in a beneficial way.

Taoist theory suggests that suffering occurs under several conditions:

- When we separate themselves from nature and its cyclical patterns
- When we deny our internal self and place too much attention on external conditions
- When we lose our sense of safety and spontaneity
- When attachment to things is more important than developing spiritual strength and meaningful relationships with others and nature
- When we are not open and present-minded
- When we believe that technology and materialism will solve all difficulties
- When we become rigid and unwilling to change
- When one creates and nurtures negativity
- When busyness and complexity are preferred over stillness and simplicity
- When we live in the past and the future

Suffering occurs when we separate ourselves from nature and its cyclical patterns, especially through willful interference. The origin of all human suffering is in believing the illusion that humans are separate from the natural world. Anxiety, dangerous beliefs, troubles, and feelings of loneliness, emptiness, and weaknesses are all results from the illusion that humans are separate from nature.[175]

Suffering occurs when we deny our internal self, and place too much attention on external chaotic conditions. Humans suffer when they let outside pressures and complications reside within them, and when they concentrate on what one does rather than knowing who one is.[176] The Tao is the origin of all things, both happiness and distress. Nevertheless, when people are free of yearning and conflict, suffering is less.[177] By implication, people would lessen their suffering by curbing their ambition, slowing down the tempo of their lives, simplifying their lives, and by working with their hands as well as their heads.

Suffering occurs when people rely upon the writings, thoughts, and beliefs of others rather than listening to their internal intuitive selves.[178] When people abandon their personal responsibility for happiness and become reliant upon government, medicine, psychotherapy, religion, etc., they become disconnected from the internal self and become frustrated and sometimes angry. No one other than ourselves can know what is best for us. When clients tune in to their intuitive selves, they realize that they have known all along what they need in order to be happy.[179]

When we rely upon our intuitive nature, we remain connected to our true self. Decisions are based upon our truth rather than someone else's way of being. When we do not respect our intuitive nature, we become easily distracted and influenced by others' opinions. We gain control over our lives as we work with our own thoughts and feelings.[180]

Suffering occurs as the result of disharmony between yin *and* yang *principles*.[181] *Yin* is manifested as the internal, nourishing, and motherly energy; and *yang* is considered the external, protective or fatherly type of energy. *Yin-yang* principles emphasize harmony and balance. Each person develops his or her own disharmony based upon his or her constitutional, social, spiritual, and environmental relationships. The source of the imbalance, however, may not be apparent immediately from the symptoms.[182] In other words, there may not be a linear cause and effect between symptoms and the origin of distress.

Harmony is not an absolute state to achieve; rather, therapy assists the client in increasing flexibility, adaptability, acceptance, and humbleness in relation to one's self and the environment thereby decreasing distress. Therapy helps clients to become aware of their own unique strengths and weaknesses, their attitudes and beliefs, and to develop a healthy perspective of their life situation.[183] The goal is to help the client achieve internal and external harmony by working from the inside out to increase personal flexibility, acceptance, adaptability and humbleness.

Suffering occurs when we lose our sense of safety and spontaneity. This is a very serious condition for a follower of Tao. When we work in a job because we feel we "must" in order to obtain the salary to buy the things we think we need to make us happy or to maintain benefits, we let the "shoulds" and "musts" interfere with our peace and happiness. "Shoulds" and "musts" are often our interpretations of others' beliefs about what is necessary for self-fulfillment.

Suffering occurs when we interfere with wu wei *and push to get things done, rather than letting ourselves follow our natural rhythms and the rhythms of life around us.* We forget that we need to balance action with nonaction. At times, doing nothing can be more productive than plowing ahead. Suffering develops when spiritual and natural laws are ignored.[184]

Suffering occurs when attachment to things is more important than developing spiritual strength and meaningful relationships with others and nature. Wealth can come and go, but the peace of mind created in a strong spiritual self that is supported by others will last a lifetime. Attachment to feelings and the dictates of society also produces suffering and interferes with natural occurring adaptation.[185] As a consequence, people learn to mistrust their "gut," and they attempt to control their feelings and thoughts.[186] Attachment to things, stereotypes, and preconceived thoughts covers over the genuine self, stifles creativity, and interferes with this ability to adapt.

Suffering occurs when we are not open and present-minded. When thinking is restricted, we cannot see what is in front, beside, behind, above, or below us. Thinking gets stuck in "what ifs," in fears of the future, or in sadness about the past. Consequently, anxiety and misery result from worry about what might be and what might have been. Enjoyment of the moment is lost. As we look back, we realize we have not experienced life fully, and this realization leads to feelings of despair and inadequacy.[187]

Misperceptions can create suffering. Our mood, health, and contentment depend on how we look at things. Often people are dismayed that a person who has committed a heinous crime does not look like someone who could do "such a thing." Preconceived notions of what someone or something "should" look like can lead to misperception, misunderstanding, and distress as illustrated in the following story by Lieh-tse as retold by Hoff.

> A man noticed that his axe was missing. Then he saw the neighbor's son pass by. The boy looked like a thief, walked like a thief, behaved like a thief. Later that day, the man found his axe where he had left it the day before. The next time he saw the neighbor's son, the boy looked, walked, and behaved like an honest, ordinary boy.[188]

Misperceptions in our ability also create suffering as in the following story from Chuang-tzu, retold by Hoff.

> An archer competing for a clay vessel shoots effortlessly, his skill and concentration unimpeded. If the prize is changed to a brass ornament, his hands begin to shake. If it is changed to gold, he squints as if he were going blind. His abilities do not deteriorate, but his belief in them does, as he allows the supposed value of an external reward to cloud his vision.[189]

What is humbling and perhaps encouraging for those of us who are not yet Sages, is that irrational beliefs interfere in the perceptions of even the wise. Humans often misinterpret situations and fail to notice anything but the unusual. For example, we do not notice how much shade a tree provides until it is blown down by the wind. We overlook the chatter of our children until they have grown up and moved away. We do not notice the everyday things in our lives until their presence or absence is emphasized.[190]

Suffering occurs when we believe that technology and materialism create happiness and solve all of our difficulties. Many people in industrialized societies have come to desire and value things for what they represent to others, not for what they truly are. When they do not satisfy this purpose, the material possessions are discarded. Consequently, the West has become a throwaway culture. We get rid of what is no longer useful, trendy, or prestigious. Unfortunately, we do not even appreciate or pay attention to what is acquired because we are too busy rushing after different things and reportedly more efficient technology. We fail to see what we have, where it has come from, and where both it and we may be going. The wisdom of the natural world needs to be recognized, respected, and understood by us and not merely viewed through distorted lenses of our illusions that nature exists to serve our personal needs.[191]

It is not possible to achieve personal happiness and peace by increasing material possessions. Accumulated things are fragile and transient sources of pride and ego, which only serve to cover up negative self-feelings.[192]

Suffering occurs when we become rigid, unyielding, and unwilling to change. We often refuse to look at something that appears to be negative, and consequently, lose out on the opportunity to turn something negative into something positive. A crisis can be an opportunity for growth and transformation.

The dragon is the Chinese symbol for transformation, and Taoism is often referred to as the Way of the Dragon. For centuries, Taoists have been associated with transforming negatives into positives and attracting positives with positives. It is one reason why Taoism has been associated with magic, mysticism, and alchemy.[193]

We need to be flexible to adapt. As the saying goes, it is a waste of energy to ". . . push through a porthole."[194] By joining forces with the situation encountered, we can see what is truly there as opposed to what we want to see. When there is nothing we can do to adapt to a situation, we must recognize that fact and move on without regret, frustration, or anger.[195]

Suffering occurs when we create and nurture negativity. The more we believe in the negative, the more negativity occurs in our lives (a self-fulfilling prophecy). Life would not be very interesting without struggle and difficulty. Coping with problems promotes personal growth. The nature of problems is not as important as what we do with the problems encountered.[196]

Suffering occurs when busyness and complexity are preferred over stillness and simplicity. Over achievers appear self-motivated, but in reality, they are pulled in many directions and by whatever appears most sensational or interesting. They seem to have endless energy, and they love to be busy all of the time, but their busyness is a way of avoiding being still, being with themselves, and being spiritual.[197] Though they seem in control of their lives, they are really not. They nurture the illusion of control.

It is very easy to be edgy, impulsive, insensitive, and absent minded. It is just as easy to look for a miracle cure or instant relief. Those who receive instant relief, however, often become disappointed when it does not frequently recur.[198] Their ability to tolerate frustration appears to decrease and may limit their creativity and adaptability.

If you live to satisfy your impulses, your impulses will control you because as soon as one impulse is satisfied, another is likely to arise. Sustained satisfaction comes from working through a solution and remaining true to your inner self. The impulsive fulfillment of desires is not satisfying in the long term, because they lack feelings of accomplishment that come when one persistently works toward attaining long-range goals.[199]

Concentration, prolonged effort, and pleasure in the process significantly increase the probability of attaining a goal. Wisdom and happiness cannot be pursued; both are recognized when we are still enough to notice them. When our hearts and minds are open, and when we stop trying so hard, wisdom and contentment naturally arise.[200]

Suffering occurs from living in the past and the future. Most people spend 95 percent of their waking moments in the past or the future. Worrying about past actions and future "what ifs" makes peace and contentment unattainable.[201] At the end of life, people wonder where the years or time have gone? They do not remember it because they did not live it as it occurred. They were too busy berating themselves for past indiscretions or worrying about what might happen in the future, hence they missed what was going on in the present.

Symptoms of Distress

The Tao is "The Way" to dynamic peace. It is eternal and the source of creation and fulfillment.[202] If we lose "The Way," we become alienated from others and nature, and many difficulties ensue. We begin to suffer from anxiety, confusion, distorted thinking, depression, anger, and lethargy. The symptoms of distress occur when busyness is used to avoid problems; frantic doing displaces authentic being.

Frustration and distress also occur when we take things apart under the guise of gaining greater understanding. In other words, the knowledge of the whole is discounted for a limited analysis of selected parts. Names and labels are applied to personality that do not reflect the complete experience of the individual. Analytical approaches of personality can lead to misunderstanding and misinterpretation of the universal. Concentrating on select aspects of one's personality can lead to imbalances in life that, in turn, can lead to physical, psychological, social/environmental, and spiritual distress. Balance and moderation of the biopsychosocial/environmental and spiritual realm need to be maintained in order to live a long and peaceful life. When analytical philosophy and Western science limit and confuse the understanding of the universe through the use of words and statistics, the wholeness of personality, the experiences of the person, can be forgotten. Care needs to be taken so not to confuse the games or rules we contrive in an effort to further understanding with the genuine patterns of nature. The wholeness of the human being should not be forsaken in the name of scientific achievement.[203]

THEORY OF THERAPY

The biopsychosocial and spiritual models of Taoism are comprehensive, unifying, and holistic theories. By contrast, Westerners have a tendency to separate the biological, psychological, social, and spiritual aspects of personality formation and human suffering. Therapists and clients often look for a magical cure, such as correction of a low serotonin level, which has been implicated in a variety of mental disorders, including but not limited to substance abuse, depression, aggressive, and impulsive behaviors.[204] Biopsychosocial and spiritual models, however, are more likely to support therapeutic gains than a biomedical approach. Medication often alleviates symptoms of DSM-IV Axis I disorders, but outcome studies usually support a combined or interactive treatment of medication and therapy. In addition, psychotropic medications have had limited effect on Axis II disorders. Finally, understanding the client's experience is more important than attempting to diagnose according to DSM-IV criteria. The goal of the therapist, therefore, is to understand the client's distress in consideration of his or her internal and external situation and assist the client in obtaining greater peace, contentment, and happiness.[205]

Purpose of Taoist Therapy

A basic Taoist principle is that personal growth and transformation is continual.[206] The major goal of Taoist therapy is personal growth. The purpose of Taoist therapy is to assist clients on a spiritual journey that touches the heart and encourages personal transformation. It is a path in which meditation and increased awareness and mindfulness encourage goodness and love, acceptance, and adaptability in life. Increased awareness allows identification of fears, judgments, and attachments that have limited us from living a full and loving life. Awareness is the first step in learning to go of efforts to control naturally occurring rhythms and letting natural rhythms occur without fear.[207]

Personal transformation is a major purpose of Taoist psychotherapy. Transformation means working with whatever comes your way. It means *becoming aware of the ordinary moments and valuing them,* when we can connect with another person in a caring, loving way. Transformation also means that when you are stuck in life (as in a traffic jam), you do not throw away your energy by becoming angry, blaming, and judgmental; rather, you can use the time to relax and reflect, increase self-awareness, or to identify moments in which you positively connected with another, and to recognize that for which you are truly grateful. If someone throws rocks, use the rocks to build a garden wall or house foundation. By changing your perceptions and attitudes you can change the outcomes of situations.[208]

Helping clients to accept that change, impermanence, and transitions are natural is a virtual component in Taoist therapy. With change comes reassurance that there will always be new experiences.[209] Once the client becomes accustomed to ceaseless change, he or she is free to be in a state of relaxed alertness, always open to new opportunities, and ready for growth and transformation. [210]

Personal growth and transformation occur when egocentricity and life's "shoulds" are abandoned.[211] Many negative personality traits can be transformed. Self-centered stubbornness can be changed into selfless devotion to altruistic causes. Desire to control others can be turned into improving one's inner-self and helping others to do the same. A proclivity to become lost in complexity can be transformed into connecting things carefully; exclusiveness can be developed into a more balanced point of view. Taoism encourages cooperative work with all aspects of mental, emotional, physical, and spiritual health to promote a long, peaceful life.[212]

"Taoists seek to dig deep under all the layers of cultural and psychological silt that has accumulated in us humans over the millennia in order to bring forth the shining pearl that lies beneath."[213] The purpose of Taoist therapy is to assist clients in being comfortable with their genuine self so that they feel free to "sprout, blossom, and yield fruit as they sway and dance in the breeze of life."[214] Change, however, does not occur according to a preconceived or prescribed timeline. Change occurs when it is in its nature to do so.

Other purposes of therapy are: (1) to increase client genuineness and trust in one's innate, intuitive ability; (2) to honor internal and external physical and emotional rhythms; and (3) to increase cooperation between others and nature. As their skills increase, clients experience greater peace, contentment, and joy.

The Taoist approach argues that we are always doing the best we can at any given moment and that there is no point in judging what is best or less than best. Behavior and actions simply occur and labels are self-limiting. There are many books explaining methods of how to become one with Tao. There are also many books on how to be successful in the therapy arena. A Taoist therapist realizes that therapy cannot be fully explained because it is as illusive as describing the Tao. Therapy cannot be reduced to a series of tangible steps; rather, it must be intuited, experienced, and practiced without being knotted in words and procedures.[215]

Taoism has survived in China for thousands of years because it has proven to be useful. The Chinese do not respect a philosophy or theory that does not work. Taoism is a philosophy that can be applied to everyday life. If Taoism is distilled into its essential elements it would tell us to look and listen, figure out, and apply what is learned.[216] Taoism teaches that what is most important is to observe what is around you, set aside your preconceptions, look at a situation as though you are seeing it for the very first time, trying to see its essential elements. The goal is to seek simplicity in complexity through the use of logical and intuitive thought processes,[217] uncovering relationships by going to the core, and then taking action as indicated by what was observed and deduced. A Taoist observes the natural laws that surround him or her and lives by those laws. Taoist therapy helps clients to live in a manner that promotes survival, harmony, and participation in life, regardless of the situation.[218]

Taoism is psychotherapy that frees the spirit.[219] Psychotherapy is a dialectical process that is essentially reflective. Reflection involves stepping back from appearances, studying them, and developing a new relationship with them.[220] In contemplative Taoist therapy, the therapist includes moments of nonreflective presence that facilitate a shift into a deeper dimension of being.[221] Peace and acceptance of self and others develops when one lets go of anxiety and begins to follow the course of nature and the line of least resistance. No textbook can completely explain "The Way" of Taoist therapy. It is something that must be intuited and felt.[222] Taoist therapy cannot be explained completely in words.

There are no textbooks that can completely explain either "The Way" or the way of Taoist therapy, despite attempts of several authors, including this one.[223] Nevertheless, some characteristics of this approach can be described. Taoist therapy is *holistic, intuitive,* and *integrative.* It is holistic in that health, integration, balance, and harmony of mental, physical, emotional, and spiritual components is of paramount importance. The whole of the individual is greater than the sum of its parts. Any attempt to separate aspects of the individual from the whole negates complete understanding of the person. The human condition must be looked at as a whole system, and not through a reductionistic separation of the mind, body, and spirit.[224]

The integrative purpose of Taoist therapy is to help clients find a path that promotes mental, physical, emotional, and spiritual integration and balance. It is a path in which meditation and increased awareness allow goodness and love to permeate life. Increased awareness allows identification of fears, judgments, and attachments that limit living a full and loving life. Awareness is the first step in learning to let go of frantic efforts to control naturally occurring rhythms, and to let natural rhythms occur without fear.[225]

Taoist therapy is an intuitive approach, and not a way of technique or gimmick. Techniques, per se, can lead to pain and suffering.[226] Learning to navigate life intuitively with all of its twists and turns contributes to a long and contented life. If technique is relied upon in therapy, it will likely fail in the long run. By gently guiding the client in understanding and awareness of what is genuine and relevant versus illusory and artificial via technique, he or she gradually will be able to navigate life more efficiently in the long term.

The Taoist theory of personality and therapy is truly integrative. It is not simply eclectic but skillfully integrative. It considers a client's social, psychological, biological, cognitive, spiritual, and emotional strengths and weaknesses. Therapy is based in empathic nurturing, but is also directive and gently confrontational when in the best interests of the client. Knowing what therapeutic stance will be most beneficial for the client is based on training, experience, and intuition.

As a psychotherapist's skills mature, he or she naturally moves into *wu wei*. In *wu wei,* the clinician no longer needs to stop and think which therapeutic intervention may be most appropriate, it arises spontaneously. The Taoist therapist acts spontaneously and unconsciously, without scheming, planning, or doubt. The clinician acknowledges his or her strengths and weaknesses and carefully chooses clients that fit with that skill and nature. Those clients who are not appropriate for the Taoist therapist are referred to a clinician who has the skill, experience, and nature to work with the client.

After *wu wei* has been achieved, the clinician continues to hone therapeutic skills through reading, experiential process, and additional training, but he or she is no longer worried about providing the basics of therapy. *Wu wei* comes with wisdom, maturity, experience, knowledge of the self and others. Until the state of *wu wei* is achieved, guidance and support from psychotherapists who are more knowledgeable and skilled in the practice of psychotherapy are sought in order to provide the care that is in the best interest of clients.[227]

Tao Therapists

"Knowing steps to create living growth: that is an art."[228] Taoist masters are often elusive because they cannot explain the secrets of their craft.[229] As with Taoist masters, Taoist therapists cannot always explain how or why therapy works. What may be beneficial for one client may not be for another client. Therapy is an art.

The most important quality of the Taoist therapist is unconditional presence. This helps clients to relax and be open to their deep internal experience.[230] The concept of unconditional presence means that the therapist meets each client with open-mindedness, compassion, creativity, and patience. The Taoist therapist is patient and willing to persevere because he or she knows things will change because that is the nature of life; change is constant. The therapist acts naturally and spontaneously in harmony with the ever-constant change that occurs within the client, the environment, and within the therapist. Similar to water, the therapist develops an internal and external state of harmony where he or she "flows with life," realizing that he or she can manage whatever the client places before him or her.[231] With fear and other emotions set aside, the therapist is better equipped to be accepting and nonjudgmental. The therapist who is unconditionally present,[232] practices psychotherapy with empathy and ease[233] without concern for self, emotions, or previously learned theories. He or she is truly with the client during the session.

The Tao is the mother of the ten thousand things, and within the ten thousand things is therapy in all of its unique forms. Therapists learn to recognize intuitively when a therapy session has been helpful because the therapist is in tune with the client. With nonjudgmental attentiveness, the therapist listens to understand the underlying meaning of what the client is saying and experiencing. The therapist attempts to remain impartial, as with the unconditional presence of the sun. Warmth and light are extended to each client from the therapist's spiritual center.[234] The therapist listens with all of his or her attention and body, noticing what emotions, thoughts, sensations arise. The therapist is aware of body language and postures of both self and client, and gently observes where the mind wanders during the therapy session.

The therapist becomes one with the client without losing his or her self. Through this therapeutic bond, the therapist can understand the client's suffering more completely, and is able to gently guide the client toward greater harmony, balance, and centeredness. Within a nonjudgmental atmosphere, the therapist, as with the Sage,[235] is compassionate, clearheaded, honest, and when necessary, direct and to the point.

Taoist therapy is practical and reflective. In traditional Western psychology, relationships to experiences are always mediated by theoretical constructs. Theoretical constructs can be useful in understanding the client's distress, but if the therapist is thinking about theory and not being fully with the client, understanding of the client's experience is missed. Most clients easily detect this lack of understanding.[236] Western psychologists try to explain or change the problematic contents of a client's experience rather than working with the client's overall process of experiencing. In Taoist therapy, the whole of clients' experiences, as well as theoretical explanations of the clients' distress, are intricately interwoven.

The ancient Sages advocated acquisition of skills and their continual refinement. Their writings remind us today that what appears magical is the result of continued learning and inner growth.[237] Therapists who are followers of Tao build their skills continually in order to maintain a sharp mind. Eventually, the Sage therapist will practice therapy so skillfully that client difficulties "fall away as simply as fruit falling from a tree."[238] The goal of a Tao therapist is to have the work of therapy be a smoothly flowing, harmonious, and joyous event. As the ancient Sages conducted government, the therapist of today guides people back to a state of harmony with Tao.[239]

Tao therapists realize that expertise is gained through practice. Followers of Tao work toward excellence by beginning on the path of learning, rather than simply longing for proficiency. They take pride in the work they do for the sake of their clients, the clients' families, the public, and the environment in an effort to increase connectedness and harmony among all of nature. They know that the more work on the self, the less needs to be done, but that personal work is never done.[240] Balance and harmony are the "core of all healing."[241] These conditions must occur first within the therapist.[242] The therapist works at not pushing clients to improve within his or her time frame. Clients are allowed and encouraged to make the changes they need to make in their own time. Tao therapists also realize that learning comes from their clients' wisdom. Work is part of the Tao therapist.[243]

Tao therapists also know that progress can be obtained only by persevering and by building upon the skills clients bring with them. All of these resources must be collected to go the distance with the client. With persistent effort, the important tasks in therapy can be completed. Tao therapists remain concentrated and focused, and realistic about what they can take on.

Development of the relationship between client and therapist is essential in order for a client to achieve therapeutic goals. Nurturance, empathy, positive regard, and unconditional acceptance from the therapist are crucial in development of the client-therapist relationship and to personal growth.[244] Furthermore, therapy cannot be rubber-stamped or follow a standardized mold. It must have spirit. It must have the therapist's own handmade style obtained by skillfully integrating knowledge and insights obtained through education, therapeutic experience, and from knowing the inner-self. These abilities need to be honed and integrated until they become second nature. This integration creates the healing spirit clients sense as they walk into the therapy room.

Tao therapists realize it can take a long time to overcome obstacles to personal growth. Sometimes quick fixes will result in only temporary resolution or relief, and the client will be faced with working through the same difficulty in the future. It is far better to be honest with the client in the beginning, and to fully explain the benefits of short- and long-term changes and interventions. Tao therapists work for what lasts a lifetime.[245]

Followers of Tao realize that life is ever-changing and that nothing is static. All of life is part of Tao, and client difficulties must be considered in the entirety of one's genetic make-up, environment, psychological characteristics, and personal and work relationships. Separating problems into separate categories is only an intellectual effort, which ultimately does not create greater understanding of the client. The study of the client needs to include how one functions and feels in all domains of life. Dissection of a client's life is of limited usefulness because life overall is dynamic and interactive. To understand your client's personal life, inquire into all of it; be curious. Whatever you want to know about your client, you can learn by being with him or her.

Therapists maintain respectful boundaries between themselves and their clients, but they also realize that they are not separate from their clients.[246] Tao therapists know that given similar life circumstances, they too, may have similar difficulties as their clients. Tao therapists remain balanced and centered within the constant movement of the Tao. Oftentimes, clients' stories and difficulties can feel overwhelming to therapists, especially if therapists do not know themselves well, or fail to maintain healthy emotional boundaries. Tao therapists realize that in order to be fully present for their clients, it is essential to honor their own physical and emotional rhythms, and to care for themselves. A therapist whose empathic reserves are exhausted has no room for the worries of the client. Only by keeping to their hearts, remaining truthful, and respectful of themselves, can therapists maintain the equilibrium needed to face the immensity of what the Tao brings to them. Helping others leads to greater self-understanding, which in turn leads to assisting clients on their spiritual journey.[247]

Tao therapists realize that "all spirituality begins and ends with the self."[248] All of the answers that we seek are within ourselves. All of the answers that clients are seeking are within themselves. The heart is the center of the body from which all truth originates. Tao therapists understand there is no separation between the heart and the mind. Heart and mind are one in the same. Moreover, they realize that there is neither separation between thinking and emotion nor between intuition and logic. The body is the foundation for the mind. There is no duality between the mind and the body. The body and the mind are indivisible parts of the whole. Following the Tao is integrative and intuitive, rather than analytical or intellectual.[249]

Therapy Process

The therapy process is spontaneous, flexible, fluid, compassionate, and gently interspersed with humor. A central aspect of this process is the client's experience of compassion. Compassion does not mean simple acceptance of a client's condition and perceptions. Passive sympathy merely fosters continued anxiety and suffering. In therapy, the client is continually encouraged to explore answers to his or her dilemmas, and to increase understanding of his or her self and the universe. Immediate resolutions are not anxiously sought out; rather, solutions are allowed to arise spontaneously through contemplation and study. Neither science nor religion is viewed as having all or the definitive answer to questions, nor does the therapist claim such authority.

The focus in therapy is on developing awareness and mindfulness. As in psychoanalysis, Taoist therapy emphasizes the importance of bringing the unconscious into conscious awareness. As in cognitive therapy, Taoist therapy also emphasizes the importance of becoming aware of distorted cognitions and the busy mind. Taoist therapy focuses on developing awareness, the acceptance of self and others, developing balance and centeredness, learning the benefits of both action and nonaction, and developing and maintaining compassion for self and others. It is also nondirective in the sense that it allows clients to choose what they need to work through. The therapeutic process is experiential, collaborative, intuitive, cognitive, respectful, occasionally confrontive, educational, and, hopefully, enjoyable.

Taoist therapy is an informal learning process fashioned after the ancient teachers. Therapy may be brief or long term. Longer-term therapy is advisable when separateness from others and nature is great. For example, if there is a significant lack of social support, conflict between partners, problematic anger, depression, impulsiveness, substance abuse and/or history of emotional, psychological, sexual, physical abuse, etc. The length of therapy is often left up to the client. When assisted to rely upon his or her internal knowledge, the client will realize how long the guidance of a therapist is needed. In the beginning, therapy sessions are used to prepare and to get to know the client so that his or her defensiveness is softened, fears are reduced, and strengths are identified, acknowledged, and fortified. Once this occurs, the rest of the therapy will go easily and often quickly.

Tao therapists assist clients through experiential exercises, gentle Socratic questioning, modeling, observation and reflection, and teaching meditation and visualization. "Homework" is often given to enhance learning and to provide additional opportunities to test and rework limitations. Clients are advised that change takes both time and perseverance; in other words, it does not occur magically. Therapy sessions may occur in an office, outside under a tree, or in another environment that is comfortable for the client and is growth-promoting. Therapists realize they are also fallible human beings and do not dictate remedies for the client. They believe in the client's ability to make his or her own decision and are sensitive to the client's perceived needs and desires. The work of therapy is to uncover a client's genuine spirit and develop life skills that lead to peace and contentment, and greater connections with life in an atmosphere of safety and collaboration.[250]

Intermediate Process Goals

The general goal of Taoist therapy is to translate conceptual theories into real-life practice in order to nurture a healthy human spirit. This general goal is pursued through intermediate goals related to the therapeutic process. Process goals include centering, emptying, and grounding the mind, and reestablishing the connections of the mind with the heart.[251]

Centering the Mind

Times of solitude allow the defenses, which are designed to protect the ego, to be gently relaxed. The mind is quieted so that one can tune into the whispers of the higher self.[252]

Emptying the Mind

When the mind has been quieted in silent solitude, it can be emptied of negative thoughts, perceptions, or attitudes, which obstruct one's attention and block one's potential.[253]

Grounding the Mind

After the mind has been emptied, cultivation of intuition, imagination, and intellect begins.[254]

Connecting the Mind and Heart

After the mind has been centered, emptied, and grounded, unity, insight, creativity, and compassion can be realized for self and others. Through this process the mind and heart become reconnected and lead to increased interconnections with others.[255]

PRACTICE OF THERAPY

These intermediate therapeutic goals can be achieved through a variety of therapeutic strategies including focusing-oriented psychotherapy,[256] reflective therapy,[257] creativity and attachment exercises, meditation, yoga, t'ai chi ch'uan, cognitive behavioral, gestalt, existential, or experiential therapies.[258] Effective therapy always keeps the best interests of the client in mind, with what appears to be effortless skill. In other words, the therapeutic process appears natural and uncomplicated. When therapy is done by the "book" and consists only of methods and technique, it can lack heart and clients can become frustrated. Therapy requires a teacher who is not only wise and trustworthy, but who is willing and able to model freedom and joy.[259]

Centering the Mind

The mind governs the body. In Taoism, however, the mind is part of the heart, which commands all mental powers. When the mind is agitated, confusion ensues. When the mind is quiet, insight emerges. Taoism teaches the importance of sitting calmly, collecting the mind, and detaching from desire and other attachments. By calming and freeing the mind, it becomes free to merge with the Tao. Maintaining a calm mind leads to serene stabilization.

As serene stabilization is maintained, distress eases, and one becomes free to be open and genuine. When nothing is obscured, concealed, or ambiguous, mental disorder is banished.[260]

Meditation can be used to achieve serene stabilization (calm mind and body). Quietness is needed "to hear the whisper of the Tao."[261] The original purpose of meditation and t'ai chi ch'uan was to join the energies of the body, mind, and spirit with Tao in order to achieve the greatest human potential.[262] As external concerns are eliminated from the mind, one becomes immediately aware of thoughts as they arise. Letting them go results in peaceful calmness throughout the body. Obsessive fixations and random thoughts soon leave the mind. Calmness is maintained without shutting the mind down.

Habit determines whether the mind is agitated or calm. Disciplining the mind takes regular practice. Diligent practice quiets the unsettled mind and allows it to empty and open up. After a period of intense work, the mind will come under control. Eventually, it will become calm spontaneously. The key to governing the mind is to choose to let go of random thoughts (positive or negative) as they arise so that the mind does not become agitated. When problems or doubt arise, one must take the time to understand the difficulty, solve the problem, and then empty the mind.[263]

Emptying the Mind

Emptying the mind requires learning to let go of the negative thoughts, which imprison us and undermine our well-being. We can appreciate the dialectical quality of experience (*yin* and *yang*), gain insight, and recover our genuine self in the process.

Letting Go

"Because of desire and craving, stress and anxiety arise. Because there are anxiety and stress, body and mind are afflicted by tensions."[264] We must learn to let go of personal cravings. Moreover, tensions are reduced when situations are accepted for what they are, and when we stop pretending to be someone other than our true self.[265] Situations mold personality, but they do not define personality. The objectives of this experience of "letting go" are to learn the futility of trying to change something that cannot be altered (the past), to realize our strengths and weaknesses in a given situation, and to work with the them and the situation, rather than against them.

In therapy, clients learn that displaying ability, virtue, intellect, or wealth to build self-esteem only yields temporary gains. These motives prevent true action and need to be relinquished. Excess is not necessary to attract others, and we do not need to emulate others in an effort to feel connected. Setting limits and having personal and physical boundaries that support our true, genuine self and the Three Treasures are what are ultimately important. Desire for reputation and social status are all excesses of emotional desires and rarely enhance life for the long term. Those that pursue these things bring about their own confusion.[266]

Moreover, attachment to habitual ways of thinking and seeing interferes with our ability to think and see clearly. Perceptual filters impede understanding of our environment. The Sage, however, is not attached to stereotypes and is free to respond creatively and freshly to all of life's circumstances.[267]

Negative, Destructive, Judgmental Thoughts Can Imprison Us

Addiction to negative, judgmental thoughts needs to be broken. This takes great discipline and effort. Taoist therapists believe all people are intrinsically pure, but that their pureness is covered over by education, pretense, and experiences.[268]

Random thoughts fill the mind constantly, and many of them are negative and judgmental. They need to be abandoned as soon as one is aware of them. Criticism and praise need to be ignored and not allowed to take refuge in the mind. If these thoughts are allowed to infiltrate the mind, it soon will be filled. An empty mind void of thoughts and judgments, leaves room for Tao.[269]

The empty mind is not preoccupied with external conditions. It is peaceful when empty and uncluttered by judgments and evaluations. When the mind is empty, one will be free to acknowledge the Tao.[270] Once the inner mind is free of attachment, external actions, and pretense, it will not be disturbed or altered by either rigorous religious standards or irreverent values. One goes along centered, and able to vary thoughts, feelings, and behavior according to the demands of each unique situation. A calm mind that is balanced and centered will always be spontaneously in tune with the situation.[271]

At times one cannot avoid getting dragged down in self-defeating, destructive thoughts. Acknowledgment of these thoughts provides the opportunity to work with them, to contemplate their validity in light of one's strengths and weaknesses, and to choose a course of action appropriate to the situation. Through this process, one can return to feeling greater emotional and physical balance. If the mind is too intensely controlled (e.g., as in denial or repression of thoughts and impulses) psychological illness can occur. Not all mental activity can be extinguished, or one would lose the ability to distinguish between right and wrong. Nevertheless, cravings and ruminations need to be extracted. Attachment, subjectivity, judgments, hopes, and rivalries must be culled. When one is free of these traps, the mind is light and exhilarated.[272]

Ingrained habits and biased thoughts need to be relinquished. When they are cleared away distress diminishes. Thoughts come and go throughout the day and night. If we make attempts to dismiss them, they are harder to get out of our mind. It is important to review these thoughts and determine whether they are true or false. If they are false, they need to be let go. If they are true, action may need to be taken. False thoughts and worries need to be identified and clarified to uncover the source of the distress, but first the mind must be calmed so that the source can be revealed. Once the source of distress is revealed, choices can be made regarding the appropriate action or nonaction.[273]

Thoughts and Perceptions Affect Our Well-Being

Sometimes we experience events over which we have no control. Our strength lies in how we react to life's circumstances, and how we react to situations often depends upon our thoughts.[274] We can control our response to events. Life and death, fortune and misfortune, can occur at any time. These exigencies are not under our control. It does not make sense to worry over things for which we have no control.[275]

Energy follows the mind; therefore, wherever you place your attention your energy will follow, both positive and negative. Consequently, it is very important to be aware of the energy we attract and create within ourselves.[276] Positive energy, similar to that which occurs during reframing or disputing negative thoughts, can act as an antidote to negative emotions such as anxiety, anger, and depression.

Yin-Yang

Perception requires duality. In order to perceive anything, one needs to recognize the polarity of *yin* and *yang*. Nothing can be perceived without contrast.[277] For every action there is a reaction between the self and in the situations and environment that surrounds one, for example aggression begets aggression.[278] By being aware of the shifts in our *yin-yang* qualities and in the environment, we are better able to make decisions that are individually, socially, and environmentally appropriate and congruent. To promote internal and external harmony, Taoists encourage moderation so that the action and reaction "wave" is kept within reasonable and manageable limits. Each person needs to develop his or her understanding of the dualistic nature of *yin* and *yang* in themselves, others, and nature. Through the understanding of the rhythmic dance between these two opposites, balance and harmony can be found.[279]

Intuition and logic are used to understand the polarities that are observed and sensed. During observation, we need to look for connections, patterns, and relationships, and study the natural laws that are in operation. When the practice of "observing, deducing and applying"[280] becomes a habit, we begin to sense or intuit a pathway through troubles that often leads to greater understanding of self and others. As this realization deepens, we will understand that events are not "either-or" conflicts, but combinations of many different complementary events.[281]

We all need goals along with the energy and determination to meet those goals. Goals give us meaning and direction, but it is the process of working toward goals that provides meaning and enjoyment. We also need to know when to stand up and when to go along. Following the Tao does not mean simply going along with life. It also means knowing when to do the hard stuff, when to separate from the group, and when to fight for a cause. It is critical to have good judgment and inner resources in addition to remaining open, wakeful, and aware of our surroundings in order to choose the most appropriate action.[282] Each of us perceives situations differently, albeit slightly, based upon previous experience.[283] One needs to know the self through experiencing rather than depending upon others' observations or opinions. Study of the Tao allows people to learn to act wisely within a constantly shifting environment. Clients need to become sensitive to the ever-shifting changes in their internal self and in their surroundings.

The balance between *yin* and *yang* suggests the principle and virtue of moderation. Moderation in food, drink, sleep, and activity are also required for contentment. Moderation in lifestyle helps to maintain an empty mind. Consequently, problems slip away and the basic, genuine spirit is able to appear spontaneously.[284]

Insight

When the mind is empty and quiet, insight is uncovered. Insight is derived from our heart. Genuine insight occurs spontaneously; when we do not hunt for it. It is not something that is acquired.

Insight provides knowledge of The Way, but it is not attainment of the Way. Those who know The Way nurture intelligence, and they use their intelligence to nurture serenity. As serenity and intelligence nurture each other, reason and harmony emerge. Serene intelligence allows knowledge of Tao.[285] Once insight emerges, it needs to be cherished.[286]

Return to the Genuine Self—The Uncarved Block

Therapists assist clients in uncovering, understanding, and returning to their genuine self. The genuine self is the "uncarved block" that exists before being carved into something by circumstances and by the socialization process. In Taoist therapy, clients learn that the names given to them are not necessarily who they are. Their birth names, accomplishments, culture defeats, career, and social position do not define their true identity.

Taoist therapists assist clients in undoing the constraints experience and society have placed upon them. Therapists work to uncover clients' original nature, the nature with which they were born. Clients learn to understand they have public persona and personal selves. Underneath the public person is the core self that has existed since birth. In therapy, the client reconnects with his or her core self and begins to "trust his or her gut," that is, one's natural intuition or instinctive knowing.

The Taoist therapist assists clients in the difficult task of identifying and trusting his or her own feelings. Distrust of feelings leads to self-doubt and difficulty in not knowing one's genuine feelings. Self-doubt is often the result of internal chatter that clouds the core with negative messages, for example being wrong, inadequate, or not having the right to feel as they do. Through acceptance and honoring of our genuine feelings and perceptions, we "feel" our way along life's path, gradually building understanding and vision of who we are and what we are meant to do.[287]

The genuine person is called the "True Person."[288] In order to know ourselves, change, and thrive, we must go to the root. Moreover, if we do not understand ourselves, we cannot understand others. Minds must be active, open, and constantly in search of the true self. By gaining self-understanding, we learn our deepest longings, what is good for us, what is bad for us, and where our talents lie. Journey to self discovery is not easy or quick work. It requires diligence, perseverance, and patience.

Self-discovery must be taken on the client's own level. The therapist guides the client to discover the self to reduce distress, but self-exploration cannot be forced. The therapist assists the client in setting aside the need to please parents, teachers, employers, and others to do what he or she was meant to do. The client learns not to let others control him or her.[289]

Grounding the Mind

Grounding the mind involves present-mindedness, awareness, problem solving, effortless action, concentration, and connecting the mind and heart. The consequences are increased cooperation and connection with others, clear boundaries, and a responsible application of Taoist principles to life.

Present-Mindedness

Refining the mind is an hour-to-hour, moment-to-moment activity. Peace and clarity of mind and heart are the goals of Taoism. We can achieve both goals by being mindful of the present. Attention is focused on the present moment, and, consequently, worries of the future and the past are set aside. By concentrating on the moment, we see and hear what is actually occurring, anxiety is reduced, and greater peace and contentment can be achieved.[290]

According to Parr, present-mindedness is the vital therapeutic mechanism in rational-emotive behavior therapy.[291]

Unfortunately, many people live as Sisyphus, the ancient King of Corinth, did. Sisyphus was condemned by the gods to rolling a huge boulder up a hill. When he reached the top of the hill, the boulder always rolled back down and Sisyphus had to repeat the struggle back up the hill. This struggle was Sisyphus' eternal punishment. As with Sisyphus, we all have "boulders" to push up the hill day after day. We torture ourselves, however, through complaining, moaning, and believing that goals can never be achieved, that the situations we find ourselves in are unfair, that our problems are much worse compared to others, or that we can never have what we want or need.[292]

Attention to each present moment in whatever activity we are participating in leads to a stronger sense of purpose, meaning, and happiness in life. Performance anxiety, self-other comparisons, and worries about past failures and future goals need to be set aside so that full attention is available for the task at hand. What happens when we are working on a task and simultaneously think of something else? We become distracted from what we are doing and have missed the present, our chance to experience purpose and meaning in the here and now. Purpose, meaning, and happiness will remain an elusive goal, until we learn to be fully present.[293]

When our thoughts remain in the past or the future, the experiences and opportunities of the present are forever lost. If we have trouble remaining in the here and now, future plans are meaningless because when they arrive, we will not be cognitively or emotionally available to experience and enjoy them. The more we concentrate on the past or the future, the more we will miss what is occurring in the here and now. How often have we heard clients regret not telling a family member he or she was loved before he or she died because they were too busy thinking about future events? To live mindfully requires paying attention to what we do, giving our full attention to each and every activity, moment by moment.[294]

Mindfulness must not be confused with the psychological concept of awareness of either intentional self-instructions or silent thoughts surrounding activities or experiences. A silent, verbal narrative is assumed in Western theories of motivation and decision making. Awareness or mindfulness does not mean internal chatter before, during, or after completing a task. That type of silent verbal narrative is considered mindless.[295]

Eastern mindfulness is nonverbal, nontheoretical, and nonintellectual. The mindful individual appears to act effortlessly and gracefully as an accomplished musician who gives his or her best performance. For example, when Itzak Perlman is playing in the present moment, he is not consciously aware of how to play the violin or a particular piece of music. The best performance occurs when the musician, instrument, and music become one in the present moment, moving fluidly and elegantly together. This concentration is what makes the activity meaningful and enjoyable.[296]

Some of the most rewarding times in life are when we are participating in an activity of our own choosing that is worthwhile, but yet somewhat difficult.[297] As we become fully immersed and absorbed in the project, all thoughts of the future, past, and self are forgotten and we feel happy. This state of mind is described as flow, an optimal experience.[298]

When in flow, involvement in the activity is complete and void of distraction. Actions are spontaneous, automatic, and separation from the self and the activity are lost. We become "one" with the activity being performed. When these experiences occur, they are usually intrinsically rewarding. Life in the present is rewarding because it is not attached to thoughts of past failures or future desires.[299]

Only the present exists. The past and future are only illusions. Unfortunately, many people spend the majority of the time working through the events of the past and avoiding the anticipated pains of the future. The ideal present-minded state is when 75 percent of one's life is spent in the present moment and the remaining 25 percent is spent equally in the past and the future. We learn from the past what to repeat and what to avoid.[300]

Pleasant memories are reviewed to bring us comfort. Reminiscing can be enjoyable and enhance life as long as it is not excessive, greater than approximately 12 percent of our time. Thinking of the past does not mean beating ourselves up over what we "should" have done, or lamenting over lost opportunities or past loves. Reflecting on the past can help us learn to navigate life more effectively. The key question to ask ourselves as we are reminiscing about the past is, "What did I learn from this experience?" Furthermore, thinking about troublesome times also needs to be balanced with thoughts about wonderful times.[301]

We think about the future to set goals and to make plans to achieve those goals. We do not worry or dwell on "what ifs," but may anticipate meeting our goals. The more we practice being present minded, the less time we spend on thoughts about the past and the future. Enjoyment on the present does not allow us to dwell in the past or future, thereby reducing or eliminating feelings of loss, regret, and anxiety.[302]

If the moment is not enjoyed, life cannot be enjoyed.[303] Training ourselves to stay in the moment with unconditional acceptance of self and others leads to happiness. Joy comes from concentration on whatever we are doing. If we are similar to Sisyphus pushing a boulder up a hill, joy can still be found in concentrating on the process of completing the difficult task. In so doing, feelings of perhaps not liking the task or feeling overwhelmed and defeated are set aside. Furthermore, life often presents us with difficult and unpleasant tasks. So, rather than complaining about it, the Taoist concentrates on the process of completing the task moment by moment, and similar to Sisyphus, pushes his or her boulder up the hill.[304]

Awareness

A second element of the grounded mind is freedom from fear and development of wisdom, which ultimately comes from intelligent awareness.[305] Successful psychotherapy requires increased awareness of self and environment. The journey to self-awareness and self-discovery can be consciously chosen; however, we often choose the easier or less painful route of letting others tells us what to believe, feel, or do. In therapy, clients are given the opportunity to uncover their own unique self in order to gain deeper understanding of who they truly are.[306] Even though the process can be painful when personal limitations are explored and ingrained behavioral patterns are being brought into awareness, the end result can lead to a stronger sense of self that is better able to successfully navigate whatever life presents.

In therapy, clients work to be more like the Sage and see beyond social conditions. Without the weight of habit and stereotypes, thinking becomes more creative and we discover our well of inner resourcefulness that assists us while solving problems. Clinging to the past is nonproductive and narrows awareness and insight into new possibilities. By not being attached to a certain way of life, we are able to transform ourselves to a given situation, and as a result, we are in harmony with the constant changes that occur in life and no longer need to fret about what is to come.[307]

Awareness is dialectical. The principle of the *yin* and *yang* polarity tells us that every action has both positive and negative aspects to it. Words and actions can be the origin of disaster and the beginning of fortune. Loss and gain are inherent in everything, but are not to be contemplated as we strive to fulfill our goals. Our greatest task is to keep our minds at rest whether or not there is a task to complete.[308]

We can strive to attain goals, but without excessive attachment or greed. Money needs to be earned but it should not be hoarded. By avoiding greed, we can be free of anxiety, and loss. Let your outward appearance be similar to others, but let your mind be clear and calm and free of threat. Once the mind and body are calm, we are free to observe what is truly happening in and around our self. Taoism promotes cultivation of our internal state rather manipulating external conditions. It is a practice that takes diligence.[309]

Problem Solving

A third element of the grounded mind involves problem solving. Most problems can be solved through accurate observation and intelligent awareness without emotional misperception. Before a problem can be solved, however, it must be clearly seen. The best time to observe a problem is when it begins. Lao-tzu advised tending to small matters before they become big matters, and prevent difficulties before they start.

When situations are not seen for what they are, we may struggle against difficulties that are not there, create problems, or turn small problems into large ones. When emotion is added to problems or problems are perceived as threats, they become even larger problems. To a Taoist, this type of problem solving is seen as a useless waste of energy.[310]

The first step in problem solving is to set aside as much emotion as possible and discern whether the situation presents a real difficulty. What appears to be problematic may not be truly a difficulty. Americans consider illness to be bad; however, many people have responded to such conditions by examining their lives and changing their lifestyle, thereby building up their health and strength to remarkable degrees. All situations have many valuable lessons to teach us. "Even death itself may not be necessarily bad,"[311] especially when it ends intractable, excruciating pain, and when it encourages others to reexamine their priorities and improve their own lifestyle.

In order to live fully, we need to look at ourselves and life around us. Life's tribulations need to be examined rather than avoided to determine what they are attempting to teach us. Perhaps the tests life presents us, even the difficult ones, are gifts to help us grow personally and spiritually—gifts perhaps designed to help us increase our problem-solving skills and/or understanding of our self, others, and nature. Problems provide opportunities to achieve greater wisdom, happiness, and truth.[312]

Effortless Action (Wu Wei)

This fourth element of the grounded mind involves learning to accept change rather than working against it.[313] Clients learn to find strength in flexibility and yielding. Clients learn that softness equals resilience, as with the young bamboo in the spring that is flexible enough to bend back and forth in a heavy gale, but unlike the massive oak that rigidly resists the wind and is blown over and uprooted.[314] *Wu wei* is effortless action. The solution to a problem often cannot be found by purposely looking for it. The "right" answer arises, when we remain in an open quiet state of mind that is neither passive nor dull, a relaxed state of alertness that is tuned to the ever-changing nature of life.[315]

"That which is old grows stiff and then decays. That which is young is pliant and soft. Therefore, those who follow Tao follow the way of softness in order to avoid death."[316] We all need stiffness of the bones to hold our bodies upright. Our bodies, however, are not so stiff so that they do not allow movement.[317] Difficulties arise in life often because we have grown inflexible in our thinking, actions, and being. In therapy, clients learn to rediscover their innate flexibility of mind, heart, and spirit and to combine both the hard and the soft of themselves to avoid withering away. Following the Tao also requires going to the heart of one's thoughts, feelings, and behavior. In other words, going to the soft within (emotional core) to gain further understanding and promote personal growth. During this introspective process, it is vital for clients to remember and rely upon internal (coping skills and strengths) and external (social) supports.

The metaphor of a tree is often helpful. Its trunk and branches are still when the wind does not blow, although inside nutrients continue to move.[318] Similarly, when a stream comes to some stones in its path, it does not ask why or how the stones interrupted its journey. The stream does not become frustrated, angry, or fight with the stones to eliminate or remove them. Water simply flows around the stones. Water responds to obstacles with effortless action.[319]

People, as all things in nature, have natural cycles. Sometimes we do better in life and sometimes we do poorly. When we are in a high cycle, life is more enjoyable than when we are in a low cycle and experiencing difficulty. The key to a balanced life is to harmonize with the flow of your cycles and not to be overly excited with the highs or depressed by the lows. It is important to know that one cycle begets another. If you are in a low cycle, a high will naturally follow, just as spring follows winter.[320]

Concentration: Developing Balance and Centeredness

This is the fifth element of the grounded mind. The goal of a Taoist is to become a "nobody." A nobody is open to thoughts and ideas. His or her heart and mind is empty of preconceived notions and ideas of importance and accomplishment. A nobody adheres to the natural order of things and strives to become a happy, well-balanced person who is content with who and what they are. Taoists blend into the world around them naturally and give of themselves selflessly. By emptying the mind, they become a vessel for Tao to be continually manifested.[321]

When we can learn to control without being obsessive, to relax without being indulgent, and to accept that things do not always go our way, true awareness and concentration arise. Freedom from obsessions (yearnings, addictions, and preoccupations), allows us to follow on a true path in peaceful light. Living a balanced, centered life limits reactivity to the events one experiences, and discourages compulsive consumption of material goods. We realize that things bring neither honor nor happiness.[322]

Thinking is often filled with preoccupations and random imaginations, and people are concerned about their outward appearance and how their possessions may bring about honor or disgrace, profit or loss. This imbalance brings about craving and attachment for things, with hopes that they will bring about happiness and contentment. They forget that physical things disintegrate and ultimately return to nothingness. Once Taoists understand that physical things are ephemeral, fixation and attachment to the tangible wane.[323] Pleasure is attained in accomplishing little things and finding joy in the moment. Taoists maintain their right to live a simplified life in a complex world of material abundance.[324]

Individuals who live wisely are not concerned about the comings and goings of life because they know nothing is lasting, nothing is permanent. Everything is always in a constant state of flux; therefore, they do not cling to one thing and spurn others. The Sage concentrates on the present reality and accepts all that comes. If the present reality is unacceptable, the Sage chooses a course of action that is more suitable. He or she acts after contemplating the present situation. As we travel along life's journey of twists and turns, we remember that only the Tao remains constant and eternal.[325]

Connecting the Mind and Heart

A connected mind and heart increases self-acceptance, cooperation, and relationships with others. A grounded mind can yield healthy boundaries and increased responsibility for ones actions. As humans, we do not know ultimately where we came from, and we do not know where life will take us, but we do have the choice of what we think of ourselves and the situations we find ourselves in. Nearly all mental suffering is a consequence of how we judge others and ourselves.[326]

When searching for greater self-understanding, it is valuable to go back to the source (the Tao) to find the answer to questions.[327] Self-acceptance increases as the client realizes that an inexhaustible well of knowledge, wisdom, and creativity resides within each and every person. When the mind is cleansed of distraction, possibilities open up, potential is released, creativity flows, and a new life unfolds.[328]

Self-acceptance comes with the realization that actions are subject to natural cycles. In the natural world, all things have innate potential to succeed. To learn the natural principle of success, we need to let go of judgments and accept people, situations, nature, and ourselves as we are. Morality is not abandoned, but whatever occurs is observed and accepted as it is. With an open mind, we are better able to recognize what is really present, and to make more effective choices and decisions.[329] To become more self-accepting, we must learn to let go of good and bad self-images. Images only hide the true self.[330]

Self-acceptance involves acknowledging and experiencing feelings. In Taoist therapy, clients are encouraged to experience their emotions fully at a pace that is not overwhelming and avoids dissociation and/or emotional shutdown. As clients gradually allow their emotions into awareness, they begin to learn what they are feeling, where they are experiencing emotions in their bodies, and accept their feelings as an intrinsic part of themselves. Over time, their emotions become integrated into their personality structure, rather than remaining separated, isolated, or disowned from the whole.[331]

A relationship in which the therapist maintains unconditional positive regard and remains unconditionally present with the client is critical in promoting client self-acceptance. Nonjudgmental therapist attitudes encourage this. The result is a qualitative change in the direction of oneness with Tao, hence greater happiness.[332] Contentment and peace arise when unconditional self-acceptance combined with unconditional acceptance of others, and unconditional acceptance of the situation, while maintaining present minded.[333]

When we are free from our sense of being a separate self, we are more likely to be receptive to what occurs around us and to others. Our capacity to be receptive is obstructed if our sense of self remains paramount, and if we are driven by desires for wealth, knowledge, or fame. Selfish desires sustain the illusion of a permanent self, when in reality the self, as with all things in nature, is constantly changing and evolving. When we are free from social influence and desires for recognition and authority, greater understanding can be manifested.[334] With full presence of mind and by setting aside preconceived notions of who we "should" be, we are free to be our true, authentic self.[335]

If we are self-accepting, we recognize that the source of human worth lies deep within us in a place we share with Tao.[336] Each and every human being is both unique and extraordinary. External achievements are no measure of our complete worth as a human being. People are driven to compensate for feelings of inferiority through their achievements. Fear of insignificance leads us to compete. Genuine cooperation depends upon mutual acceptance. Only through compassionate cooperation can we expect to survive as a species.[337]

A cooperative attitude must be developed first within ourselves in order to be expressed with family, friends, colleagues, acquaintances, and strangers.[338] This type of cooperation is not merely striving toward a mutual goal, but cooperating with the course of nature. It means if nature, including human nature, is free of competition, cooperation will naturally occur.[339]

Connection with Others

Separation from self, others, and nature is the source of all suffering. Most humans have a significant need to connect with other humans. A common thread in the tragedy of workplace violence is that employees who commit a violent act often said they felt disconnected or alienated from their colleagues and the organization.[340] We all need to connect with those who surround us to gain a sense of belonging.

Connecting with others does not mean an absence of boundaries. Therapy helps clients to learn not to take responsibility for others' actions. Taoism encourages us not to take on others' problems or inappropriate actions. It also tells us not to hate those who do wrong, nor to admire those who do well because both attitudes inhibit The Way.[341] Everyone is on their own path and deserves the freedom and respect to follow their path. Self-protection can be a healthy defense. If we do not protect ourselves from all of the comings and goings in the universe, frustration, anxiety, and exhaustion ensue. The body and mind need to be protected just as the eyes must be protected in a dust storm—by closing them and not letting in the sand.[342] When feeling overwhelmed, the mind needs rest and should not move. Only the most urgent needs should be attended to peacefully and calmly. Clearing the mind gives way to options for managing the difficulties. Once options are apparent, a choice must be made. If a choice is not made, the difficulty will affect every aspect of life, and anxiety and frustration will continue. Once the mind is troubled, there can be no peace until this process is completed. It is especially important to guard the mind so that others do not influence it.[343]

We all need armor to protect ourselves from predators, but the armor must have an opening to allow us to breathe and move. We need to realize that life takes place outside of our armor, and we need to allow life experiences to penetrate our protective shields at times. Followers of the Tao look for the spaces in life, through which Tao flows, and through which will can be affirmed. As a result, we gradually become more genuine and congruent. It is important to understand that our outer shell (persona) is simply a representation of who we are, not a true reflection.[344]

Becoming aware of ourselves and our surroundings allows us to take greater responsibility for our health, emotions, relationships, habits, sexuality, spirituality, and consciousness.[345] It is the belief that it is important to concentrate and act fully in everything we do. There is no reason for sadness when we have done the most we can do. The measure of life is not how well we perform against competition, but how well we have lived our lives.[346]

To live fully, honorably, and responsibly, we must apply Taoist principles to daily living. Knowledge per se is not always helpful, but needs to be integrated into our being in order to become part of our spirit. New skills and information need to be practiced until they become reflexive. Clients in Taoist therapy learn that peace, contentment, and happiness require effort and practice, but that these goals are achievable because they, as all of nature, are part of the eternal Tao.[347]

EVALUATION

Taoist psychology meets a number of the criteria that distinguish a good theory of personality and psychotherapy. It is important, clear, and comprehensive, integrative, and practical. The present formulation awaits empirical testing, but several of its principles can be considered as both heuristic and empirically verifiable. A reduction in the number of concepts and principles might make Taoist psychology more parsimonious, but at the expense of comprehensiveness.

Taoist psychology affirms human worth and dignity, appreciates the uniqueness of each individual, and the multidimensional nature of human experience. The spiritual dimensions of experience is emphasized as it is in other religious psychologies.

POINTS OF DIALOGUE

In the interest of fostering dialogue with other religious psychologies, some of the unique elements of Taoist psychology will be emphasized, and contrasts suggested for further exploration.

Taoism emphasizes principles of natural simplicity, spontaneity, harmonious action, cyclical growth, virtue and personal power, and the dialectic of *yin-yang* polarities. Each of these principles is essential to describing Taoism both as a "religion" and as a theory of personality and psychotherapy.

In contrast to Western notions about a Creator's commandments as a foundation of a rule-oriented ethic, Taoist psychology emphasizes the fundamental oneness of all people with ultimate reality and the natural ability of people to follow the Tao because they are all an integral part of the Tao. In the absence of proof of the existence of either heaven or hell, contemplative Taoists do not believe it is realistic to affirm an afterlife, gods, ritual, or clerical authority.

Although Taoist psychology is based on sacred scripture unique to Taoism, it relies to a greater extent than some of the other approaches upon human intuition as the source of truth, insight, and wisdom. The authority of intuition is affirmed through the fundamental notion that everything that exists is interconnected and interdependent and is part of the universal Tao. An intuitive approach may be contrasted with a more intellectual approach. In Taoist psychology, book knowledge per se is not considered to be the ultimate wisdom or virtue. Formal education and intuitive knowing are both valued. In fact, it is argued that book knowledge becomes intuitive when it is learned well and integrated deeply within the self. This principle implies a unique approach to psychotherapy different from the currently popular cognitive-behavioral approaches.

With respect to personality theory, Taoist psychology affirms with other religious psychologies a biopsychosocial-spiritual model of personality structure and dynamics. A genuine self is postulated as the agent of action, in contrast to the denial of self in Buddhist psychology, and different from the universal self in Hindu psychology. The self is viewed more as a continually evolving process than as a fixed structure. The essence of all that exists, including human beings, is Tao.

Unique to Taoist psychology is the application of the *yin-yang* principle to explain how all of nature came into being and how nature continues to express itself. This includes human nature. Personality dynamics are explained in terms of both the polarities of *yin* and *yang,* and in terms of three levels of human existence: physical, mental, and spiritual.

Individual differences are accounted for largely in terms of variable degrees of harmony people experience with the Tao, but also as a consequence of varying degrees of spontaneity, inherited patterns, and life experiences. Each individual is a unique whole that cannot be comprehended analytically by focusing on particular aspects such as thoughts, feelings, or actions. The holistic emphasis seems to be common among the religious psychologies represented in this book.

Personality development is guided by the ideal self known as the Sage, an emotionally and spiritually balanced individual who relates harmoniously with others and with nature. Psychological maturity is defined in terms of characteristics of the Sage personality: humbleness, simplicity, genuineness, flexibility, adaptability, spontaneity, persistence, and acceptance. Although a number of these characteristics may be affirmed by other religious theories, the combination is unique to Taoist psychology.

In Taoist psychology human distress is viewed as the consequence of disharmony and imbalance. Disconnection from one's own essential being is presumed as central to human misery. As with the First Noble Truth of Buddhism, Taoist affirms that suffering is a natural part of life. There is not life without suffering. Taoist psychology postulates several conditions that contribute to human suffering. Among these are the denial of one's internal, genuine self; excessive attachment to external things; misperceptions; and being closed-minded, stuck in the past, and unwilling to change. In similar concepts, these causes are affirmed in other religious psychologies. An additional notion unique to Taoist psychology is that human suffering occurs as the result of disharmony between *yin* and *yang* principles that govern all of life and nature.

Similar to other religious theories, the purpose of Taoist therapy is to assist clients on a spiritual journey that encourages personal transformation. Perhaps unique to Taoist therapy are the goals of (a) increasing clients' trust in their intuitive abilities, and (b) honoring cyclical rhythms. Increased awareness, reflection, and self-acceptance are considered essential therapeutic processes similar to other religious theories of psychotherapy. Moreover, Taoist psychology shares with other religious theories an emphasis on the qualities of both the therapist and the therapeutic relationship.

The therapeutic process is described as spontaneous, flexible, fluid, compassionate, and gently laced with humor. The intended outcome is to gently guide clients in uncovering their true self and increasing consciousness of the cyclical nature of life, and interconnections among all within the universe. Through a process that focuses on centering and grounding the mind, emptying the mind, and opening the mind, clients become free of negative thoughts that impede their goals, become open to what can be, and let go of egocentricity. As clients connect their heart and mind, they find interconnections with others more rewarding and purposeful.

As with other religious psychologies, Taoist therapy is integrative and eclectic. Among the techniques that distinguish Taoist practice are meditative exercises for emptying and centering the mind, developing present mindedness, and learning to let go, especially of negative and judgmental thoughts. Other strategies seem to be common across religious theories of psychotherapy: acquiring insight, uncovering the genuine self, increasing awareness, problem solving, and connection with others. Unique to Taoist therapy is teaching recognition of the polarity of *yin* and *yang* in all of life, connecting the mind and heart, and effortless action.

CASE STUDY*

In an atmosphere of compassion and unconditional positive regard, the Taoist therapist gently guides clients to greater levels of awareness, mindfulness, self-understanding, self-acceptance, and acceptance of others. Through this process clients become more genuine, emotionally balanced, and compassionate with self and others. The exquisiteness of the Tao and Taoist therapy is that it is all encompassing (i.e., all of nature, including all forms of therapy, are within the Tao). By analyzing the case study reported by Madill and Barkham we can uncover the Tao implicit within the process of psychodynamic-interpersonal psychotherapy. To that end, the authors' discourse analysis of the psychodynamic-interpersonal psychotherapy will be compared with a Taoist case formulation and therapy.

Diagnostics in Taoist therapy are not viewed as helpful in furthering client understanding. In this case study, the diagnosis of a major depressive episode was assigned to the client. The label described her symptoms according to the DSM, but the label certainly did not fully appreciate the reality of her circumstance. Madill and Barkham also realized this and provided carefully delineated text that described the situations from which the client's distress appears to emanate.Therefore, it seems that even though the authors do not explicitly state the limited usefulness of DSM categorization, it appears to be implicitly acknowledged.

---

*The case selected is the analysis of a forty-two-year-old, married, employed, Caucasian woman suffering from a major depressive episode. Madill and Barkham (1997). From "Discourse analysis of a theme in one successful case of brief psychodynamic-interpersonal psychotherapy," *Journal of Counseling Psychology, 44* (2), 232-244.

Taoist therapy posits biopsychosocial and spiritual paradigms. Since the initial component of this theoretical perspective is biological, the biological aspect is considered. Therefore, when a client presents with a high moderate degree of depression, as indicated by the Beck depression inventory score of 29 in the case study, the Taoist therapist would discuss with the client if she would consider psychiatric evaluation to determine whether medication would assist in alleviating some of her discomfort. A referral to a medical doctor to determine whether an underlying physical disorder is causing or exacerbating the client's symptoms would be discussed as well.

Taoist therapy can be brief or long term, depending upon the needs of the client. The therapist and client discuss a length of time that is mutually agreeable. Ultimately, the length of therapy is left to the client; therapists or third-party payers do not predetermine it. As self-awareness increases, the client becomes more able and willing to determine the amount and length of assistance he or she requires. Therapists and clients discuss the ongoing nature of change realizing that it occurs both inside and outside the therapeutic arena. In the case study, the client's symptoms appear resolved within eight sessions. It seems the client ended therapy not only when she reached the goals described at the onset of therapy, but also when she achieved awareness or insight into her life situation. In Taoist therapy, this process is carried somewhat further to supplement the development of the client's intuitive ability, to uncover her genuine self, and then to share her insights and gifts with others. It does not appear from the case study that these objectives of Taoist therapy were achieved.

One of the initial goals in Taoist therapy is to calm the client's confused, agitated mind. Once the mind is quiet, insight becomes possible. Meditation, grounding exercises, and quiet reflection are the therapeutic methods the therapist may employ to assist the client in calming the mind. Calming and centering the mind would allow awareness and insight to arise. Learning and practicing meditation, focusing, grounding, or quiet reflection would likely not only give the client the skills she needs to work through her current difficulty, but those in the future as well.

Part of the process of calming the mind involves reviewing how any ordinary person would handle a similar situation to determine how the client's responses to her current situation are similar to or different from others. In the case study, the client appears to be beginning the grieving process of her mother's eventual death. From a social perspective, it does not appear unreasonable, that others in similar situations may be confronted with similar thoughts and feelings, especially those who experienced similar childhood, parental issues. Suffering occurs when one feels disconnected from others, a situation that appears fundamental in this case. It may be very beneficial, therefore, for the therapist to assist the client via Socratic questioning to reflect, observe, and deduce what she perceives her losses and worries consist of, whether she is currently grieving, how she usually grieves, if she believes she is grieving, how she sees herself in comparison to others, the stages of grieving, etc., to help her make sense of her suffering.

Understanding of life circumstance is also enhanced through the acknowledgment of *yin* and *yang*. When difficulty and sadness enter one's life, one needs to be mindful that happiness will emerge. The client in the case study appeared to have experienced this *yin-yang* cycle. She felt depressed when faced with the decision to place her mother into a nursing facility, but felt enormous emotional relief after doing so, and appears to have been able to "let go" of many destructive self-beliefs. Learning and believing in the cyclical nature of life can often provide hope for the future. Realizing the cyclical nature of life also allows clients to grieve change and begin the process of accepting it by living in and finding comfort in the present.

Taoist therapy assists clients in releasing negative thoughts or clearing the mind of destructive influences. The client appears to suffer from low-ego strength. In conjunction with calming the mind, the client in Taoist therapy would also utilize cognitive strategies to identify negative or destructive thoughts, challenge their rationality, and dispute or reframe them in an effort to let them go. Clients are further encouraged to use meditation, focusing, and other reflective methods to clearly identify their strengths and weaknesses. Once identified and acknowledged, strengths can be bolstered and weaknesses can be turned into positives or at least managed more effectively. Changes can be achieved by learning new skills, honing current skills, and changing one's perspective. Energy and actions follow the mind (positive or negative); therefore, if one thinks positively, anxiety, anger, and depression often begin to melt away.

Goals give us direction and meaning. The goals established in the case study appear to have been sensitively and cooperatively established between the therapist and the client. In fact, the tape recording of the session appears to have provided both client and therapist the information needed to develop goals that were appropriate and achievable. Taoist therapy is also goal oriented and collaborative. Therapeutic strategies are selected consistent with the chosen goals of treatment. Once goals are attained, the strategies are practiced to enhance learning so that they do not gradually dissipate. In the case study, it appears that treatment goals were achieved, suggesting that there is no exclusive treatment of choice. Similar to the Tao, the results of therapeutic strategies cannot be fully explained, whether by discourse analysis or Taoist principles. It is possible, therefore, that the methods described in this chapter on Taoist therapy would have similar therapeutic effects as those applied in the case study.

"Homework" and experiential exercises are important components of Taoist therapy. Experiential exercises would be especially helpful insofar as they aid the client's understanding of herself and her identity after separation from her mother, her experiences of loss and grief, and how others respond to similar situations. "Homework" provides opportunities for clients, not only to practice newly acquired skills, but to enhance their understanding of life situations and how others have found peace in their situation, and what gives the client peace. In "homework," clients "try on" the skills learned in therapy sessions.

As in the case study, the therapy process in both psychodynamic-interpersonal and Taoist therapy relies upon observations and deductions to aid the uncovering process. In Taoist therapy this would be accomplished by Socratic questioning, suggestion, metaphor, and experiencing, perhaps visiting nursing facilities, exercises that clarify and enhance appropriate expression of emotions and attachments to others; for example, participating in group therapy for adult children who are experiencing similar difficulty. Therapy sessions held in a nursing facility could be utilized to explore feelings surrounding the placement of a loved one in a nursing home. Experiential exercises, however, do not need to be performed in vivo. Imagination, visualization, and reflection can also be used to further understanding, emotional balance, and well-being.

Reconnecting with others and with one's environment are vital components of Taoist therapy. Part of the therapeutic process is to help clients recognize their significance to the whole of life. Oftentimes, this can be accomplished by encouraging them to gradually reintegrate with family, friends, and eventually their community. Group therapy is often a useful adjunct in this endeavor. By being with others who face or have faced similar circumstances and distress, clients learn they are not alone, not "crazy." They find comfort and receive care from others. As they begin to find greater emotional centeredness, they are able to give comfort and assistance to others, the environment, and nature, and so complete the circle and find balance and connectedness in life. Through this therapeutic process, life purpose and meaning can be revealed.

NOTES

1. Feng, G. and English, J., translators. (1997, Twenty-fifth Anniversary Edition). *Lao Tsu: Tao Te Ching.* New York: Vintage Books, A Division of Random House, Inc., Chapter 62.

2. Watts, A. (1994). *Tao: The Watercourse Way.* New York: Quality Paperback Book Club, p. 51.

3. Hoff, B. (1982). *The Tao of Pooh.* pp. 50-55; Watts, *Tao: The watercourse way.* New York: Dutton, pp. 33, 53.

4. Watts, *Tao: The watercourse way,* pp. 54-55.

5. Hoff, B. (1992). *The Te of Piglet.* New York: Dutton, pp. 130-140; Watts, *Tao: The watercourse way,* p. 55.

6. Watts, *Tao: The watercourse way,* pp. 88, 90.

7. Ibid.

8. Ibid., pp. 54-55.

9. Ibid., pp. 88, 90.

10. Hoff, *The Te of Piglet,* pp. 2, 106-110; Watts, *Tao: The watercourse way,* pp. 54-55; Dreher, D. (1990). *The Tao of peace: A guide to inner and outer peace.* New York: Donald I. Fine, Inc., p. 26.

11. Dreher, *The Tao of peace,* pp. 28-29.

12. Ibid., pp. 25-67.

13. Heron, J. (1990). *Helping the client.* London: Sage; Shirley, D. and Langan-Fox, J. (1996). Intuition: A review of the literature." *Psychological Reports, 79*(2), 563-584.

14. Shirley and Langan-Fox, "Intuition: A review of the literature," pp. 563-584.

15. Williams, D. I. and Irving, J. A. (1996). "Intuition: A special kind of knowing?" *Counseling Psychology Quarterly, 9*(3), 221-228.

16. Gregory, R. L. (Ed.). (1987). *The Oxford companion to the mind.* Oxford: Oxford University Press.

17. Williams and Irving, "Intuition: A special kind of knowing?", pp. 221-228.

18. Heron, *Helping the client,* pp. 563-584.

19. Williams and Irving, "Intuition: A special kind of knowing?", pp. 221-228.

20. Ibid.

21. Kirschenbaum, H. and Land Henderson, V. (Eds). (1989). *The Carl Rogers Reader,* pp. 414-415.

22. Watts, *Tao: The watercourse way,* pp. 44-46.

23. Maddux, J. E. (1997). "Habit, health, and happiness." *Journal of Sport and Exercise Psychology, 19*(4), 331-346.

24. Ibid.

25. Ibid.

26. Ibid.

27. Ibid.

28. Csikszentmihalyi, M. (1990). *Flow: The psychology of optimal experience.* New York: Harper and Row.

29. Gross, P. L. and Shapiro, S. I. (1996). "Characteristics of the Taoist sage in the Chuang-Tsu and the creative photographer." *The Journal of Transpersonal Psychology, 28*(2), 175-192.

30. Seaward, B. L. (1995). "Reflections on human spirituality for the worksite." *American Journal of Health Promotion, 9*(3), 165-168.

31. Watts, *Tao: The watercourse way,* p. x.

32. Hoff, B. (1992). *The Te of Piglet.* New York: Dutton, p. 2.

33. Watts, *Tao: The watercourse way,* p. 36; Hoff, *The Tao of Pooh,* pp. 20-21.

34. Huang and Lynch. (1992). *Thinking body, dancing mind: Tao sports for extraordinary performance in athletics, business, and life.* Walpole, New Hampshire:

Bantam Books, pp. 18, 31-33; Hoff, *The Te of Piglet*, p. 107; Watts, *Tao: The watercourse way*, p. 98.

35. Huang and Lynch. *Thinking body, dancing mind*, pp. 37-47.

36. Ibid.

37. Covey, S. (1990). *The seven habits of highly effective people*. New York: Fireside Books, pp. 205-206.

38. Huang and Lynch. *Thinking body, dancing mind*, pp. 37-47.

39. Seaward, "Reflections on human spirituality for the worksite," pp. 165-168.

40. Feng and English, *Lao Tsu: Tao Te Ching*, chp. 1.

41. Watts, *Tao: The watercourse way*, pp. 12, 37-41.

42. Ming-Dao, D. (1990). *Scholar warrior: An introduction to the Tao of everyday life*. San Francisco: Harper, p. 183.

43. Hoff, *The Te of Piglet*, pp. 18, 23; Watts, *Tao: The watercourse way*, pp. 3-38, 43-46.

44. Dreher, D. (1990). *The Tao of peace: A guide to inner and outer peace*. New York: Donald I. Fine, Inc., p. 26; Hoff, B. (1982). *The Tao of Pooh*, pp. 4-5; Watts, *Tao: The watercourse way*, p. 42.

45. Watts, *Tao: The watercourse way*, pp. 41, 47-49.

46. Kryder, R. P. (1997). "A modern way of the eternal Tao, a commentary." In G. Feng and J. English (translators), *Lao Tzu: Tao Te Ching*. New York: Random House, p. 2.

47. Watts, *Tao: The watercourse way*, p. 32.

48. Hoff, B. (1982). *The Tao of Pooh*, pp. 64, 78, 153; Watts, *Tao: The watercourse way*, pp. 13-14, 19-21, 32, 43-44, 51.

49. Dreher, *The Tao of peace: A guide to inner and outer peace*, p. xiii; Durant, W. (1963). "The Far East." In W. Durant (1963) *Our Oriental heritage*. New York: Simon and Schuster, pp. 636-693; Hoff, *The Tao of Pooh*, pp. 19-20; Watts, *Tao: The watercourse way*, pp. xxii-xxv.

50. Hoff, *The Te of Piglet*, pp. 19-20; Durant. "The Far East," pp. 636-693.

51. Watts, *Tao: The watercourse way*, pp. 23, 36; Bolen, J. S. (1982). *The Tao of psychology: Synchronicity and the self*. San Francisco: Harper, pp. 86-94.

52. Hoff, B. (1982). *The Tao of Pooh*, pp. 5-6, 13, 20-21, 24-26; Watts, *Tao: The watercourse way*, p. 123.

53. Durant, "The Far East," pp. 636-693.

54. Watts, *Tao: The watercourse way*, pp. 46-49.

55. Ibid.; Hoff, *The Tao of Pooh*, pp. 24-35; Watts, *Tao: The watercourse way*, pp. 24, 55, 88, 90-91, 97, 115, 117.

56. Durant, "The Far East," pp. 636-693; Hoff, B. (1982). *The Tao of Pooh*, pp. 24-26; Watts, *Tao: The watercourse way*, pp. 24, 55, 88, 90-91, 97, 115, 117.

57. Ming-Dao. *Scholar warrior*, p. 179.

58. Ibid., pp. 177-178. 59. Ibid., p. 177; Watts, *Tao: The watercourse way*, p. xxv.

60. Hoff, *The Te of Piglet*, p. 19.

61. Kryder, "A modern way of the eternal Tao," p. 2.

62. Ibid.; Hoff, *The Te of Piglet*, pp. 13-21.

63. Hoff, *The Te of Piglet*, pp. 20-21.

64. Ibid.

65. Ibid., pp. 13-21.

66. Ibid.

67. Ibid.

68. Watts, *Tao: The watercourse way,* pp. xxii-xxiii.

69. Ibid.

70. Ibid., p. 78.

71. Dreher, *The Tao of peace,* pp. xiii-xv; Watts, *Tao: The watercourse way,* p. 115.

72. Watts, *Tao: The watercourse way,* pp. 27-29.

73. Ibid., pp. 19-122; Hoff, B. *The Tao of Pooh,* pp. 1-158; Hoff, B. *The Te of Piglet;* Dreher. *The Tao of peace,* pp. xiv, 11-15, 77, 111-112, 161-168, 212-225.

74. Hoff, *The Tao of Pooh,* pp. 10-11; Watts, *Tao: The watercourse way,* pp. 34-35.

75. Ibid.

76. Dreher, *The Tao of peace,* pp. 122-124.

77. Watts, *Tao: The watercourse way,* pp. 42-44, 53.

78. Kryder, "A modern way of the eternal Tao," p. 2; Watts, *Tao: The watercourse way,* pp. 35-43.

79. Watts, *Tao: The watercourse way,* p. 43.

80. Ibid., pp. 43-44.

81. Ibid.

82. Ibid., pp. 42-48.

83. Watts, *Tao: The watercourse way,* p. 41.

84. Hoff, *The Tao of Pooh,* pp. 67-90; Watts, *Tao: The watercourse way,* pp. 75-98.

85. Watts, *Tao: The watercourse way,* p. 76.

86. Hoff, *The Tao of Pooh,* pp. 67-90; Watts, *Tao: The watercourse way,* pp. 75-98.

87. Watts, *Tao: The watercourse way,* p. 76.

88. Hoff, *The Tao of Pooh,* pp. 75-98; Dreher, *The Tao of peace,* pp. 77, 213-222.

89. Dreher, *The Tao of peace,* pp. 35-36, 218; Hoff, *The Tao of Pooh,* pp. 71, 101-106; Watts, *Tao: The watercourse way,* pp. 51-52.

90. Watts, *Tao: The watercourse way,* p. 76.

91. Ibid., pp. 54, 82-84; Hoff, *The Tao of Pooh,* p. 4.

92. Hoff, *The Tao of Pooh,* pp. 67-90; Watts, *Tao: The watercourse way,* pp. 75-98.

93. Ibid.

94. Ibid.

95. Ibid.

96. Ibid.

97. Feng and English, *Lao Tsu: Tao Te Ching,* Chp. 55.

98. Watts, *Tao: The watercourse way,* p. 107.

99. Ibid, 106-122.

100. Hoff, *The Te of Piglet,* pp. 184-188; Watts, *Tao: The watercourse way,* pp. 106-122.

101. Hoff, *The Te of Piglet,* p. 186.

102. Ibid.

103. Dreher, *The Tao of peace,* pp. 12-37; Hoff, *The Te of Piglet,* pp. 3, 160, 191-196.

104. Kryder, "A Modern Way of the Eternal Tao," p. 2.

105. Dreher, *The Tao of peace,* pp. 14-18.

106. Watts, *Tao: The watercourse way,* p. 119.

107. Dreher, *The Tao of peace,* pp. 12-24; Hoff, *The Te of Piglet.*

108. Watts, *Tao: The watercourse way,* pp. 19-21.

109. Dreher, *The Tao of peace,* pp. 31-37; Watts, *Tao: The watercourse way,* pp.19-36.

110. Feng and English (translators). *Lao Tzu: Tao Te Ching,* chp. 2.

111. Watts, *Tao: The watercourse way,* pp. 19-36, 114.

112. Ibid., 19-36.

113. Ibid.

114. Feng and English, *Lao Tzu: Tao Te Ching,* chp. 11.

115. Watts, *Tao: The watercourse way,* pp. 32-36.

116. Ibid., pp. 19-36; Hoff, *The Tao of Pooh,* pp. viii, 12, 68-79.

117. Hoff, *The Tao of Pooh,* p. 6.

118. Ibid., pp. 6-7.

119. Lam, D. J. (1991). "The Tao of clinical psychology: Shifting from a medical to a biopsychosocial paradigm." *Bulletin of the Hong Kong Psychological Society, Jan-July 26-27,* abstract.

120. Engel, G. L. (Fall, 1992). "The need for a new medical model: A challenge for biomedicine." *Science, 10*(3), 317-331; Zubin, J. and Spring, B. (1977). "Vulnerability: A new view of schizophrenia." *Journal of Abnormal Psychology, 86*(2), abstract.

121. Dreher, *The Tao of peace,* pp. xv, 8, 205-206; Seaward, "Reflections on human spirituality for the worksite," pp. 165-168; Watts, *Tao: The watercourse way,* p. 112.

122. Watts, *Tao: The watercourse way,* p. 53.

123. Stone, M. H. (1993). *Abnormalities of personality: Within and beyond the realm of treatment.* New York: W. W. Norton and Company, p. 4.

124. Bolen, *The Tao of psychology,* p. 92.

125. Feng and English, *Lao Tsu: Tao Te Ching,* chp. 42.

126. Towler, S. (1997). *Embarking on the Way: A guide to Western Taoism.* Eugene, OR: The Abode of the Eternal Tao, pp. 94-101.

127. Ibid., pp. 94-95.

128. Ming-Dao, D. (1996). *Everyday Tao: Living with balance and harmony.* San Francisco: Harper, pp. 139, 141, 144; Towler, *Embarking on the Way,* pp. 95, 100, 104, 106, 108, 149-151.

129. Towler, *Embarking on the Way,* pp. 95-96.

130. Ibid.

131. Ibid., p. 95.

132. Ibid.

133. Watts, *Tao: The watercourse way,* pp. 110-112.

134. American Psychiatric Association. (1994, Fourth edition). *Diagnostic and Statistical Manual of Mental Disorders:* DSM-IV. Washington, DC: American Psychiatric Association.

135. Gross and Shapiro, "Characteristics of the Taoist sage in the Chuang-Tsu and the creative photographer," pp. 175-192.

136. Ibid.

137. Towler, *Embarking on the Way,* pp. 51-54.

138. Ibid.

139. Ibid., pp. 10, 21-23, 50-55, 145.

140. Ibid., pp. 29-30, 42, 45-47, 151.

141. Ibid., pp. 5-6, 34, 94, 145, 150.

142. Ming-Dao, D. (1996). *Everyday Tao: Living with balance and harmony.* New York: HarperSanFrancisco, pp. xiii, 31, 145-146, 228, 244.

143. Towler, *Embarking on the Way,* p. 46.

144. Ming-Dao, *Everyday Tao,* p. 244

145. Ibid., pp. 86-87, 220, 244, 247.

146. Ibid., p. 124.

147. Towler, *Embarking on the Way,* pp. 51-57, 85, 101, 113, 144-147.

148. Parr, V. E. (1997). "How to feel good without feeling good about yourself (or the art of living)," *Journal of Rational-Emotive and Cognitive-Behavior Therapy, 15(1),* 5-17.

149. Ibid.

150. Towler, *Embarking on the Way,* pp. 55-59.

151. Dreher, *The Tao of peace,* pp. 31-37; Towler, *Embarking on the Way,* pp. 55-59.

152. Dreher, *The Tao of peace,* pp. 32-37; Towler, *Embarking on the Way,* pp. 55-59.

153. Dreher, *The Tao of peace,* pp. 32-37, 77; Ming-Dao, *Everyday Tao,* pp. xiii, 92; Towler, *Embarking on the Way,* pp. 55-59, 101, 118, 122.

154. Ming-Dao, *Everyday Tao,* pp. 59, 82.

155. Ibid., pp. 110, 178.

156. Ibid., p. 83.

157. Towler, *Embarking on the Way,* pp. 4, 25-28, 31, 57, 58, 87, 119, 125, 145.

158. Ming-Dao, *Everyday Tao,* pp. 35, 95, 158, 161, 190, 247; Towler, *Embarking on the Way,* p. 99.

159. Ming-Dao, *Everyday Tao,* p. 59; Towler, *Embarking on the Way,* p. 33.

160. Ming-Dao, *Everyday Tao,* pp. 172, 183, 216.

161. Ming-Dao, *Everyday Tao,* p. 181; Dreher, *The Tao of Peace,* pp. 61-62.

162. Gross and Shapiro, "Characteristics of the Taoist sage in the Chuang-Tsu and the creative photographer," pp. 175-192.

163. Ming-Dao. *Scholar warrior,* p. 200.

164. Hoff, *The Tao of Pooh,* pp. 108-109, 150-151.

165. Ibid.

166. Ibid.

167. Ibid.

168. Gross and Shapiro, "Characteristics of the Taoist sage in the Chuang-Tsu and the creative photographer," pp. 175-192.

169. Ibid.

170. Ibid.

171. Gross, P. L. and Shapiro, S. I. (1993). "Leap into the boundless: Knowledge, wisdom, and liberation in the Chuang-tzu." *International Journal of Transpersonal Studies, 12*(1), 1-21.

172. Towler, *Embarking on the Way,* p. 100.

173. Ibid., 92-110.

174. Ibid.

175. Hoff, *The Te of Piglet*, p. 69.

176. Hoff, *The Te of Piglet*, pp. 195-201; Hoff, *The Tao of Pooh*, pp. 91-113.

177. Kryder, "A modern way of the eternal Tao," p. 2.

178. Hoff, *The Tao of Pooh*, pp. 84-85, 104, 120, 132; Hoff, *The Te of Piglet*, p. xiv; Dreher, *The Tao of peace*, pp. 28-29.

179. Dreher, *The Tao of peace*, p. 206.

180. Ibid., pp. 28-29, 206.

181. Towler, *Embarking on the Way*, pp. 55-59.

182. Ibid.

183. Ibid.

184. Kryder, "A modern way of the eternal Tao," p. 2.

185. Doeffinger, D. (1992). *The Kodak workshop series: The art of seeing*. New York: Kodak Publication KW-20.

186. Dreher, *The Tao of peace*, pp. 66-67; Watts, *Tao: The watercourse way*, p. 118.

187. Hoff, *The Te of Piglet*, pp. 107-109.

188. Ibid., p. 109.

189. Ibid., p. 110.

190. Ibid.

191. Hoff, *The Te of Piglet*, pp. 107-141; Hoff, *The Tao of Pooh*, pp. 69, 120-122; Watts, *Tao: The watercourse way*, pp. 20-21.

192. Parr, "How to feel good without feeling good about yourself (or the art of living)," pp. 5-17.

193. Hoff, *The Te of Piglet*, pp. 53-106, 233-234.

194. Doeffinger, *The Kodak workshop series: The art of seeing*, p. 76.

195. Ibid.

196. Hoff, *The Te of Piglet*, 53-81.

197. Ibid., pp. 113, 242-243.

198. Ibid., pp. 83-106.

199. Ibid., pp. 94-99.

200. Ibid.

201. Parr, "How to feel good without feeling good about yourself (or the art of living)," pp. 5-17.

202. Kryder, "A modern way of the eternal Tao," p. 2.

203. Watts, *Tao: The watercourse way*, pp. 42-43.

204. Goodman, S. and Levy, S. J. (1999). The biopsychosocial model revisited: A psycho dynamic view of addiction. <http://www.rocklandpsych. com/ biopsychosocial.htm>, pp. 1-18.

205. Ibid.

206. Ming-Dao, *Everyday Tao: Living with balance and harmony*, pp. 65, 220.

207. Dreher, *The Tao of peace*, pp. 130, 62-64, 210; Kornfield, J. (1993). *A path with heart: A guide through the perils and promises of spiritual life*. New York: Bantam Books, p. 42.

208. Dreher, *The Tao of peace*, pp. 38-46, 237; Hoff, *The Te of Piglet*, pp. 234-235.

209. Gross and Shapiro, "Characteristics of the Taoist sage in the Chuang-Tsu and the creative photographer," pp. 175-192.

210. Ibid.

211. Ibid.

212. Ibid.

213. Towler, *Embarking on the Way,* p. 7.

214. Ni, Hua-Ching (1990). *The Book of Change and the Unchanging Truth.* Santa Monica, CA: Seven Star Communications as quoted in Towler, *Embarking on the Way,* p. 7.

215. Towler, *Embarking on the Way,* p. 7; Watts, *Tao: The watercourse way,* p. 112.

216. Hoff, *The Te of Piglet,* pp. 145-153.

217. Ibid., pp. 153-154.

218. Ming-Dao. *Scholar warrior,* pp. 125, 209, 177, 187.

219. Watts, A. W. (1961). *Psychotherapy: East and West.* New York: Pantheon, pp. 1-160.

220. Gross and Shapiro, "Characteristics of the Taoist sage in the Chuang-Tsu and the creative photographer," pp. 175-192.

221. Welwood, J. (1997). "Reflection and presence: The dialectic of self-knowledge." *The Journal of Transpersonal Psychology, 28*(2), 107-128.

222. Watts, *Tao: The watercourse way,* p. 42.

223. Ibid.

224. Seaward, "Reflections on human spirituality for the worksite," pp. 165-168.

225. Kornfield, *A path with heart,* pp. 42-43.

226. Cleary, T. (1996). *Practical Taoism.* Boston: Shambhala, p. 2.

227. Ming-Dao. *Scholar warrior,* pp. 185-210.

228. Ming-Dao, *Everyday Tao: Living with balance and harmony,* p. 94.

229. Watts, *Tao: The watercourse way,* pp. 111-112.

230. Welwood, J. (1997). "Reflection and presence: The dialectic of self-knowledge." *The Journal of Transpersonal Psychology, 28*(2), 107-128.

231. Gross and Shapiro, "Characteristics of the Taoist sage in the Chuang-Tsu and the creative photographer," pp. 175-192.

232. Welwood, "Reflection and presence: The dialectic of self-knowledge," pp. 107-128.

233. Herrigel, E. (1953). *Zen in the art of archery.* New York: Random House.

234. Ming-Dao, *Everyday Tao: Living with balance and harmony,* pp. 7-8.

235. Feng and English, *Lao Tzu: Tao Te Ching,* chp. 58.

236. Ibid.

237. Ming-Dao, *Everyday Tao: Living with balance and harmony,* pp. 27, 94.

238. Ibid., p. 114.

239. Kryder, "A modern way of the eternal Tao," p. 2.

240. Ming-Dao, *Everyday Tao: Living with balance and harmony,* p. 116.

241. Ibid., p. 98.

242. Ibid., pp. ix, 95, 98, 136, 137, 245-247.

243. Ibid., pp. 210, 222.

244. Ibid., pp. 194, 195, 196.

245. Ibid., pp. 42, 113.

246. Ibid., pp. 84, 201.

247. Ibid., pp. 98, 122, 128-129, 133-139, 235.

248. Ibid., p. 200.

249. Ibid., p. 202.

250. Ibid., pp. ix-x, 116-117.

251. Seaward, "Reflections on human spirituality for the worksite," pp. 165-168.

252. Ibid.

253. Ibid.

254. Ibid.

255. Ibid.

256. Gendlin, E. T. (1996). *Focusing-oriented psychotherapy: A manual of the experiential method.* New York: The Guilford Press.

257. Welwood, "Reflection and presence: the dialectic of self-knowledge," pp. 107-128.

258. Seaward, "Reflections on human spirituality for the worksite," pp. 165-168.

259. Watts, *Tao: The watercourse way,* pp. 110-111; Kornfield, *A path with heart,* p. 228.

260. Cleary, *Practical Taoism,* p. 4.

261. Ming-Dao, *Everyday Tao: Living with balance and harmony,* pp. 20, 17, 35, 85, 113, 137, 158, 221, 246.

262. Seaward, "Reflections on human spirituality for the worksite," pp. 165-168.

263. Cleary, *Practical Taoism,* pp. 1-19.

264. Wong, Eva. (1992). *Cultivating stillness: A Taoist manual for transforming body and mind.* Boston: Shambala, pp. 141-142.

265. Ibid.

266. Ibid.

267. Gross and Shapiro, "Characteristics of the Taoist sage in the Chuang-Tsu and the creative photographer," pp. 175-192.

268. Ming-Dao, *Everyday Tao: Living with balance and harmony,* pp. 9, 31, 63, 487, 223.

269. Cleary, *Practical Taoism,* pp. 1-19.

270. Ibid., pp. 9, 16, 18-19, 24, 37.

271. Ibid., 1-19.

272. Ibid., pp. 6-7.

273. Ibid.

274. Towler, *Embarking on the Way,* p. 33.

275. Ibid.

276. Ibid., p. 111.

277. Ming-Dao, *Everyday Tao: Living with balance and harmony,* 217.

278. Ibid., p. 74; Dreher, *The Tao of peace,* p. 173.

279. Towler, *Embarking on the Way,* pp. 55-58.

280. Hoff, *The Te of Piglet,* p. 153.

281. Ibid., pp. 72, 153-154.

282. Ming-Dao, *Everyday Tao: Living with balance and harmony,* pp. 83, 86, 88; Ming-Dao, *Scholar Warrior,* pp. 200-208.

283. Ming-Dao, *Everyday Tao: Living with balance and harmony,* p. 217.

284. Ibid., 136-140, 146, 151, 31, 40, 45, 89, 99, 105, 190.

285. Ibid., pp. 10-11.

286. Ibid., pp. 39, 67, 123, 161, 190.

287. Ibid., pp. 171, 196, 208.

288. Ibid., p. 99.

289. Ibid., pp. 102, 130.

290. Cleary, *Practical Taoism,* pp. 14, 22.

291. Parr, "How to feel good without feeling good about yourself (or the art of living)," pp. 5-17.

292. Ibid.

293. Maddux, J. E. (1997). "Habit, health, and happiness." *Journal of Sport and Exercise Psychology, 19*(4), 331-346.

294. Ibid.

295. Ibid.

296. Ibid.

297. Csikszentmihalyi, *Flow: The psychology of optimal experience,* p. 4.

298. Ibid.

299. Maddux, "Habit, health, and happiness," pp. 331-346.

300. Csikszentmihalyi, *Flow: The psychology of optimal experience,* pp. 43-163.

301. Parr, "How to feel good without feeling good about yourself (or the art of living)," pp. 5-17.

302. Ibid.

303. Ibid.

304. Ibid.

305. Watts, *Tao: The watercourse way,* pp. 40, 90, 117, 120, 121.

306. Towler, *Embarking on the Way: A guide to Western Taoism,* pp. 41, 48, 89, 116.

307. Gross and Shapiro, "Characteristics of the Taoist sage in the Chuang-Tsu and the creative photographer," pp. 175-192.

308. Cleary, *Practical Taoism,* pp. 7-8.

309. Ibid., p. 8.

310. Hoff, *The Te of Piglet,* pp. 171-173.

311. Ibid., pp. 176-177.

312. Ibid., pp. 178-179.

313. Towler, *Embarking on the Way: A guide to Western Taoism,* pp. 57-58, 144.

314. Ibid.

315. Gross and Shapiro, "Characteristics of the Taoist sage in the Chuang-Tsu and the creative photographer," pp. 175-192.

316. Ming-Dao, *Everyday Tao: Living with balance and harmony,* p. 221.

317. Ibid, p. 220.

318. Ibid., p. 221.

319. Hoff, *The Te of Piglet,* p. 157.

320. Towler, *Embarking on the Way: A guide to Western Taoism,* pp. 2, 4, 23, 26, 100.

321. Ibid., pp. 25-28.

322. Cleary, *Practical Taoism*, pp. 1-12, 36.

323. Ibid., pp. 8-9, 54.

324. Towler, *Embarking on the Way: A guide to Western Taoism*, pp. 6-8, 25, 43-44, 54-53.

325. Ming-Dao, *Everyday Tao: Living with balance and harmony*, pp. 79, 80, 90.

326. Parr, "How to feel good without feeling good about yourself (or the art of living)," pp. 5-17.

327. Ming-Dao, *Everyday Tao: Living with balance and harmony*, pp. 204, 206, 225.

328. Ibid., p. 225.

329. Towler, *Embarking on the Way: A guide to Western Taoism*, pp. 9-10.

330. Hoff, *The Tao of Pooh*, p. 158.

331. Welwood, "Reflection and presence: The dialectic of self-knowledge," pp. 107-128.

332. Parr, "How to feel good without feeling good about yourself (or the art of living)," pp. 5-17.

333. Ming-Dao, *Everyday Tao: Living with balance and harmony*, p. 26.

334. Gross and Shapiro, "Characteristics of the Taoist sage in the Chuang-Tsu and the creative photographer," pp. 175-192.

335. Ming-Dao, *Everyday Tao: Living with balance and harmony*, pp. 150, 209-211, 223.

336. Towler, *Embarking on the Way: A guide to Western Taoism*, pp. xii, 22, 84, 124.

337. Covey, *The Seven Habits of Highly Effective People*, pp. 262-284.

338. Seaward, "Reflections on human spirituality for the worksite," pp. 165-168.

339. Ibid.

340. Ibid.

341. Cleary, *Practical Taoism*, pp. 8-9.

342. Ibid., p. 16.

343. Ibid., pp. 4-19.

344. Ming-Dao, *Everyday Tao: Living with balance and harmony*, pp. 145, 244, 252.

345. Towler, *Embarking on the Way: A guide to Western Taoism*, pp. 5-11.

346. Ming-Dao, *Everyday Tao: Living with balance and harmony*, p. 223.

347. Ibid., p. 225.

Chapter 4

Jewish Anthropology: The Stuff Between

Elaine E. Hartsman

INTRODUCTION

Everyone has an explicit or implicit belief system to explain human nature. This system is an interrelated set of principles, axioms, and hypotheses used to explain, understand, and interpret a range of topics. A belief system provides the parameters in which to explore an array of issues from what motivates human behavior to what is the meaning of an individual's existence. This belief system also provides boundaries within which a person experiences a sense of identity and relationship to his or her world.

Judaism offers such a belief system. It provides a container or prism for understanding the nature of humanity, how and why people behave as they do, the array of differences among people, how people develop, the reasons for their suffering, and their hope to reach toward meaningful life in relation to the Transcendent.

The relationship between a religious and psychological belief system is indeed complex and open to a wide range of interpretation. This chapter is one interpretation of the relationship of Judaism to psychological theories. It is offered as *a* Jewish psychology, not *the* Jewish psychology.

Historical Context and Content of Judaism

The first seeds of Judaism occurred approximately 4,000 years ago. According to the Hebrew Bible, Abraham, the first patriarch in Judaism, left his familial home in the Mesopotamia region.[1] After rejecting his parents' gods, he traveled to the town of Haran and encountered Adonoi (God) for the first time. The background of this encounter is critical. The people in the dominant surrounding culture had religious beliefs that included worshiping a multitude of gods, each one influencing an aspect of the human experience. These deities had their virtues and serious shortcomings, and were represented as statues. They were worshiped with great pageantry.

Abraham, who was the patriarch of a small nomadic tribe, espoused religious beliefs that clearly separated them from their neighbors. What made the God of Abraham so different was that among the pantheon of ancient deities, Adonoi was One.[2] God was also experienced as ethical, invisible, and omnipresent.

Monotheism is the core foundation of Judaic theology. This is a belief in one universal God, who cannot be represented by an idol or statue. In addition, God is present in every aspect of the world and in every aspect of a person's life. Most important, with Abraham, God had entered into a relationship with humankind,[3] in which God revealed standards for holy and ethical behavior.

God and Abraham entered into a covenant, a unique, reciprocal, and pivotal relationship. Abraham and his tribe were committed to worship only God and follow his ways. In return, God would make Abraham the father of a mighty nation to dwell in the Promised Land. Furthermore, Abraham and his descendants would receive God's blessing.[4]

This divine-human covenant is once more explicated and elaborated approximately 400 years later. After God delivered the Israelites from bondage in Egypt, Moses ascended Mt. Sinai and received God's commandments to live justly, mercifully, and to follow in his ways.[5] If the people did so, they would multiply and prosper in their land. If they did not, they would face certain hardship including exile.[6]

However, when Moses was receiving the divine commandments, the people rebelled against God. Because of this lack of faith and obedience, they were forced to wander in the desert for forty years.[7] At the end of this time, the Israelites, under the leadership of Joshua, crossed the river Jordan into the land of Canaan, the Promised Land. According to Jewish history, a loosely knit kingdom was established to rule over the twelve tribes of Israel.[8]

This was a chaotic period of history for the fledgling nation. Two major sets of interrelated events affected the kingdom. First, it was a time of military battles with other powerful nations over possession of the land. Second, it was a time for gathering scriptures and understanding their meaning and importance in the evolution of Jewish theology and its impact on every day life. Through military conquest, the Israelites acquired Jerusalem, and it became both the capital of the nation and the place where the Temple was built. The Temple became the central and holiest of places in religious life. It was here that the locus of God's presence among the people was established. In this sacred place, the priests conducted the prescribed rituals until the Temple was destroyed.

Two temples were destroyed. The first was in 586 B.C.E. (before the common era), when the ten tribes residing in the northern part of the kingdom were defeated by Babylon and forced into exile. The second was in 70 C.E. (common era), in Israel's defeat in the war with Rome.

This second Temple destruction is critical for several reasons: the Temple was never rebuilt, and the people lost their holiest and central place of worship and communal life, a place where they were able to perform all of God's *mitzvot* (commandments). In addition, the people faced exile and expulsion from their Holy Land.

After the final destruction of the second Temple, the rabbinic period ensued. Rabbis replaced the priests of the Temple and became the guardians of religious authority. Synagogues, community centers for worship and study, became the places of religious activity. During this time sacred writings continued to be compiled. According to one source, the most sacred of these writings, the *Torah,* was scribed.[9] This work represented the word of God. It contains the five books of Moses that were written on parchment in the mid-sixth century. The *Torah* was canonized as early as 50 B.C.E.,[10] and tradition asserts that this most sacred work has always existed in written form. One of the significant aspects of the written *Torah* was that the people could carry God's word with them, which assured the mobility of Judaism.

The sacred scriptures evolved during a time of religious revival as well as political upheaval, both from within the Jewish nation and in relation to external forces. Within the nation, the people were turning from God, and emulating their neighbors' beliefs and practices. Prophets arose to warn the wayward to return to the ways of God.[11]

External forces continued to mount. Parallel with the destruction of the second Temple, Christianity was forming, and the Promised Land was once more the battleground for the powerful nations of that time. As political and religious wars raged, the majority of tribes of Israel gradually disappeared. In the southern part of the land, the tribe of Judah survived the longest. The people who became known as Jews descended from this tribe.

In spite of the external turmoil and internal threats of destruction, Judaism continued to develop. During the latter part of the Rabbinic period, other sacred works evolved and were eventually written. Two works were codified, the *Mishna,* which started as oral commentary of the *Torah* and the *Gemara,* which was a further elaboration on the *Mishna.* Together, these two documents comprise the *Talmud,* which provides the basis for the interpretation of Jewish law, referred to as *halacha.*[12]

As wars continued to rage, persecution of the Jews became commonplace. To escape such persecution, Jews began migrating to other parts of the world—to northern and central Europe as well as Spain. As Jews lived in other cultures, they were influenced by that culture, and in turn influenced it. In addition to their religion, they brought their knowledge, skills, and wisdom to their new homes.

There were times when the Jewish people prospered, such as in the Golden Age of Spain, which began in the seventh century C.E. Jews, Muslims, and Christians lived harmoniously, each appreciating the value and gifts of each other. However, this type of living ended with the Spanish Inquisition in the late fifteenth century when Jews, as well as Muslims, were exiled and/or forced to convert to Christianity on pain of torture and/or horrible death.

The Jews who migrated to northern Europe fared somewhat better than those who settled in central Europe. However, both groups suffered persecution. Certain times were easier than others, but antisemitism has always been a force with which to be reckoned, either in the forefront or the background; but never gone.

In the contexts of persecution and suffering, another sacred work, the *Kabbalah* emerged. This text, developed over time in Central Europe in the eighteenth century, offers people understanding and solace through mysticism rather than logic. An approximate understanding of its message is that every Jew must seek a close, personal relationship with God through both prayer and adherence to the commandments. After this is accomplished, the Messiah will appear to bring salvation to the world.[13]

Suffering and persecution continued to occur in modern history. Hitler attempted to systematically obliterate the Jews in the mid-twentieth century. It was indeed a very black period of Jewish history. It is also important to note that this Holocaust could have only emerged from centuries of sanctioned persecution.

After World War II, many Jews emigrated to the United States and to Palestine, which in 1948 became the State of Israel. For Jews, those who live in Israel, as well as those who live around the world, Israel is the Promised Land, the fulfillment of hope their for returning home.

Jews are now living in Israel as well as every corner of the globe. There is wide diversification among Jewish people. There are Jews who are ultra-observant of Jewish law, and those who identify with Judaism as a culture rather than a religion. I once heard a rabbi illustrate this by describing Judaism as a very wide, very deep meandering river that nourishes much life. Even the trees at the edge of the water receive sustenance from the river.

Sacred Sources

There are three Jewish theological resources: the *Torah,* the *Talmud,* and the *Kabbalah.* The *Torah* is comprised of the five books of Moses, which are Genesis, Exodus, Leviticus, Numbers, and Deuteronomy. The Jewish Bible, the *Tanakh,* contains the *Torah,* and the Prophets and the Writings. The *Torah* is interpreted as the word of God. Interpretation of the *Torah* varies, with some asserting that its meaning is literal and others claiming its meaning is metaphorical. However, study of the *Torah* is revered by all adherents and is considered crucial because it is the foundation of Judaism.

Beginning as an oral rabbinic commentary on the *Torah,* the *Talmud* was later put into writing. It is the codification of Jewish law. The written organization of it is unique. In the center of the page is the tract of the *Torah* to be commented on. Surrounding this tract are the various rabbinical interpretations of this tract.

The *Kabbalah* represents a body of works representing Jewish mysticism. It delves into the mystery and the complexity of the Divine Spirit and what this means for humankind. Rabbis caution that one must be at least forty years of age before attempting to grasp the wisdom of the *Kabbalah*.

By virtue of its sacred scriptures and history, Judaism is known for its monotheistic beliefs, for its ethical principals, its rich contributions to other cultures, and its ability to sustain its people in diverse and harrowing conditions.

Cautionary Statements of Limitations

Judaism offers a rich and varied tapestry from which psychological theories do emerge. It would be very presumptuous to state that there is a Jewish psychological theory. However, it is important and valid to examine what Judaism states about the nature of humanity, how people develop and function, and how help can be offered to those in psychological distress.

It is also important to appreciate the experience and limitations of this writer. As a psychologist, much of my formal training was informed by psychodynamic and behavioral theories. Both of these orientations imply that human behavior is essentially a product of upbringing or a result of how an individual has been reinforced by his or her environment. For me, both stances were incomplete and did not answer important questions such as "What is the meaning of life, my life?" After receiving my PhD, I wandered into the more humanistic/existential camps of psychological theory, which seemed to hold more promise to explore these meaningful questions.

As a Jew, I was raised in a secular home where the cultural, political, and social aspects of Judaism were very important. I learned as a very young girl that my Jewishness was a core part of my identity. In addition, my family nurtured independent thinking and I learned to question everything, beliefs about religion, any religion, beliefs about God, beliefs about human nature, and how people should value and interact with one another. As a result of this continuous soul searching, I became a "wandering Jew." After almost forty years, I wandered back to my historic roots, where I continue my questioning; and where I find hopefulness that I may find some answers.

This chapter is an attempt to illustrate how psychological stances can emerge from a religious ground and impact how one does psychotherapy. It is critical to acknowledge that this chapter represents my interpretation of how these two sources of knowledge interact. My interpretation of Jewish theology and values is just that, my interpretation. I am not a scholar on Judaism. I am a psychologist who is Jewish, with a growing awareness of the role my religious beliefs play in my professional life. However, I know for me, Judaism provides the mortar, the glue, and the bond between individuals and for people who are reaching out for more in the universe. For me, it represents "the stuff between."

By way of anticipation, the major themes of a Judaic psychological theory, which will be addressed in this chapter, are the crucial role of relationship (covenant), the role of obligation *(mitzvot),* the role of choice, and the opportunity for repair *(t'shuva).* Within these parameters, people discover the meaningfulness of their lives.

PERSONALITY THEORY

As one explores major themes of Judaism and their implications about the nature of humankind and its functioning, it appears that Judaism is compatible with more than one psychology. The core of Judaism revolves around humans' relationship with God and with each other. Within the parameters of these relationships, Judaism also concerns itself with every aspect of a person's life, and on all levels: behavioral, cognitive, affective, and interpersonal.

Motivation for practicing Judaism does vary among people. For those who are more observant of Jewish law, it is driven by *halacha.* For others, it is value-driven. However, its message is clear—to bring holiness into the world, vigorously encouraging each individual to reach out to others. It asserts that people are accountable for their actions. Its concern with the multifaceted nature of humanity suggests a holistic psychology. However, to understand the whole, it is necessary to understand its parts—behavioral, cognitive, affective, intentional and moral, and the commitment to struggle for holiness.

On the behavioral level, the practice of *halacha* is important to understand. These rules regarding religious ritual that the observant Jew is obligated to follow, are critical to the practice of Judaism. There are 613 *mitzvot,* which instruct the person on how to behave. These *mitzvot* address ethical behavior as well as behavior concerning religious ritual. The more observant the Jew, the more commandments that are followed concerning religious ritual. These commandments cover every aspect of life, from birth to death. For many, how one behaves as a Jew is more critical that what one believes.

The cognitive aspect is likewise important. The study of *Torah,* the *Talmud,* and other Jewish sources is vital for its intrinsic value and in order to gain insight and guidance about decisions. People have the ability to decide how they will act, what choices they will make. Jewish scriptures are available to all who choose to study them. Religious education is highly valued. For many, this value for education had also transferred to the pursuit of secular education. To make correct, righteous decisions, one must have knowledge.

In addition to beliefs and behavior, the importance of intention is also clearly recognized. To be in relationship with God and with each other, it is necessary to perform *mitzvot,* to observe the commandments. However, those who perform *mitzvot* with feeling *(kevanah)* perform them more fully and their experience becomes richer. They are elevated to a higher plane than those who perform *mitzvot* by rote *(keva).*

Factors which influence feelings and values are also noted in a Jewish psychology. Unconscious feeling and motivation are reflected in the *Kabbalah,* which addresses the mystery of God. David Bakkan (1958) puts forth a convincing argument that Freud was strongly influenced by the mysticism of the *Kabbalah.*[14] He argues that there is a strong parallel between Freud's theory of human sexuality and how the different mystical aspects of God are described in the *Kabbalah.*

The ultimate goal of Judaism, to bring holiness into the world, implies a commitment to struggle. To follow God's commandments regarding ritual and ethical behavior requires vigilance and self-awareness. The *Torah* has many stories in which the heroes are continually struggling to fulfill God's commandments as well as their own humanity.

In summary, the importance of relationship is pivotal in a Jewish psychology. The covenant—the relationship that God has with humanity—is the core of Judaism. Also important is the relationship people have with each other, for this reflects their relationship with God. The importance of relationship and the willingness to struggle with relationship are keys to finding meaning, and they are important concepts that are rooted in the Jewish tradition.

Judaism offers a psychological theory in which the behavioral, cognitive, intentional, unconscious, and relational elements are intertwined to present a cogent description of human experience. To understand how these elements are interrelated, one has to appreciate that the very nature of the human experience and human development is rooted in humanity's relationship with God.

Personality Structure

In the Judaic psychology presented here, constructs that are central to understanding the personality structure include relationship, the self, the soul, the process of struggle, and the opportunity for repair *(t'shuva).*

Relationship

The relationship between God and humanity, and the relationship of people with each other is critical to the understanding of personality structure. People need God to develop their humanity, and God needs people to fulfill the Divine Other. Judaism revolves around this core relationship. This relationship is emphasized repeatedly and definitively in the *Torah* in understanding the nature of the covenant. In Genesis, God and Noah enter into a covenant.[15] But when God views the sinfulness of humanity, God decrees the destruction of the world in the form of the forty-day flood. With the exception of the one righteous man, Noah, along with his family and animals, all are destroyed. Upon experiencing such destruction, God sorrowfully tells Noah that humanity would no longer be destroyed by divine intervention regardless of how sinfully people behaved. A rainbow appears, symbolic of this divine promise.

Later, God tells Abraham, "unto thy seed will I have given this land, from the river of Egypt . . . and the Jebusite." [16] In return, Abraham will follow in God's ways. Thus, an original covenant with Noah was renewed by Abraham. However, the decisive and transforming covenant which God and the Hebrew people enter into is given later at Mt. Sinai.[17] After God leads the people, Israel, out of bondage from Egypt, God gives them the Ten Commandments and the *Torah*. These holy works describe what God expects of people in relationship to God and with each other. Later rabbinical works, such as the *Talmud,* interpret, expand, and elaborate on the covenant that is written in the *Torah*.

The sacred texts of Judaism carefully define and delineate righteous behavior expected of people. Prayers and rituals are prescribed, and people are entreated to love God with all one's "heart and might."[18] In addition to one's behavior toward God, how one treats a spouse, a parent, a widow, an orphan, or a poor person are described and elevated to a holy *(kadosh)* level. How one behaves in a business transaction, how one judges another, and how one treats a stranger are all prescribed in detail.

However, the relationship between God and humanity is not so simple as stated. The relationship between God and Israel, and God and the individual, could remain transactional. In this type of quid pro quo relationship, the individual barters with God. One performs the prescribed *mitzvot* and follows the prescribed rules, in order to be rewarded and to escape punishment. In Judaism, emphasis is put on the present life. Fulfillment of the prescribed behaviors is done with *keva,* with little feeling and/or deliberate intention. In contemporary psychological terms, one's motivation is extrinsic or instrumental. However, this divine-human relationship can evolve to a higher, transformational level, one in which there is meaningful change in the person's soul and/or personality as one struggles to learn, understand, and grow in relationship with God and other people. One of the struggles is understanding the nature of God, and humanity's relationship to the divine. As a result of such a relationship, the person has more understanding of his or her own nature and more capacity to know and appreciate how he or she contributes to the complexity of the relationship.

Rabbi Abraham J. Heschel, a modern-day scholar, discusses four attributes of God, which convey a profound impact on God's relationship with people. Rabbi Heschel states that "God is unique, alone (only), the same, and (has) the power of unity with all things."[19]

My own interpretation of Rabbi Heschel's statement is that God's uniqueness and aloneness implies that God is separate from (hence other than) humanity and nature. This expresses Judaism's monotheism in contrast to the monism of Eastern religions. However, God's sameness and power of unity implies a deep connection with humanity and nature. The divine is intimately intertwined in the world. It seems that God is both apart from the world and a part of the world. In God's relationship with the created world, God is both adamantly concerned with the welfare of people and also affected by human behavior. When God told Noah that he would not destroy humanity again, regardless of their wickedness, it can be assumed that God was affected by human suffering, which resulted from the great flood. Moreover, God's uniqueness and aloneness separate the divine from humanity and nature, and shows that God is in constant relationship with people. Further, it can be assumed that the relationships that people have with one another reflects their relationship with God. The deeper one's relationship with God, the more one's humanity is unfolded; and this relationship is transformational.

Transactional and transformational relationships occur between God and people, and also between individuals. In his classic treatise, *I and Thou,* Martin Buber states that the fundamental category for understanding human existence in neither substance, cause, time, nor space, neither personality nor experience.[20] Instead, the basic category is relation.

Buber differentiates between two types of human interaction, the I-It and the I-Thou relationship. The I-It stance refers to people viewing themselves and others in analytical or categorical terms, assessing qualities and characteristics of themselves and of others. This type of relationship fosters separateness and often functions as a shield to the impact of another. At the same time, this type of relationship can be functional since it allows people to act instrumentally, to accomplish tasks, and to utilize skills of the self and the other. This I-It relation allows one to meet basic needs and survive in the world.

By contrast, the I-Thou stance refers to a relationship in which each person is open to the impact of the other, separateness becomes blurred, and as a result of two lives intertwined, each is changed for the better. This is more a relationship of being than doing. There is more than the presence of two people; there is also a force that enhances and transcends the interaction. Could it be that this force is the presence of God, intertwined with human affairs? The stuff in between?

Rollo May discusses extensively the different relationships people have with one another.[21] As with Buber, he distinguishes various types of relationships of different qualifying value. May proposes three types of relationships: singular, plural, and dual. Both singular and plural seem to parallel to Buber's I-It relation, and dual parallels I-Thou.

In the singular mode, people are continually comparing themselves to another. Questions such as who is taller, who is richer, who is smarter, more attractive, and so on abound. The person who is operating from the singular mode is constantly comparing his or her attributes to another, but seeing neither the essence of the self or the other.

In the plural form, people interact with each other in response to the role they portray toward each other. The teacher-student, the husband-wife, the employer-employee, and the therapist-client react to each other in terms of the expectations of associated with their prescribed roles. Although the humanity of each can be more appreciated than in the singular mode, their responses to one another remain within the boundaries of their roles. These boundaries can assure a modicum of psychological safety, but also stultify personal change and growth.

In the dual form, one person is relating to another in terms of who he or she essentially is—his or her authentic self. Both parties are open to the impact of one another and are somehow transformed by the relationship. The boundaries between the two people become temporarily blurred, and each is vulnerable and open to change from being in the presence of each other. The student is changed by the teacher, and the teacher is changed by the student. Husband and wife experience themselves and each other as different because of the qualitative nature of their interaction. The boundaries between employer and employee meld, as they perceive each others' humanness. And the therapist and client are both vulnerable and open to each other as they engage in a healing relationship. This vulnerability and openness is a manifestation of one's willingness to struggle with the relationship as well as the self.

Polster and Polster suggest that the point at which a relationship is reflective of Buber's I-Thou perspective or May's concept of duality is the point of contact.[22] At this moment of the relationship, the people can experience something that is more or greater that the two who are present. And so it is that at the moment of contact there is a *something* that is present to the two people that contributes to the qualitative difference.

The Self

In order to be in an I-Thou relationship, each individual must bring one's self to such an encounter. From the perspectives of both Judaism and psychology, the individual self emerges from relationships with God and with other people. From these relationships, the self and the personhood of the individual can emerge. In his discussion on how Buber perceives the self, Gustafson explains that the development of the self evolves through different stages.[23] A young child does not perceive a boundary between him or her self, others, and the environment. With maturation, boundaries develop, along with the ability to separate his or her self from others and to develop definitions of his or her identity. This identity, this self, constitutes an individuality that creates his or her uniqueness. However, it is the capacity to relate that creates personhood.

This concept of self, which comprises uniqueness and personhood, is implicit in Rabbi Heschel's contention that God is unique, alone, and individual. Moreover, the development of self in relation to others finds a parallel between God's sameness and power of unity and the divine capacity to relate. In this Jewish psychology, a relationship with God and with others is vital for an individual's identity, one's self, to fully emerge.

The Soul: The Inclination for Evil and for Good

Personality is a manifestation of how one chooses and lives out life with respect to the moral dimensions of good and evil. Ellen Frankel tells the story (a *midrash*), of when a baby is to be conceived, an angel brings its soul before God.[24] God then decrees what type of life the child will have, rich or poor, easy or hard. God does not decree whether one will or will not live a righteous life, however. This critical part is the person's choice.

Judaism informs us that each life comes into being with a pure soul, "created in God's image,"[25] but with a dual tendency: an inclination to do evil *(yetzer hara)* and an inclination to do good *(yetzer hatov)*. Throughout one's life, there is a continual tension between choices of good and evil. Genesis states that people have been created in the image of God, and that reflection of the Holy is pure. And yet one has just to scan the *Torah* to find innumerable examples of people's destructive behavior toward one another. In Genesis, there are brothers who kill each other, sons who are forced into exile, and siblings who trick their brothers out of their birthright, and wreak havoc on one another.[26] There are fathers who definitely prefer one son to another (daughters are less important), and mothers who conspire with one child to hurt another. There is a multitude of examples of people hurting and destroying others, the *yetzer hara* triumphing over the *yetzer hatov*.

Good and evil appear to be intrinsic realities. There are innumerable ways for one do to evil, with or without intent. When people do evil things, Judaism asserts that God also suffers. Genesis states, "the Lord saw the wickedness of man was great on the earth . . . and it grieved Him to his heart."[27]

Evil is indeed a very complex matter. The rabbis of the *Talmud* discuss it at great length. The sages have stated, "There are three sins for which retribution is exacted from a person in this world and, for which he is nonetheless, denied a portion in the world to come, idol worship, forbidden sexual relationships, and murder. *Lashon horah* is equivalent to all of them."[28] *Lashon horah* is much more than mere gossip. It refers to the defaming of another's character, the willingness to transgress with the tongue against the well-being of another, and it has been viewed as a major sin.

Sins by commission or omission are an everyday occurrence. There is recognition that to be human is to follow one's evil inclination. To attend solely to one's needs and desires will jeopardize one's relationship with the divine and impair one's relationship with others. And yet, not to attend to one's needs and desires may indeed be sacrificing part of the self. The rabbis of the *Talmud* also comment that people could not have children, build cities, and conduct business if they did not follow their evil tendency.[29] The commentary points to the intricacies of good and evil. It also points out how impossible it is for anyone who engages others in the world to live a life without sin.

This analysis of good and evil, as interwoven parts of life, appears to have parallels with Buber's I-Thou and I-It relationships. Both are needed to assure the survival of humanity, even though it is the purity of the soul and the I-Thou stance that can bring holiness and transformation. Inherent in the human condition is the struggle between the different needs of one's self and others.

Struggle

The Jewish psychology presented here suggests that life is a struggle. This is preeminently a moral struggle between human tendencies and choices to do evil and to do good. These tendencies are God-given, for God created people to be similar to both "the angels above and the animals below."[30] Good and evil are intertwined in the fabric of humanity. Moreover, a person may do good but with evil intent, and a good often comes from an evil act.

In his discussion of the problem of evil in *Between God and Man,* Rabbi Heschel asserts that the more opportunity one has to deal with others, the more opportunity he or she has to do evil. "The greater the man, the more he is exposed to sin."[31] People in more powerful positions have greater potential to do harm, and thus are held more accountable by God for their behavior. Rabbi Heschel continues his commentary by pointing out that evil or destruction is often propagated by pious men. A casual reading of both history as well as current events discloses the atrocities people do to one another in the name of good. Heschel states, ". . . indeed the most horrible manifestation of evil is when it acts in the guise of good."[32]

T'shuva: *To Return, to Atone*

Although it is human to sin, it is also part of human nature to seek a better way to live. The interplay between *yetzer hara* and *yetzer hatov* results in an anxiety-laden struggle. Judaism provides a way to cope with this existential struggle: the *Torah* and *t'shuva*. The *Torah* defines what is good and evil conduct, and *t'shuva* provides the path for atonement for one's sins.

The *Torah* is God's gift to the people, Israel, which contains commandments (*mitzvot*) that direct people how to act and how not to act in their relationships with God and others. The *Torah* describes the correct life and Jewish morality. If people perform the *mitzvot*, they will be in the right relationship to God and each other. If they do not perform the *mitzvot,* they are out of sync with God and others, and more prone to do evil.

The decision between good and evil as well as between observance of religious ritual or not is essentially a decision to obey or not obey God's commandments. People are both free and capable to struggle with this decision. This struggle is continual, real, and very human. How a person chooses to cope with this struggle will affect how he or she perceives his or her self, relationship with others, and with the divine. Because a person cannot escape temptations in the world or deny the tendency to do evil, he or she is always struggling with the tension and deciding between good and evil. God has given people free will. In exercising their free will, people can choose good by controlling their tendency to do evil. Controlling this tendency is achieved through prayer, study of *Torah,* and good deeds.

Since it is human to engage in sin, God has provided people with a way they can gain forgiveness from the divine and from others. The way to return is called *t'shuva.* To engage in *t'shuva* is not only to ask for forgiveness but also to commit oneself to not repeat the offense, and to act in ways that counteract that offense. God forgives sins that are against him. But, sins people commit against other people are to be forgiven by those who are aggrieved. Also, the person who has asked to be forgiven must repair the damage that was done to the aggrieved. Reconciliation requires repentance, forgiveness, and restitution. There is a clear obligation of duty and responsibility to each other.

Personality Dynamics

The dynamics that motivate people to live a correct life by following God's commandments are indeed multilayered and complex. Promises of reward and the threats of punishment abound in the scriptures and daily prayers. The righteous are rewarded by prosperity and with a correct relationship with God and the community. The wicked suffer in many ways including being excluded from the community and separated from the divine.

The motivating factors are illustrated in the Jewish story of Passover. Passover *(Pesah)* is celebrated in the spring. During this eight-day festival, Jews throughout the world commemorate that God "with an outstretched arm" took the Israelites out of bondage from Egypt.[33] Jews, who vary in their degree of observance, mark this most important event with a seder (retelling of the story of how God led the Jews from bondage to freedom and the Promised Land) in their homes. The telling of the story is accompanied with a festive meal. As one hears this story read from the *Haggadah,*[34] one can imagine and feel that one was present at this miraculous time.

Human motivation can be inferred from this celebration. During the seder, four different children who ask about Passover are described: the wise one, the wicked one, the simple one, and the one who knows not how to ask. The wise, the simple, and the one who knows not how to ask are told that if they had been present at the time of the covenant at Mt. Sinai, they too would be included among the Israelites. However, the wicked child, because of his attitudes would not be included in the community and the covenant. There are both positive and negative consequences associated with human behavior.

Although reward and punishment motivate behavior, it is clear that this is not sufficient to explain how a Jew becomes committed. *Haggadot* written in the present day recognize that all four children are metaphors for tendencies within every person. People become committed to a holy life through study, ritual, and acts of loving kindness. These behaviors reinforce attitudes, feelings, and intent that in turn reinforce behavior. These personal dynamics occur within the context of the larger community, which supports the individual in the struggle to determine how he or she chooses his or her values. Thus, people are motivated in a variety of ways, ranging from threats of external punishment and reward from God and community to internally committing oneself to Judaic values. The meaningfulness of leading a Jewish life is also important. The goal of bringing holiness into the world by leading a pious life is viewed as meaningful to Jews.

Rollo May discusses the necessity of discovering one's values and living one's life not only in relationship with the Self, but to be meaningful—to be in relationship with each other.[35] A meaningful life is found in how we treat ourselves and each other. According to May, when we treat ourselves and others as only objects or as means to an end, we will be much less apt to discover purpose and meaningfulness in life. In contrast, if we recognize the humanity in ourselves and others, we are much more prone to find value and meaningfulness in our lives. A certain type of relationship, a certain stance toward one another, is critical for a fulfilled life.

Viktor Frankl also asserts the critical importance of the role of relationship in the discovery of meaningfulness in one's life.[36] He stated that what made his life meaningful was helping others to find their meaning. The exis-

tential therapy Frankl developed is called Logotherapy, which means healing ("therapy") through meaning ("logos").

Personality Development

Kerry Brace discusses Buber's theory. An infant has no relationship because the "I" is not yet developed; however, there is a powerful potential and
"longing" for relationship. As the child develops, he or she begins to form
his or her world through active seeing, listening, feeling, and forming. As
the child's world emerges, the longing for relationship becomes primary.
Buber states that through these very early relations with people and even in-
animate objects that are often experienced as Thou, the child confronts
life.[37] From these early relationships, a consciousness of the "I" as a separate identity takes form. The "I" representing one's identity and separateness in the world, and the It and Thou, which represent the "longing" for relationship, become more and more distinguishable. Once identity is formed,
the child, and later the adult, can enter into I-It and I-Thou relationships.
What is critical to note is the interdependence of the "I" with the It or the
Thou. One cannot exist without the other. Human existence is relational.

The importance of relationship is stressed in many psychological theories of human development. Bowlby and Winnicott, object relations theorists, discuss the importance of early relations on personality development.[38] Carl Rogers states that the child develops a trusting sense of self
when one has received care from adults who express an unconditional regard or love.[39] Rollo May expresses the necessity of developing both a relationship with oneself and with others in order to actualize one's humanity.[40]
In Judaism, one's capacity for humanity grows, and develops as the relationship with oneself, the community, and the divine deepens.

Individual Differences

Judaic theology and practice provide a rich and varied tapestry from
which many individual differences arise. The whole question concerning
what constitutes a Jew has been a prominent one. Is Judaism a religion, a
culture, an ethnic group, or a combination of all of these classifications? According to traditional rabbinic interpretations, a Jew is a person born to a
Jewish woman. Judaism is transmitted to the next generation through matrilineal lines. However, other Jews consider any person who has been raised
Jewish, regardless of matrilineal lines, or one who has converted, to be Jewish.

Many identify themselves as Jews, yet do not engage in the Jewish community or in any religious practices. Many consider themselves unaffiliated,
but "feel" Jewish. There are also some, for whom their Judaic identification
has been emotionally painful because of their family of origin issues or be-

cause they suffered blatant or subtle discrimination from the broader community in which they live. Often these people would like to deny their Judaism but cannot seem to "shake it." Throughout Jewish history, the roles of prejudice and persecution as well as assimilation have had impact on the individual's identification as a Jew. Antisemitism has often forced Jews to physically as well as psychologically cling to each other and to their traditions and beliefs. In more tolerant societies, assimilation has been the impetus for many to choose to distance themselves from Judaic practices as they no longer feel compelled to only be within the Jewish community.

There are also many differences among those who identify themselves with Judaism. An important basis for individual differences relates to how Jews observe the *mitzvot* God has commanded of them. Fewer than half deal with their relationship with God through ritual. These commandments delineate aspects of human behavior, from how and what one eats, which are the laws of *kashrut* (kosher), and observance of holidays and *Shabbat* (Sabbath), to ways of observing the life cycle and other prescriptions for Jewish practice.

The other *mitzvot* pertain to how people relate to one another, which also reflects their relationship with God. How one treats those with whom one is most intimate to how one treats the stranger is prescribed according to justice and compassion. For many Jews, it is the sense of social justice and contributing to the welfare of others that provides their bond with Judaism.

Jews differ on how the adhere to the *mitzvot* concerning ritual. Some question the relevance of observing *mitzvot* that seem not to be logical, such as the prohibition against eating meat and dairy products together at the same meal. Others counter that such observance heightens one's identity as a Jew, ennobles one, offers a discipline that increases holiness, and demonstrates obedience to God.

Rabbi Schindler states that the Jews in the United States are becoming more and more Jewish by choice.[41] He states two reasons for this phenomenon. First, there is no longer widespread prejudice in most American communities, forcing Jews to cling together for survival; and second, people are expressing a desire to understand their history and identity. Consequently, many are rediscovering the inherent value of Judaism. Within the parameters of Judaism, people are choosing to express their beliefs in a variety of ways.

The individual differences among Jews are a function of both choices they make around their self-identification as well as their level of observance of *mitzvot*. Jewish identification has many nuances. For example, there are Jews who consider themselves secular, but who can and do strongly identify with cultural and political issues that support the Jewish people. Others view their ties with Judaism mainly as historical and it has little impact on their everyday lives. But for those who observe *mitzvot,* both the ethical and ritual commandments, Judaism is interwoven in the fabric of life. A higher level of observance corresponds with the finer the weave in daily life.

THEORY OF DISTRESS

Each religious and psychological system offers an explanation for human distress and misery. For psychodynamic theorists, dysfunction and/or pathology in the individual arises when something is amiss in early relationships. Object relations theory hypothesizes that the child's connection with his or her primary caregiver, most likely the mother, is disrupted or disturbed. For Rogers, a humanist, the child and/or adult perceive a distorted view of self as a result of receiving conditional regard or love from important caregivers.[42] May, an existentialist, would argue that within Western culture, people are encouraged to develop neurotic anxiety, which cuts them off from being in relationship with themselves and/or others.[43]

In Judaism, when the person is in psychological distress or when the person has given way to one's evil tendency, something has gone awry in the relationship with either God or with other people. How the person struggles with the complexities of these relationships impacts his or her sense of self and well-being. When people are not in relationship with God, the probability that their behavior becomes sinful is high.

There are many examples given both in the *Torah* and in the Prophetic works, in which people turn to idolatry and licentious behavior when they are out of relationship with God. A classic example of this is the parable of the Golden Calf.[44] According to this story, after God performed many miracles that enabled the Israelites to escape bondage from Egypt, they erected an idol to worship, the Golden Calf, and they engaged in licentious behavior. They did so as their leader, Moses, climbed Mt. Sinai to receive the Ten Commandments. It can be inferred that the Israelites felt God had abandoned them, and thus they were out of relationship with the divine. Once the relationship was reestablished, the people returned to righteous behavior. This pattern of being in relationship with God, being out of relationship with God, and going astray, and reestablishing the covenant with God through *t'shuva,* prayer, and good works is repeated throughout the Holy written and spoken works.

Buber would contend that there is no meaningfulness apart from a relationship.[45] There is no authentic "I" apart from a Thou. Existential psychologists such as Frankl[46] and May[47] suggest that one cannot know the self except in relationship to others. Built within the very nature of humanity are both the need to be separate and the need to relate. Buber refers to this separateness as that which contributes to an individual's uniqueness, and the relatedness to one's personhood. When there is a dysfunction or glitch in one individual's relationship with another, one's personhood suffers. What often impairs or interferes with relationship is failure to confront feelings of existential guilt.

Existential or ontological guilt is a central concept in religious and psychological beliefs about human distress. There are two central factors that contribute to such guilt. The first is failure to fulfill one's potential. It is the painful recognition that one has not allowed the self to develop fully. The second factor is recognizing one's inherent shortcomings in relationships. Christianity and Judaism put different emphasis on these two factors.[48] For Heidegger, acknowledging existential guilt is confronting one's basic shortcomings, which can only be assuaged through an acceptance of and by the divine. Buber's formulation of ontological guilt is more reflective of the Judaic stance. The root of such guilt is the failure to accurately and adequately respond to the needs of another.

Buber also addresses the inherent need to be affirmed. Individuals are then caught in the painful dilemma between feeling guilty and wanting affirmation from a deity and/or each other. To escape such pain, according to existentialists, people develop neurotic guilt to ward off existential guilt. Therefore, a person may condemn one's self harshly for saying a mildly unkind remark to another. The person experiences neurotic guilt, in order not to own responsibility for the failure to respond to the needs of another (existential guilt). But it is only in confronting and taking responsibility for the guilt inherent in being human that one can find one's affirmation of humanity.

In Judaism, there is the continual struggle between being born with a "pure soul" and the "tendency to do evil." To live in the world, to marry, to have children, to do business, to risk, and to encounter are all activities that pose dilemmas—that force a person to choose right or wrong. Although the prescription for righteous behavior is clear, it is up to each individual to choose how he or she will conduct life. A rabbinic story is illustrative. There were two ships in a harbor, one coming in and one going out. The people on shore were cheering for the one going out. The rabbis comment that the cheers should be for the one coming in because people can see the state it is in at the completion of its journey, but cannot know how the other ship will be. Thus, how the person will be as one journeys in life is reflective of the day-to-day struggles with good and evil, function, and dysfunction. The choice a person has is how he or she will decide the very human struggle.

This very human struggle is also explained in psychological terms. According to May, a person chooses to confront the situations or dilemmas presented in life.[49] He was known to refer to these situations as the "throwness" of one's life. No one can control the body, culture, or time in which we are born. The examples of "throwness" are innumerable. How people influence, impact, and make conscious choices about it reflect how they will react, respond, affect, and be affected by life circumstances. To do so, to take an active instead of reactive stance in one's life implies a willingness to confront the natural pain and suffering inherent in living.

This natural pain and suffering comes not only from experiencing existential guilt but also existential anxiety. Existential anxiety is experienced when one's sense of identity is threatened. May discusses four main threats to one's identity, which he considers universal: death, loneliness, meaninglessness, and freedom.[50] As with the dynamics of neurotic and existential guilt, people develop neurotic anxiety in order to stave off existential anxiety. For example, in order to avoid the painful anxiety of death, the ultimate threat of one's identity, one can become neurotically anxious about the mere mention of death.

Existential guilt and anxiety, as with *yetzer hara,* are inherent in the human condition and are necessary for survival of a fully human and moral life. It is only in confronting existential guilt and anxiety that people can truly assert how they can take responsibility and influence their lives. Returning to the parable of the Golden Calf, it can be assumed that the Israelites, feeling abandoned and out-of-touch with God, erected the Golden Calf to stave off their pain of loneliness.[51] The worship of the idol and their resulting behavior emerged from neurotic anxiety—not being able to tolerate or confront their natural loneliness. The Israelites who remained faithful believed that God would not abandon them, and were also able to tolerate the pain of their loneliness. Each Israelite had the opportunity to choose how he or she would behave. The choice is not an easy one. Making conscious choices means having awareness of self, the capacity to confront and tolerate natural pain, and the willingness to take responsibility for one's behavior. From both a Judaic and psychological view, living a functional life is a constant struggle because it is up to each individual to choose how he or she will act and react to given situations.

Role of Choice

The role of choice is critical in Judaism. Although God knows everything that will occur, each individual exercises choice. From my interpretation, it seems that God, to use May's term, "throws" people into their life circumstances, but what decisions—what choices—are made, are within the realm of every single person.

How each person chooses affects the quality of the person's life. One who performs *mitzvot* brings holiness to one's life as well as to the world. Although it is important to perform *mitzvot,* it is also important to look at how the person does so. To reiterate what was written before, *keva* and *kevanah* explain the differences in how one does *mitzvot. Keva* refers to performing the commandments mechanically. Those who perform *mitzvot* with *kevenah* do it with feeling, reverence, with the desire to serve a greater good. This attitude of reverence is one of choice.

For example, one *mitzvah* is to give *tzedeka.* Roughly translated, this is contributing to the well-being of another. Maimonides, a teacher, a doctor, a rabbi, known for his scholarly work, espoused a hierarchy of giving *tzedeka.*[52] On the lowest rung, he said, one should give *tzedeka,* even if one is coerced to do so. On intermediate ascending rungs, *tzedeka* is given with increasing *(kevanah)* feeling. Toward the higher end of the hierarchy, one gives anonymously to help others. On the highest rung, one helps others to help themselves so they are no longer in a need of *tzedaka.* It is important to note that the person, regardless of intention, is expected to do *tzedaka.* Nonetheless, how one does the *mitzvah,* how one commits oneself to the act, and how one expresses *kevenah* is a matter of choice.

Choice is also a central concept to existential psychologists. How one chooses to confront the issues in one's life affects the ability to become a fully functioning individual. To acknowledge one's capacity to choose means acknowledging personal responsibility for one's life. It is the acceptance of life's circumstances with the courage to choose how one will act. It involves the relinquishment of blame of others and of fate. Viktor Frankl suffered unspeakable horrors in the Nazi concentration camps.[53] He acknowledged that his captors had his body, but not his mind. In this manner, he maintained his dignity and purpose of life. He also commented that he could predict when other prisoners were going to die or be killed—that they had lost their purpose or will to live. Frankl later espoused in his theory the centrality of finding meaning in one's life, which is the struggle of the human spirit.

Finding meaning in life, either from a Judaic and/or psychological viewpoint is far from easy. From a Jewish viewpoint, meaningfulness comes from bringing holiness into the world. A meaningful life is following God's commandments. It is reaching out to others through good deeds. And yet, as described previously, people are continually struggling with their pure soul, testifying that they are made in God's image, and their tendency to do evil. Study of the *Torah,* prayer, following the commandments, and good deeds provide the path through the struggle. Also when the person fails in the struggle, there is always the opportunity for *t'shuva,* to take responsibility for any harm caused, and to take steps to ensure that such failure does not happen again. This *t'shuva* is expressed toward God and/or other people. When a person expresses true *t'shuva,* God is forgiving and merciful.

For Rollo May, meaningfulness is connected with struggling, with searching, forming, and introspecting on one's values.[54] May contends that people have lost their sense of what is important. He attributes this to the many changes that occurred in the twentieth century. The horror and terror of the wars and the threat of mass destruction, the advancement of technology at an ever accelerating pace, and the changes in the institutions that traditionally transmitted values have left people in a value vacuum. To fill this existential vacuum, people have turned to an array of options. From drugs to apathy toward life, to fear of being alone, people try earnestly to avoid feeling such emptiness. A person's struggle revolves around confronting one's sense of meaningless in order to find abiding and sustaining values. For it is only in truly knowing what one values that a person finds meaning in life.

THEORY OF THERAPY

Purpose of Psychotherapy

An important goal of Judaism is to bring holiness into the world. This mission is reflected in, and is sustained by, prayers recited three times a day by observant Jews. An important goal of therapy is to empower the person to exercise his or her choice in making decisions that are in concert with his or her beliefs and values. May's concept of "throwness,"[55] coupled with one's responsibility to choose how to react to one's situation, and the Judaic belief that people are free and responsible for their moral choices are important. Both stances, psychological and religious, are emphatically stating that the actualized and/or righteous person accepts the responsibility of choice in his or her life regardless of circumstances. The biblical figure, Job, suffered tremendously without understanding God's reasons for such pain. Yet he maintained his piety and faith in God.[56] Viktor Frankl faced the horrors of the concentration camps and yet maintained his dignity and quest for the meaning of life.[57] Both a biblical and a modern man demonstrated courage for making choices that are in concert with their values. Their decisions did not alleviate their immediate suffering, but it did increase their holiness and dignity.

Principles and Processes of Psychotherapy

Three therapeutic issues emerge from the context of Judaism that are interwoven in the fabric of therapy. They are addressed throughout the therapeutic process. The first one is to explore the nature and reasons for human suffering. It is suffering that brings the client to the therapist's office. Some of this psychological pain can be relieved with techniques ranging from compassionate listening to reframing the issue, to referring the client to a psychiatrist for a medication evaluation. Other types of pain need to be further grappled with in order to understand and integrate the impact of the pain in one's life.

The second issue centers on the healing aspect of the therapeutic relationship. It is through this relationship that the client can struggle with pain and discover meaning in life. It is the healing relationship that allows the client to be open and vulnerable, thus confronting the painful issues in life.

The third issue addresses the question of the individual's obligation to Self, to others, and to his or her conception of God. The first question centers on the reasons an individual is suffering. Is one suffering because of an emptiness in life, or trying to make sense of life's circumstances, and/or experiencing failure in significant relationships? This first question begs the second question, how does the role of relationship alleviate the suffering?

Suffering and psychological pain can take many forms. It can be the result of past unresolved conflict, difficulty in interpersonal relationships, disparaging thoughts and feelings about oneself, or it can be from circumstances beyond an individual's control. A hurricane destroys property and sometimes life. One is afflicted with disease and/or disability. People with whom one has no personal relationship, such as government officials, make decisions that dramatically affect the quality of one's life. These factors can cause great pain and are part of everyone's life. The issue then becomes one of having the courage and fortitude to deal with the crisis and the ensuing psychological pain. However, this normal distress can easily become neurotic anxiety that causes the suffering to distort the perception of self and convolute one's reality.

Viktor Frankl asserts that it is not the suffering itself that causes anxiety, but the questioning of why the misfortune happened to a person.[58] Frankl talks about the importance of how the misfortune contributes to finding meaning in one's life.

Fox, in his essay on suffering and atonement, argues that personal suffering can lead to self-examination and a reconciliation with the divine.[59] Often the individual can find meaning. However, there are tragedies in life that elude meaning. At such times, comfort and empathy are offered. As with Job, people can still feel a connection to each other, even in their misery.

A *midrash,* a story or parable, enjoins others to visit the suffering to take one-sixtieth of the burden from them.[60] This *midrash* affirms the importance of relationships between people. For one person to meaningfully connect with another is inherently healing. The quality of this relationship also adds to the meaningfulness of the connection.

Within the context of a relationship, how a person's struggle is witnessed by others becomes crucial from a religious and psychological viewpoint. The story of Job once more provides a fascinating example of how a person's suffering is viewed by others.[61] Job's allegiance to God is severely tested. Job loses his family, his livelihood, and his health, and yet maintains his faith. However, he is shaken and dismayed that he has to suffer so. Three friends, who represent different types of relationships, visit him. The first two give direct advice in an attempt to help. One tells him to accept the will of God. The other tells him to look inwardly at how he must have sinned to be so punished. However, the third just sits with him in his misery. It is with the relationship of this friend that Job finds comfort and the will to continue his struggle and affirm his faith. Such a relationship is healing because this friend affirms Job's reality, which is his misery.

Buber discusses the need for affirmation.[62] Friedman discusses the importance of "restoring relational trust."[63] Affirmation is necessary to confirm the person's uniqueness and relatedness for one's personhood, one's perception of reality. The therapist serves as a witness to the struggle to find uniqueness and experience relatedness. The therapist becomes a partner in a relationship that allows the person to examine his or her life and to make choices that are in concert with his or her values. The effective therapist is open to the client's suffering, to be present, to be able to tolerate the client's alternative worldview, and to be able to authentically share oneself with the client.

Both Buber[64] and May[65] differentiate between the I-It and the I-Thou relationship. May further differentiates two different I-It stances, the singular and the plural. As mentioned earlier in this chapter, the singular stance is one in which one compares oneself against another on any given characteristic, from one's physical attractiveness, to one's wealth, to one's intellectual abilities. This comparison denies the intrinsic value of the people involved in the comparison. The plural stance is one in which people relate to each other through their prescribed roles such as husband-wife and student-teacher. Although the intrinsic value of the individual is not as blurred as in the singular, the essence of each person remains obscured. It is only in the I-Thou relationship that each person reveals one's essence and is vulnerable and open to the impact from the other.

Nonetheless, it could be argued that each type of relationship has its functional and nonfunctional properties. The singular relationship allows an individual to differentiate from the other, a task that is vital to the development of the uniqueness of the self. However, to be "stuck" only in this mode impairs the development of relatedness, which is also vital for personhood. The plural relationship allows each individual to express uniqueness and relatedness, but these expressions are in prescribed ways. It is this mode of relatedness that allows people to engage in activities that facilitate functioning in the world, such as employment. It allows people "to do." This "doing" in the Judaic paradigm allows people to engage in the world but also permits them to be vulnerable to *yetzer hara*.

The I-Thou relationship, in which two individuals are open and vulnerable to one another, facilitates a change in one's being, one's essence. The individuals experience who the other is essentially. Their relationship becomes the container or the context in which each person can experience both the self and the other. Most people have experienced being "touched" by another in a way that has impacted their lives. These encounters are by their very nature transitory. One cannot sustain such a relationship before one is "pulled back" to one's role and perceives the other in a prescribed way. These different types of relationships permit people to individuate, to do, and to experience. All are necessary to further one's humanity.

The issue of obligation to the self, to others, and to God is the third issue to be considered. The role of obligation is deeply anchored in Judaism. Not fulfilling one's obligations or acting according to what one values can cause psychological distress.

Much suffering is rooted in unfulfilled obligations in relationships, either with other people or with God, or in concordance with one's value system. When faced with disappointment, a person must explore his or her contribution to the disrupted relationship or the unfulfilled obligation, and then take responsibility toward its repair. This process closely parallels the Judaic process of acknowledging wrongdoing, feeling remorse, and repairing the relationship with another person and/or God.

Stages of Psychotherapy

From the moment a client calls for the initial appointment with a psychotherapist to the moment of termination, the person is on a journey of self-exploration that can lead to various end-points from resolution of an issue to the acceptance of the self and/or a situation. The role of the therapist is to foster an atmosphere and to create a relationship with the client that empowers him or her to travel this psychological journey.

Such a journey is marked by various stages. These stages are framed within the context of a relationship model instead of a linear one. This implies that there can be much overlap between stages and a forward and backward flow of the work done within each stage. However each stage, the beginning, middle, and the end, is characterized by the way the client is negotiating the journey and the role that the therapist plays.

The client begins therapy to seek relief from psychological pain. The client's hope is that therapy will provide an answer that will alleviate the suffering. At this stage, he or she may feel that the painful circumstances can be changed if and only if external variables are changed. An example of this is a client who expresses pain regarding his or her spouse's behavior and wanting such behavior to change. However, another client may express an awareness that something needs to be changed from within in order to bring relief and discovery of self.

The therapist's initial role is twofold. First, it is to understand the client's perception of how the person frames the psychological distress and how the person copes with it. The therapist listens very closely not only to what the client's story is but also to how the story is told. The second task, which incorporates the first one, is to start building a relationship of trust and rapport that will enable the client to explore issues with more depth.

At this stage of therapy, the relationship between the therapist and client is mainly transactional. The therapist is able to encourage the client to reveal more of the story in return for compassionate and accurate understanding of his or her perceptions. In this manner, therapy begins.

The middle stage of therapy is where the client does most of the psychological work. Viewing the issue from another angle in order to shift one's perceptions, assuming more personal responsibility for reactions and behavior, confronting painful issues, and learning to appreciate personal qualities are some of the varied tasks associated with psychological change. To engage in such a process implies a commitment to struggle. To change something about oneself means to give up something. Although this "something" may be highly dysfunctional, it is still a part of the self. This process can provoke anxiety.

The therapist's role at this stage of therapy is a willingness to become involved in the client's struggle. Commitment to compassionate listening, confronting, supporting, and suggesting creative strategies to facilitate the client's process are some of the therapist's tasks. However, the most important task is the willingness to be in a relationship where both client and therapist are open and vulnerable to the impact of the other. Such a relationship becomes transformational, and enables change to occur.

The final stage of therapy occurs when the client is working to integrate new learnings, insights, and a behavior into established perceptions of the Self and environment. It is a time for sharing reflections, thoughts, and feelings between client and therapist. The client may speculate on how these changes will impact the self and others who are important in the client's life. Differences in viewing and coping with psychological pain before and after therapy may be discussed. There is an acknowledgment that the process of struggle will continue, for it is woven into the fabric of human nature. However, this struggle will continue with more awareness, more courage, more appreciation of the self, and more confidence in one's coping skills.

The therapist's role is to support such integration, cheer on the client, be a witness to the client's journey, and perhaps even share how the process has impacted him or her on a personal as well as professional basis. The importance of honoring the struggle is emphasized. The relationship between client and therapist can be both transactional as well as transformational.

This process of personal struggle with a fellow human being as well as with God permeates Judaic tradition. Abraham pleaded with God to spare the people of Sodom and Gomorrah, Jacob wrestled with the angel, and Moses begged God to be merciful with the people Israel. It is out of struggle that transformation occurs in the divine-human relationship.

PRACTICE OF THERAPY

The alliance that occurs in psychotherapy can often have characteristics of the I-Thou relationship. All therapists, regardless of theoretical orientation, agree to the importance of providing an atmosphere that encourages the client to explore personal issues. The degree of this importance varies, depending on the conceptual perspective of the therapist. Those who have a cognitive-behavioral orientation, view the importance of relationship as a necessary catalyst for the appropriate techniques to work. Those who are psychoanalytically inclined, view relationship as an indispensable conduit to provide the corrective experience for the client. Finally, existential therapists view the relationship between client and therapist as the key ingredient to successful therapy.

The relationship is also critical from a Judaic viewpoint. The therapist brings his or her personhood to the relationship. The therapist, as with Job's third friend, witnesses the client's suffering, encourages self-exploration, and shares reactions to the client's process. There is a willingness to engage in the I-Thou relationship.

The therapy is process-oriented. Witnessing the client's struggle, the therapist helps facilitate the client's exploration of his or her experiences on a behavioral, cognitive, and affective level. Both Judaism and psychology address the different aspects of human experience. Both client and therapist assess what the client's issues are and what he or she wants to achieve. Based on this mutual assessment, the therapist can intervene on a behavioral, cognitive, and/or affective level.

The goal of therapy is to empower the client to be able to engage in the process of struggling with what it is to be human and to be in concert with one's values. In the Jewish tradition, the ultimate purpose of any life is "to bring holiness into the world." According to Maimonides, the highest form of help one can give another is to enable the person to live a life with dignity and self-sufficiency.[66]

EVALUATION

Many clinicians draw a clear and defined boundary between psychotherapy and religion. Psychology students and new therapists are encouraged to refer their clients to clergy when "spiritual" issues arise. To do otherwise could be seen as practicing outside one's competency, a violation of the Professional Code of Conduct.[67]

The clear separation between therapy and religion started when Freud declared that religious beliefs were merely part of one's neuroticism or something to be cured.[68] However, it is interesting to note that Bakken hypothesizes that Freud's rejection of his religion, Judaism, as well as the religion of others was a result of the wide spread antisemitism in his home of Vienna.[69] In fact, Bakkan argues that despite Freud's negative view of religion, his own religious background influenced the development of psychoanalysis. Psychological theory and practice are based on the scientific method. A scientific theory has clear and precise tenants, it is comprehensive as well as parsimonious, and most important, and it is empirical and heuristic. The function of such a theory is to understand, explain, predict, and, at times, modify human behavior.

Some of the functions of a religious system, such as Judaism, are similar to a psychological system; however, the main tenant in Judaism, the significance of the divine-human covenant, is not subject to experimental controls, as it affirms a nonempirical dimension of experience. Herein lies the conflict between religion and psychological theory that is rooted in scientific methodology. Despite their methodological differences, both can contribute to the understanding and welfare of humanity. Both seek to understand human nature and to influence human destiny. Clergy and psychologists can overlap in their work with an individual, recognizing that a person's issues are not dichotomized into the psychological and spiritual realm, but can be addressed from a holistic stance. The psychological stance emanating from Judaism is the self and the other—the "I" and the Thou—are separate and intimately related.

Although scientific theory cannot and probably should not be applied to a religious system, how religious beliefs explain and affect human behavior can be studied. The pivotal and healing nature of the relationship, the role of obligation and choice, the manifestation of distress, and the opportunity to make amends, are important concepts in Judaism that can be studied. Quantitative as well as qualitative research can be done to discover how these different concepts impact a person's mental health. For example, one could study the conditions that affect how the observance of *halacha* enriches one person's life and is experienced as restrictive to another.

Scientific evaluation of a Judaic psychological approach to therapy can be very useful. However, it is important to recognize that much of a religious system transcends the scientific method.

POINTS OF DIALOGUE

The major themes of the following have been the crucial role in Judaic psychological theory: relationship (covenant), obligation *(mitzvot)*, choice, and the opportunity for repair *(t'shuva)*. Within these parameters, people discover the meaningfulness of their lives.

These themes appear to be addressed by other religious and psychological systems. However, there are differences in the importance of a given theme and how it is expressed in the system. A word of caution is important here. The similarities and differences between Judaism and other religions are based on the perceptions of this author. I have stated earlier in this chapter that I am not a scholar in Judaism. I am also clearly not an expert in other religions. With this in mind, I offer some comparisons of Judaism with other religions and their impact on psychology.

Christianity and Islam

Both Christianity and Islam have strong historical and cultural bonds with Judaism. The Christian Old Testament is the Jewish Bible, and Jesus of Nazareth, the accepted Messiah in Christianity, was a Palestinian Jew. Islam shares many of its roots with Judaism. The patriarch of Judaism, Abraham, is also a patriarch in Islam.

A striking similarity between these three prominent religious traditions in the western world is that they are monotheistic and are based on a covenant between the divine and humankind. For Christians, the covenant between God and people is mediated or reconciled through the acceptance of Jesus of Nazareth as the Messiah. For Muslims, the covenant is between Allah and people. This sacred relationship is explicated in the Scripture, the Koran, as told by the prophet Mohammed. Another similarity between these religions is that each exhorts its followers to treat each other in such a manner as to reflect that relationship between the divine and people. This treatment reflects the importance of ethical standards and of choosing to lead a "good life."

Although the manifestation of the divine-human relationship seems to vary, the concept of covenant is crucial to these three faiths. It would follow that the psychology that emanates from each emphasizes relationship and one that is reflective of the divine-human connection. The understanding of the individual is possible in the understanding of the relationship with the other which, is both separate and connected to the individual.

Buddhism and Hinduism

In Western religions, the concept of relationship is based on a dyad, the self and the other. In Eastern religions, such as Buddhism and Hinduism,[70] the aspiration of the individual is to lose the self or to submerge one's individuality into the totality of being. An interpretation of this belief is that the self and the other become one with no separation ("That Thou Art"). The relationship seems to be how a person is experiencing the totality of being at that moment. Enlightened detachment to others and events allows the person not to be stuck with any one perception, and to participate in the free flow of experience. It is important to note that this detachment does not mean not caring. It is believed that each person's behavior impacts the experience of all. A person who does good or harm brings that into the world.

Buddhism, Hinduism, and other Eastern religions have a different impact on psychology than the Western ones. The emphasis would not be to develop the self through meaningful relationships, but to discover meaning through the submergence of self in the totality of being, experienced in the realization of oneness.

Other Theories of Personality and Psychotherapy

This chapter was written at the turn of the millennium. This is mentioned because it is important to view present-day theories within their time and culture. For many, psychotherapy is viewed as a process to treat an illness and alleviate psychological pain. Brief- or short-term therapy is used to help a person solve a given problem or to learn how to think about a problem in a certain way. Medication can be prescribed to decrease the intensity of the symptoms. Psychological pain or suffering is conceptualized as psychopathology based on a medical or deficiency model. The goal of such therapies is relieve pain and fix the problem.

Although it is true that medication can help people who have a biochemical imbalance that results in great psychological distress, medication can also be used in order to avoid the occurrences of pain and suffering that are inherent in life. The psychological theory that emanates from Judaism suggests that humans are capable of developing and growing through relationships with others and by their willingness to grapple with painful issues.

CASE STUDY*

The case example used throughout this book is about a middle-aged woman who seeks therapy for depression. For this chapter, she will be a Jewish client named Miriam. As described in the case history, she is agonizing over the decision of placing her elderly mother, who lives with her and has signs of aging dementia, in a nursing home. Miriam's struggle revolves around being a "dutiful daughter" and caring for her own needs. During the course of therapy, she realizes that her mother had indeed been very neglectful toward her during her childhood, and that her mother's presence in her home is a major contributing factor to Miriam's depression.

Based on a psychology suggested from Judaism the following issues need to be explored: (a) the importance of relationship, (b) the struggle or tension between valuing the self and the other, (c) the role of a *mitzvah* or

---

*The case selected is the analysis of a forty-two-year-old, married, employed, Caucasian woman suffering from a major depressive episode. Madill and Barkham (1997). From "Discourse analysis of a theme in one successful case of brief psychodynamic-interpersonal psychotherapy," *Journal of Counseling Psychology, 44* (2), 232-244.

obligation, (d) commitment to accepting responsibility for one's actions, and (e) assigning and understanding the meaning to life experiences.

Importance of Relationship

The cornerstone of Judaism is the covenant, the relationship between God and humanity. This sacred bond is often reflected in how people relate to each other. This sacred covenant manifests in relationships that serve to deepen an understanding and appreciation of the self as well as the other.

Judaic scriptures emphasize the crucialness of the parent-child relationship with the fifth commandment: "Honor thy father and mother . . . all the days of their lives."[71] The fourth commandment revolves around the divine-human relationship. Five others focus on relationships between people. It is important to note that the commandment of the parent-child relationship is of prime importance, positioned immediately after addressing the relationship of God and humanity, but before addressing other relationships among people.

Stories throughout Judaic teachings emphasize the pivotal nature of parent-child relationships. The Story of Ruth is a lovely parable of how Ruth, after the death of her husband, declares her devotion and loyalty to her mother-in-law, Naomi.[72] It serves as a model of a loving relationship between a mother and daughter.

However, the relationship between Miriam and her mother is not that loving. As the therapy progresses, the client reveals more and more unhappiness over how her mother treated her during childhood. Nonetheless, she still struggles with her guilt about placing her mother in a nursing home and giving up her role as the primary caregiver.

The therapeutic relationship issues are twofold. The first is for the therapist to create an atmosphere in which there is the potential for the I-Thou relationship to facilitate client change. The second is acknowledging and exploring the importance of Miriam's relationship with her mother, with all of its joy and pain. The child-parent issues in this case may be construed ontologically and theologically as reflections of the struggles between humanity and God.

Tension Between Valuing Self and Other

The ontological nature of the parent-child relationship suggests that when there is a disturbance in such a relationship, either party, parent or child, will feel guilt. Rollo May refers to this as normal guilt.[73] However, normal guilt can become disproportional to the disturbance, hence neurotic guilt. Miriam's normal guilt (that she may not be happy on how she is fulfilling her obligation to her mother) about her relationship with her mother has become disproportionate. She is agonizing over whether she is a "good enough" daughter and at the same time, realizing that her mother was not a "good enough" mom. This conflict of feelings is contributing to neurotic guilt.

At this juncture of therapy, the therapist's task is to provide a relationship that helps the client sort out what the client thinks is a normal reaction toward the event (mother's illness) and what is disproportionate. The therapist listens carefully to the client's view as well as confronts values and assumptions. Such a therapist could listen compassionately to Miriam's concern that she is a good daughter, and yet challenge the implicit belief that being a good daughter means sacrificing her own mental health for the benefit of the mother.

Role of Mitzvot *or Obligation*

Relationship is central to Judaism, and central to relationship is reciprocity. In order to assure reciprocity, one must feel an obligation to perform basic tasks to maintain the relationship. *Mitzvot,* commandments from God, serve to maintain the divine-human bond as well as the relationship between people.

In addition to giving in a relationship, one is reminded to care for oneself, "Love thy neighbor as thyself."[74] Obligation to oneself as well as the other person is important. Thus, the therapist could inquire as to what Miriam sees as her obligations to her mother as well as herself. Assuring good physical care for the mother and visiting on a regular basis may indeed fulfill the obligation of honoring one's parent. Committing oneself to a relationship because of obligation but not self-sacrifice, could also lead to a more fulfilling relationship. This result could be a fortunate by-product rather than a goal in therapy.

Responsibility for Action

Authenticity in a relationship, with God or a fellow human being, requires responsibility for one's own feelings, thought, values, and actions. To do otherwise would sabotage any attempt to have an open, clear relationship that is vulnerable and open to change. The therapist, working with Miriam, shares feelings and thoughts about their relationship, creating authenticity. To create this, Miriam must accept responsibility for her actions.

The genuine, open relationship that the therapist establishes with the client can assist the client in fostering other authentic relationships in life. When Miriam first entered therapy, she did so because her doctor told her that caring for her mother at home was contributing to her depression. Miriam was able to use this injunction as a springboard to explore her feelings about her struggle of being a dutiful daughter.

However, to be authentic with herself, Miriam needs to wrestle with and to decide what a dutiful daughter is and how she does and does not conform with this image. Fulfilling an obligation to the other as well as to oneself with *kevanah* or feeling, requires accepting responsibility for personal reactions and behavior.

Creating Meaning

Miriam's relationship with her mother had been filled with vague, unspoken conflict. As an adolescent, she learned from her sister-in-law that her conception was a mistake—that her mom did not want her. She also had feelings of being ignored and not recognized by her mother. She felt "in the way." As an adult, she cares for her mother at home and feels torn between her guilt about being a "dutiful daughter" and recognizing her desire to care for herself. Miriam has suffered, both as a child and as an adult.

As Madill and Barkham explain the progression of this case, the client's suffering is ameliorated in the following manner. Her desire to attend to her needs is augmented and her feelings of neurotic guilt are decreased by her gradual awareness that her mom was neglectful and critical of her. As a result, her depression is resolved.

The resolution of depression is indeed a satisfactory result for psychotherapy. As Madill and Barkham describe the case, the client came "to peace" with the notion that she could feel less obligated to her mother because her mother was an inadequate mom. This resolution is based on the transactional model or quid pro quo of human relationships, and many clients as well as therapists, would feel satisfied.

However, Miriam's suffering, which is a part of normal anxiety and guilt, may not be relieved by such a conclusion. Her struggle may center on understanding the impact her mother had on her personhood. Exploring and creating meaning of her suffering and making decisions, with awareness, on how she wants to behave toward her mother can be of utmost importance. Seeking such understanding and meaning enhances one's personhood, creating the potential for an I-Thou or transformational relationship. Even though the possibility of having such an encounter with her mother is low, the potential for having this type of interchange with others in her life increases. Such a conclusion not only resolves her current depression, but it increases her ability to cope with normal anxiety, normal guilt, and the pain that is part of everyone's life. As she accomplishes these tasks, she gains a fuller appreciation of her personhood and more meaningfulness in relationships.

Miriam can accomplish these tasks because she and her therapist developed a relationship that has characteristics of the I-Thou stance. The therapist can hear Miriam's pain, and Miriam can be open to the therapist's support and confrontations. It is through relationship that individual issues can be resolved and struggles can be honored.

NOTES

1. In Genesis, 12:1. Biblical references throughout are from, *Tanakh—The Holy Scriptures.* (1985). Philadelphia: Jewish Publication Society (often cited as NJPS).

2. The Sh'ma, a prayer central in the liturgy, declares Adonoi is God, Adonoi is One.

3. In Genesis 17:10.

4. Ibid.

5. In Exodus 18:27.

6. The *Torah* as well as the liturgy is replete with admonitions of what would occur if the people did not in God's way. God would turn away from them.

7. The central story in Exodus is how God delivered the Israelites from bondage in Egypt, God's giving of the Ten Commandments, the people rebelling against God, resulting in their forty years of wandering in the desert before entering the Promised Land.

8. The history of the Jews is told in several books. See Mack, S. (1998). *The story of the Jews.* New York: Random House; Dimont, M. (1984). *The amazing adventures of the Jewish people.* New York: Behrman House; and Wylen, S. (1989). *Settings of silver.* New York: Paulist Press.

9. Mack, *The story of the Jews,* pp. 49-51.

10. Ibid., p. 52.

11. Ibid., pp. 56-60.

12. Dimant, Max I. (1964). *Jews, God and history.* New York: Mentor, pp. 50-85.

13. Matt, Daniel C. (1997). *The essential Kabbalah.* Edison, NJ: Castle Books, pp. 10-21.

14. Bakan, David (1958). *Sigmund Freud and the Jewish mystical tradition.* Boston: Beacon Press, pp. 271-299.

15. Genesis 8:1-20.

16. Ibid., 15:18-21.

17. Exodus 20:1-15.

18. Deuteronomy 5: 5.

19. Heschel, Abraham (1997). *Between God and man.* New York: Free Press Paperbacks, pp. 102-114.

20. Buber, M. (1958). *I and thou.* New York: Collier Books, MacMillan Publishing, pp. 53-87. Buber also discusses the presence of the Other within the I-Thou relationship in *On Judaism.* (1972). New York: Schocken Books.

21. May, Rollo (1979). *Psychology and the human dilemma.* New York: W.W. Norton, pp. 87-161.

22. Polster, Erving and Polster, Miriam (1973). *Gestalt integrated.* New York: Random House, pp. 128-172.

23. Gustafson, James M. (1993). "Mead and Buber on the Interpersonal Self." In U. Neisser (Ed.), *The perceived self.* New York: Cambridge University Press, pp. 280-290.

24. Frankel, Ellen (1998). *The five books of Miriam.* San Francisco: Harper, p. 3. This book is both a delightful and provocative. It interprets the *Torah* from a feminine perspective.

25. Genesis 1:27.

26. In Genesis Cain kills his brother Abel (Genesis 4:8); Isaac, the second son of Abraham, is preferred to Ishmael (Genesis 21:14); and, Jacob tricks his first born twin brother, Esau, out of his birthright (Genesis 25:31-34).

27. Genesis 6:5-68.

28. Maimonides, *Mishna Torah,* Dayot 7:03.

29. Ibid.

30. Genesis 1:26. The proclamation that man is above the animals but below the angels is found throughout sacred writings, such as Psalm VIII.

31. Heschel, *Between God and man,* pp. 192-193.

32. Ibid., pp. 192-193. [Loc. cit.]

33. Exodus 8:3.

34. There are several versions of *Haggadot* that tell the story of Passover. Each one may emphasize different parts of the story, but the theme of each version is that God led the Israelites from bondage to freedom.

35. May, *Psychology and the human dilemma,* pp. 25-39.

36. Frankl, Viktor (1978). *The unheard cry for meaning.* New York: Pocket Books, pp. 129-186.

37. Brace, Kerry (1992). "I and Thou in Interpersonal Psychology." *The Humanistic Psychologist, 20* (1), 52-56.

38. Ibid., 41-57.

39. Rogers, C.R. (1959). "A Theory of Therapy, Personality, and Interpersonal Relationships, As Developed in the Client-Centered Framework." In S. Koch (Ed.), *Psychology: A study of a science: Volume 3. Formulations of the person and social context.* New York: McGraw-Hill, pp. 184-256.

40. May, *Psychology and the human dilemma,* pp. 40-55.

41. Gushee, D. "Society will shape an inclusive Judaism, Reform rabbi says," Cox News Service, Saturday, January 2, 1999.

42. Brace, "I and Thou in interpersonal psychology," pp. 48-52.

43. May, *Psychology and the human dilemma,* pp. 40-55.

44. Exodus 32:1-7.

45. Buber, *I and thou,* pp. 128-168.

46. Frankl, V. (1962). *Man's search for meaning.* Boston: Beacon Press, p. 154. See also Bulka, Reuven P. (1975). "Logotherapy and Talmudic Judaism," *Journal of Religion and Health, 14* (4), pp. 277-283; Crumbaugh, James C. (1977). "The Seeking of Nooetic Goals Test (SONG): A Complimentary Scale to the Purpose in Life Test," *Journal of Clinical Psychology, 33* (3), 900-907; Crumbaugh, James C. and Maholick, Leonard T. (1964). "An Experimental Study in Existentialism: The Psychometric Approach to Frankl's Concept of Noogenic Neurosis," *Journal of*

Clinical Psychology, 20(2), 200-207; Sahaklan, William S. (1985). "Viktor Frankl's Meaning for Psychology," *The International Forum for Logotherapy, 8* (1), 11-16.

47. May, *Love and will.* (1969). New York: W.W. Norton and Co. A central theme of this book is about a person's ability to choose to develop one's self.

48. Kaufmann, Walter (1980). *Discovering the mind: Nietzsche, Heidegger, and Buber,* Vol. II. New York: McGraw-Hill.

49. May, *Psychology and the human dilemma,* pp. 55-83.

50. Ibid., pp. 111-120.

51. Exodus 32:1-7.

52. From Maimonides, *Laws of Tzedaka,* 10:7-14.

53. Frankl, V. (1962). *Man's search for meaning.* Boston: Beacon Press.

54. May, *Psychology and the human dilemma,* pp. 25-52.

55. May, *Love and will,* pp. 267-270.

56. Book of Job, 31.

57. Frankl, *Man's search for meaning.*

58. Frankl, *Man's search for meaning,* pp. 159-181.

59. Fox, David (1987). "Suffering and Atonement as a Psycho-Judaic Construct," *Journal of Psychology and Judaism, 11* (22), pp. 91-102.

60. A *midrash,* a parable, is told to reinforce an ethical point. Visiting the sick is an important *mitzvah.*

61. Kish, Jeremy (1990). "Job's friends: Psychotherapy, Precursors in the Ancient Near East." *Psychotherapy, 27* (1), 46-51.

62. Buber, *I and thou,* pp. 53-74.

63. Ibid., p. 63.

64. Buber, *I and thou,* pp. 123-128.

65. May, *Love and will,* pp. 304-322.

66. Maimonides, *Mishna Torah,* Law of Charity, 10.1, 7-14.

67. Minnesota Board of Psychology: Rules of Conduct, State Document, 1990, p. 5.

68. Gay, Peter (1987). *A godless Jew: Freud, atheism, and the making of psychoanalysis.* New York: Hebrew Union College Press.

69. Bakken, David (1987). *Sigmund Freud and the Jewish mystical experience.* Boston: Beacon Press, pp. 27-29. See also Spero, Moshe H. (1992). *Religious objects as psychological structures.* Chicago: University of Chicago Press.

70. Kementz, Roger (1995). *The Jew in the lotus.* New York: HarperCollins, pp. 79-90.

71. Exodus 20:1-14.

72. Ruth, 1:16-17.

73. May, *Psychology and the human dilemma,* pp. 168-181.

74. Leviticus 19:18.

Chapter 5

Christian Humanism

R. Paul Olson

INTRODUCTION

This overview of Christian anthropology consists of a brief description of its historical context and content, a contemporary expression in the form of Christian humanism, and comments about sacred scriptures and primary sources.

Historical Context and Content

About 2,000 years ago, Christianity emerged as a movement in Palestine at the beginning of the Common Era (C.E.), which marks the start of the calendar for Western civilization.[1] The central historical figure, Jesus of Nazareth, was born to Hebrew parents and lived in the region of Galilee, roughly 100 miles north of Jerusalem and about twenty miles inland from the Mediterranean Sea. Under the tyranny of imperial Rome in the time of Caesar Tuberous, and during the spring celebration of Passover in Jerusalem in about 30 C.E., Jesus was crucified for sedition as "King of the Jews."[2] The epithet was both religious and political, and it reflected the threat he posed to both the religious establishment and to Roman rulers, who perceived him as a religious rebel and political insurgent.[3]

Christians have turned to the teachings of the historical Jesus for answers to questions about the meaning of life and how it ought to be lived. His message and the story of his life constitute the essential core of the Christian faith. From a historical perspective, Jesus of Nazareth was the decisive catalyst of the Christian movement. His teaching is the primary criterion for assessing all later theological developments. Moreover, without Jesus of Nazareth, the Christ of the Creeds would be an ideal archetype or an empty metaphysical doctrine.[4] The title "Jesus Christ" stands for "Jesus the Christ," which expresses the Christian conviction that the historical Jesus was the Messiah (Christ),[5] the one "anointed by God," whom Israel hoped would eventually come to usher in a messianic age of redemption and peace.

The history of how Christianity developed[6] and the periodic quests for both the historical Jesus and his authentic message[7] are beyond the scope of this chapter, but constitute relevant background for anyone who wants to learn more about this religious tradition. Jesus' liberating covenant of reconciliation expressed in his religious symbol of the kingdom of God[8] is an important part of human history and especially Western civilization. Moreover, the evolutionary transformation of Christianity from Hebrew to Greek soil, and from the religion of a persecuted minority to the dominant religion of the Roman empire by the early fourth century is itself a historical phenomenon. It is worthy of study for that reason alone. It is included here by virtue of its compelling insights into the human condition.

Christian Anthropology

Although there are various forms of Christian anthropology, they share a characteristic style of thought. Christian anthropology is trinitarian, dialectic, holistic, multidimensional, paradoxical, spiritual, and Christocentric. The central propositions of Christian humanism[9] presented here can be summarized as follows: The human person is

- a created, unique, multidimensional unity,
- whose life is experienced in time and space in biological, psychological, social, spiritual, moral, and historical dimensions,[10] who is
- conditionally free,
- alienated from God, self, and others,
- reconciled in love by Grace through faith in Jesus as the Christ and sustained in hope by the power of the Spirit of God, and
- whose dignity and final destiny transcend finite roles and temporal life.

Christian humanism suggests that the dominant biopsychosocial model in secular psychology must be informed and completed by another trinitarian portrait: the spiritual-moral-historical model of the Christian faith. The two are contrasted here as a natural versus an existential psychology. The latter includes the former, but the reverse is not the case.

Basic themes of Christian humanism are presented in the following sections: personality structure is understood as a multidimensional unity symbolized by the self; the concept of the will is central to personality dynamics; faith formation, character formation, and spiritual transformation are central to understanding personality development; individual differences are discussed in terms of six dimensions of life that are organized uniquely in the self-structure of individuals; human suffering is understood in terms of a multidimensional diagnosis; psychotherapy is informed by the general goal of attaining a more reconciling life; and the primary mechanism of change is compassionate confrontation in a therapeutic relationship that is experienced through several stages of therapy utilizing a variety of techniques.

Sacred Scriptures and Primary Sources

There are differences among Christians over the relative authority of scripture, tradition, reason, and experience as the sources and criteria for theological formulations and ecclesiastic decisions.[11] Some consider scripture the infallible Word of God to be taken literally as God's own words, while others consider Scripture inspired, but to be human literature, culturally and historically bound, and much more inspiring in some parts than others. Among liberal Christians, with whom this author identifies, scripture is taken too seriously to take it literally.[12]

Although there are some differences among Roman Catholic, Eastern Orthodox, and Protestant Christians about which writings belong in the sacred canon, they are united by a shared collection of sixty-six "books" called the Bible. It includes thirty-nine books of Hebrew scripture (commonly called the Old Testament, but more appropriately termed the Tanakh). Some Bibles include the Apocrypha—those books of the Catholic Old Testament not found in Jewish Bibles—but as a distinct section. The biblical canon expressing the Christian faith emerged as the New Testament by the late second century.[13] By the mid-fourth century, it consisted of twenty-seven books: four narrative Gospels; the book of Acts, which describes early missionary activity; and several epistles, especially the letters of the apostle Paul to the earliest churches he established and/or encouraged in Rome, Corinth, Galatia, Thessalonia, and Philippi.[14]

The New Testament was written originally in Greek. Since the dawn of historical-critical research in the nineteenth century, the Synoptic Gospels of Matthew, Mark, and Luke have been considered the most accurate accounts of Jesus' teachings, as descriptions of how his life issued in the service of his mission, and as testimonies to the impression that he made upon his disciples.[15] These earliest editions and interpretations of Jesus' teachings were written from forty to sixty years following Jesus' death.[16] In addition, the earliest version of the Gospel of Thomas has been dated between 50 and 60 C.E. A later translation in Coptic language of the Gospel of Thomas dated about 350 C.E. was discovered in 1945 at Nag Hammadi in Egypt. This has been evaluated as an authentic, independent source of some of Jesus' sayings and parables.[17]

Basic sources claimed by most Christian anthropologies are the books that comprise the New Testament of the Bible. *The HarperCollins Study Bible: New Revised Standard Version* has been the primary source for the anthropology of the New Testament presented here. *The NRSV Concordance Unabridged* by J. R. Kohlenberger is a second major source for identifying salient constructs and where they appear throughout the New Testament. *The Interpreter's Dictionary of the Bible* and several commentaries have served as supplemental sources.

For contemporary interpretations of the teachings of Jesus, I have relied primarily upon Mark Saucy's *The Kingdom of God in the Teachings of Jesus in 20th-Century Theology,* Beasley-Murray's *Jesus and the Kingdom of God,* and Marcus Borg's books on *Jesus: A New Vision: Jesus in Contemporary Scholarship,* and *Meeting Jesus Again for the First Time.*[18] Other primary sources are listed in the footnotes and references. I am indebted especially to the Christian existential anthropologies of Paul Tillich and Rudolph Bultmann, and to the Christian personalism of Ernst Troeltsch.

PERSONALITY THEORY

Personality Structure: A Multidimensional Unity

Proposition One: *Christian humanism supports a holistic, relational, self theory of personality structure, which is multidimensional, idiographic, and personalistic.*

The major assertions about personality structure from the perspective of Christian humanism can be summarized as follows:

1. The human person is essentially a created, multidimensional unity.
2. The unity of personality structure consists in the integration of six dimensions: three natural dimensions (biological, psychological, and social) and three existential dimensions (spiritual, moral, and historical). The concept of "person" expresses the oneness, totality, and unity of personality structure. Synonyms include the individual or the self. These terms highlight human agency.
3. Although the six dimensions can be studied as if they were independent and distinct, all six dimensions of life are interrelated and interdependent, both directly among them, and indirectly through the self-structure.
4. The dimensions are not related hierarchically as if separate levels, layers, or compartments of life. The relations among dimensions are better symbolized by a series of increasingly inclusive, concentric circles than by a pyramid divided into separate levels or layers. The concept which encompasses all dimensions is the "person" or "self."
5. That mode of existence that is most inclusive of others and presupposes them is valued more highly, but not absolutely. By this criterion, human being is of higher value than animal or plant life by virtue of the power of being, to include a maximum number of potentialities in one living actuality.[19] Moreover, the spiritual dimen-

sion within the human realm is more inclusive, hence of higher value relative to other dimensions. The highest value is the person as a whole in the image of God, affirmed as the infinite value of the soul.

6. Although all six dimensions are actualized in the human realm, personality structure is determined ultimately and primarily by the existential dimensions (spiritual-moral-historical) in accordance with the principle of functional autonomy of higher dimensions.[20] Short of actualizing these three dimensions, authentic human life is not possible.

7. Because the essential structure of human being is its multidimensional unity, the life of an individual cannot be comprehended by reducing it to any one of the six dimensions, nor to any one domain within a particular dimension. Thus to describe human beings in terms of the cognitive domain within the psychological dimension is a partial truth, but also incomplete and inaccurate when affirmed as the sole dimension or domain.

8. By speaking of personal life and personality structure as the unity of multiple, interacting dimensions, Christian humanism emphasizes first the essential unity of the personality over any hypothesized divisions; second, it appreciates the multiple and unique expressions of life both in whole persons and in diverse dimensions or realms; third, what conflicts exist among these dimensions is inherent to the ambiguous union of essential and existential being in life; and finally, these conflicts can be reconciled and must be reconciled without the destruction or absorption of one dimension by another. The reconciling agency is the self transformed by Grace.

9. Just as one can speak of a multidimensional life, so we can speak of one individual life lived in different realms.[21] A "realm" is a metaphor to indicate an aspect of life in which a particular dimension is predominant. Thus we may speak of life in a psychological realm or spiritual realm, and so forth. Although a spatial metaphor, the concept of "realm" is primarily relational or social, pointing to the central Christian emphasis upon relationships within and between realms, and to the essential self-world structure of being.

10. Christian humanism defines the good life as a reconciling life. The reconciling life is a threefold experience: (1) a spiritual experience of liberation grounded in faith in God's creative and providential Grace; (2) a moral experience of fulfilling one's vocation in a labor of love for the kingdom of God; (3) a historical experience of finite existence grounded in the hope for eternal life.

Personality Dynamics: The Human Will

Proposition Two: *Christian humanism supports a voluntaristic and teleological theory of motivation: purpose is paramount; conscious strivings count; intentions, goals, and hopes are important. The human will is central in personality dynamics.*

Numerous terms have been used in academic and clinical psychology to express personality dynamics: instincts, drives, desires, dispositions, traits, inclinations, needs, motives, strivings, goals, anticipations, expectancies, incentives, and reinforcers.[22] "Depending upon one's point of view, a motive may be construed physiologically as a drive, cognitively as an expectancy or as a reason for doing something, affectively as a felt need or emotional inducement to act, behaviorally as reinforcement, or teleologically as purposeful striving. These are some of the common ways motivation is construed in the field of psychology."[23] These terms have replaced the older concepts of "demons," "humors," "instincts," and to some extent the concept of "will."

The concept of will fulfills both of the theoretical functions of a motive.[24] By willing something, we are both energized to act and directed to act toward a particular goal. These connotations of will make it relevant to psychotherapy because the latter involves human volition and intentional change. Joseph Rychlak defined "will" as a verb: "To will is therefore to opt, decide, affirm one meaning-alternative from among the many possible." He notes that willful reasoning need not be entirely conscious, as illustrated by Freud's concept of the unconscious "counterwill." More than other motivational terms, the concept of will denotes human agency and preserves human freedom as in the concepts of "freedom of will" or "free will."[25] Finally, the concept of will and the experience of willing are also consonant with Jesus' teaching about the kingdom of God as the realm wherein the "will of God" is actualized to reconcile broken relationships and to liberate the oppressed. According to Jesus, what counts with God is not merely doing good deeds, but why one does them, that is, a person's intentions. Transformation of the human will is essential, not just outward conformity in action. The will of God constitutes a claim upon the whole self and requires intentional decisions and deliberate actions.[26] Jesus was unique because he was a man who made God's liberating covenant of reconciliation his own life purpose. Consequently, he revealed what God intends for humankind, namely a liberating realm on earth transformed by reconciling relationships characterized by love, justice, and peace.

As a summary statement,

> the concept of will integrates both unconscious wishes and conscious decisions; it affirms enough freedom to make finite choices; sufficient

rationality to make discriminating and moral judgments about alternatives; the capacity to envision a future determined in part by one's present decisions; and the ability to bring about outcomes one intends through conscious commitments and selected actions.[27]

A behavioral theory that attempts to explain motivation in terms of eliciting, discriminative, and reinforcing stimuli originating externally in one's environment is not compatible with Jesus' emphasis upon inner intentions and human motives. He rejected particularly a moralistic meritocracy in which motivation is understood in terms of earned rewards or deserved punishments. Moreover, Jesus was critical of behavioral conformity to religious and moral commands based upon formal obedience, that is, performing only because it is commanded.[28] That is the error of legalism expressed religiously in one's quest for holiness as a form of works righteousness and self-justification.

In the entire New Testament the most common motivational terms are cognates of will, want, desire, need, choose, and wish.[29] Three primary terms—want, will, and desire—appear about 255 times in the New Testament, and more than all other motivational terms combined. These terms suggest that persons are motivated beings in the process of becoming.[30] Consequently, to comprehend human behavior we must understand what a person wants and intends to do.

The presence in the New Testament of the motivational concepts "choose" (sixty-three times) and "decide" (twenty-two times) suggests that Christian humanism presupposes human freedom in its theory of action. Consequently, it may be characterized as a *voluntaristic theory*. These same terms in the New Testament, and particularly, purpose and intention, suggest a *teleological theory of motivation*. Cognates of purpose and intention combined occur about fifty times in the New Testament. The presence of these terms suggests that the basic unit of action in Christian anthropology would be more like the "telosponse" in phenomenological theory[31] than the concept of "response" in learning theory and behavioral psychology. A *telosponse* is the integrated, triphasic act of (a) consciously reasoning about various options, and (b) choosing one of the alternatives as one's purpose for the sake of which (c) behavior is intended and enacted. A telosponse may involve cognitive, affective, volitional, and behavioral elements as well as interpersonal dimensions.

Joseph Rychlak advocated this construct to integrate the insights about human nature found in psychodynamic, phenomenological, and behavioral theories of psychotherapy. The concept serves equally well to incorporate Christian existential theory that highlights the spiritual, moral, and historical dimensions of human experience and action. To say that human behavior is telosponsive is to affirm that it is an act of will and as such, the consequence of conscious deliberations and decisions, purposeful and intentional. Conscious plans in the present are emphasized over unconscious dynamics from the past, but not exclusively. Gordon Allport agrees:

> A full understanding of the adult cannot be secured without a picture of his goals and aspirations. His most important motives are not echoes of the past, but rather beckonings from the future. In most cases, we will know more about what a person will do if we know his conscious plans than if we know his repressed memories.[32]

Human behavior is both willed and goal-directed. In the specialized discipline of psychology known as personality theory,

> a major trend has become the representation of personality in terms of dynamic processes, emphasizing how individuals strive for personally defined goals, construe daily opportunities for the realization of these goals, and regulate their behavior in an attempt to progress toward that which is personally meaningful and self-defining.[33]

The voluntaristic and teleological theory of motivation in Christian humanism seems compatible with an accent upon the future more than the past. Although the cardinal Christian virtues of faith, love, and hope all involve a remembered past, an experienced present, and an anticipated future, it is particularly the concept of hope that expresses the future orientation of human strivings. We may savor a fond memory or regret something in our past; what we hope for lies in the future.[34] Christian psychology is a *future-oriented psychology of hope.* It is a hopeful psychology because it is both a psychology of reconciliation and a reconciling psychology.

Although hope is a central category in Christian humanism, the primary category of the spiritual dimension is not hope, but faith. Moreover, since faith subsumes the concepts of will and meaning, a theory of motivation that suggests the primacy of the "will to meaning" is compatible with Christian humanism. Perhaps faith itself could be construed as an expression of the will to meaning, if not a medium of its fulfillment. In other words, *as with hope and love, faith is itself a motive and motivating.*

A popular term in contemporary theories of motivation is *needs.* This concept can be included in a voluntaristic and teleological theory of motivation by associating it with the various dimensions of life. In the *biological* dimension are the homeostatic needs of the cardiovascular, respiratory, digestive, muscular, and endocrine systems, sexual needs, and needs for physical safety, food and water, and shelter and clothing. In the *psychological* dimension are the needs for personal security, identity, and self-esteem. In the *social* dimension are the needs for belonging and healthy relationships characterized by genuine mutuality, liberty, equality, and justice. In the *spiritual* dimension are the needs for transcendence and meaning, authenticity and reconciliation. We may speak also of the spiritual needs for faith, hope, and love. In the *moral* dimension are the needs for integrity of character, the need to abide by one's conscience, to fulfill one's sense of duty, to be virtuous, and to act ethically. In the *historical* dimension are the needs to remember one's collective heritage and personal past, and to anticipate a meaningful future while living fully in the present.

Personal integration requires that these various needs be harmonized and balanced. Abraham Maslow's principle of a hierarchy of needs is helpful here, but the ultimate need is not self-actualization as advocated in secular humanistic psychology.[35] In Christian humanism, the need for a reconciling life with God, self, and others constitutes the overarching need and the primary purpose by which all other motives are ordered by the individual to achieve personal integration, self-transcendence, and healing.

Personality Development: Faith, Character, and Spiritual Gifts

Proposition Three: *The development of character is central in Christian humanism. Primary virtues include faith, hope, and love. Faith formation and character formation are both prerequisites for spiritual transformation into a more reconciling life.*

Developmental theories provide a way to think about the dynamics of change and transformation, and simultaneously appreciate issues of equilibrium and continuity throughout time. Stage theories of development attempt to describe predictable changes in individuals throughout the life cycle in largely formal terms. Their approach to personality is *nomothetic,* that is, a descriptive outline of general features and patterns of growth applicable to all people.

The development of the self is one of the defining characteristics of human growth. Development of a healthy self-concept and self-esteem are considered essential to mental health and to adaptive functioning. In Christian humanistic theory, the self is presumed to change over time in a continuous process of becoming. In general, both changing and enduring attributes of the self are affirmed. The self develops and changes, yet it does not cease to exist. A self that does not change does not endure. Our ideas, sensations, feelings, and volitions may change, even our concept of our real and essential selves (who we truly are), yet our real selves continue through time to be a primary datum directly apprehended, if not always accurately comprehended. The self develops as a multidimensional unity. It is experienced not as a static substance, but as a dynamic movement. To be is to become.

A developmental theory affirms that "what humans are depends in large part on experience; we become who we are through learning and development."[36] In the natural realm of human experience, which includes the biopsychosocial dimensions, developmental theory has focused on stages of psychosexual development (e.g., Freud), psychosocial development (e.g., Erikson), and cognitive development (e.g., Piaget). In the existential realm of human experience, which includes the spiritual, moral, and historical dimensions, stage theories have been offered to describe and understand moral development (e.g., Kohlberg), faith development (e.g., Fowler, Oser), and historical developments (e.g., Teilhard de Chardin). Christian developmental theories have focused on (1) faith formation, (2) character formation, and (3) spiritual transformation and growth.

The utility of understanding *faith formation* within the context of a developmental perspective has been demonstrated by James Fowler's theory on the stages of faith. Building upon the undifferentiated trust of infancy, Fowler describes the six stages of faith development in terms of the various forms faith takes: intuitive-projective, mythical-literal, synthetic-conventional, individualistic-reflective, conjunctive, and universalizing faith. Comparable to other stage theories of human development, both risks and limitations, and strengths and potentials are associated with each stage of faith development. Likewise, there are conditions specified for the emergence of one stage from another.[37]

As with the developmental theories of Erikson and Kohlberg, Fowler's theory of faith development is not merely descriptive, but normative. The higher stages of faith development are also judged of greater value in terms of multiple criteria such as the use of reason, empathy, moral reasoning, objectivity, self-reliance, self-responsibility, choice, awareness, and commitment.[38] These values constitute criteria for assessing both religious and secular forms of faith.

According to Christian humanism, discussion of faith development needs to be complemented with discussion of the *moral development of character.*[39] Moral development from a Christian perspective involves considerations of moral reasoning, ethical principles, the divine moral imperative to love, and the development of conscience and virtues as primary determinants of character. Both legalism and moral license are rejected in favor of life in the Spirit, characterized by the three cardinal Christian virtues of faith, hope, and love. In general, Christians address the ethical question, "What should I do?" by asking first, "What has God done?" Christian ethics are grounded in historical theology, the imperative in the indicative.

Faith development and character formation are related to *spiritual transformation.*[40] Faith, hope, and love are domains relevant to the spiritual dimension since all three express and provide meaning. Moreover, the moral and spiritual dimensions are inseparable. It would be irrational to obligate people to do what they cannot do. Liberal Christian anthropology acknowledges that "ought" implies "can." Christian humanism encourages the development of spiritual gifts and fruits of the Spirit to enable believers to acquire the requisite virtues, and thereby to empower individuals to fulfill their divinely ordained duty to love God and one another. Christian virtues are sustained by spiritual gifts bestowed by the Holy Spirit active in the life of a genuine disciple of Jesus.

In the Catholic tradition, *spiritual gifts* are described as dispositions of character that make one receptive to the promptings of the Holy Spirit.[41] As with the three cardinal virtues, these spiritual attributes dispose Christians to be led by the Spirit of God and to be guided by divine inspiration. Catholic Christians affirm seven spiritual gifts: wisdom, understanding, counsel, fortitude, knowledge, piety, and reverence for God.[42] These gifts of the Spirit function to enable and sustain the Christian moral life. They complete and perfect the virtues of believers who are blessed with these gifts.

The concept of spiritual gifts reflects the basic notion that Christian virtues are less human achievements than they are creations of the divine Spirit in communion with the human spirit. While human efforts are involved in their development, faith, hope, and love are ultimately creative inspirations of the Spirit of God and empirical indicators of God's active presence in human life.[43] God is the source of all that is good and its present power.

As one grows in spiritual maturity, becoming more sanctified, perfections are acquired as *fruits of the Spirit.* Christian anthropology describes the following personality characteristics as fruits of the Spirit: charity, joy, peace, patience, kindness, goodness, generosity, gentleness, faithfulness, modesty, and self-control.[44] These fruits of the Spirit are the consequence of a life of holy obedience to the will of God, and they are manifested particularly in compassionate care for the poor and in liberating acts of justice for the oppressed. Through the process of spiritual transformation one experiences these fruits of human efforts as the blessings of God. In the Catholic tradition, human nature has always been graced nature, and human history is a graced history. Christianity is a religion of second chances and new beginnings.

Within the Protestant tradition, Paul Tillich suggested that spiritual transformation is experienced as the power of reconciliation ("New Being")[45] in three ways: (1) as creation (regeneration), (2) as paradox (justification), and (3) as process (sanctification).[46] The individual experiences this spiritual transformation in and through the Christian community called the Church. The resulting change amounts to a *new spiritual identity.* One actualizes the image or likeness of God, which constitutes essential human being as created by God. The image of God *(imago Dei)* defines who we are essentially and potentially, and it functions psychologically as the Christian's self-ideal.[47] There is general consensus among Christians that Jesus as the Christ personifies and symbolizes the image or likeness of God fully actualized under the conditions of existence. To determine what God is like and what

God is doing, Christians look to the message and ministry of Jesus as the Christ.

Individual Differences in Six Dimensions of Life

Proposition Four: *Individuals are unique and different in many ways. Neither heredity nor environment are primary considerations in explaining individual differences. Of primary importance is the quality of one's conscious relationship with God in Christ by the power of the Holy Spirit experienced and expressed in varying degrees as faith, hope, and love.*

The developmental approach to personality is nomothetic, that is, it provides a descriptive outline of general features and patterns of growth applicable to all people. Occasionally neglected in such theories are the significant individual differences in rates of growth, and particular life sequences and events in unique life stories. A developmental approach needs an *idiographic* perspective to highlight the uniqueness of each and every individual and their individual differences.

According to Christian humanism, individual differences exist

1. in all three dimensions of the natural realm of life (biopsychosocial dimensions)
2. in all three dimensions of the existential realm (spiritual, moral, and historical)
3. in the relative dominance of one or more dimensions within an individual
4. in the unique organization of dimensions and their domains within a particular person, and
5. in the changes in the relative dominance of particular dimensions within individuals through time.

A satisfactory theory of personality requires an idiographic approach in order to appreciate individual differences in concrete personal lives.

Individual differences are partly a function of the different dimensions of human experience. It is their different qualities that distinguish the separate dimensions of experience. Thus, an experience in the biological dimension (e.g., physical pain) is qualitatively different from an experience in the moral dimension (e.g., striving to fulfill an ethical obligation). Moreover, each distinct dimension of experience does not necessarily possess the same qualities as the whole of experience; rather, each dimension is defined in terms of its uniqueness, not by such commonalities as their reciprocal influence and interdependence through the self-structure.

The divergent dimensions become convergent within the mature self-structure as complementary aspects rather than conflicted factors. The *self-structure* synthesizes polarities among dimensions, hence we may speak of the self as the unity of the multiplicity of its experiences. The self-structure is both changing and enduring, simultaneously immanent within experience, and transcending experience. A classification of personality types or traits becomes possible based upon the unique organization of the dimensions and domains of experience within the self-structure of different individuals.

THEORY OF DISTRESS

Proposition Five: *Christian humanism incorporates a biopsychosocial etiology of human distress, and it adds an existential theory that emphasizes spiritual-ethical-historical dimensions. The central idea about human distress involves alienated relationships that need to be reconciled with God, self, and others.*

Consistent with the notion of the multidimensional unity of life, the symptoms, diagnosis, and etiology of human distress are viewed from a multidimensional perspective. Consequently, we may speak of biological, spiritual, and moral disorders, and so forth. The multidimensional unity of life suggests that the symptoms and disorders (as well as health) experienced in one dimension impact functioning in other dimensions.

The variety of symptoms in all dimensions reflect a common characteristic: multiplicity without unity in personality structure and functioning. The essential multidimensional unity of life is existentially distorted, resulting in a compromise of true humanity, and an ambiguous life.[48] The individual becomes alienated from one's true self, from others, and from God. Both within and among all dimensions, the symptoms of distress and dysfunction reflect personal disintegration and alienation. Human life is an existence estranged from essence. The result is a fragmented life of conflict and distress.

The correlate of the multidimensional unity of life is a *multidimensional diagnosis* of the human condition and personal life. Implicit in this approach is the view that all dimensions of life are potentially or actually present in each dimension, hence "happenings under the predominance of one dimension must imply happenings in other dimensions."[49] All the dimensions of life are interrelated and mutually influential in the unity of personal life. It follows that an accurate understanding of any client requires a multidimensional diagnosis.

This approach is analogous in form to the multiaxial assessment and diagnosis advocated in DSM-IV,[50] but different dimensions or "axes" are included here. From the perspective of Christian humanism, DSM-IV is at best an incomplete diagnostic system by virtue of both its focus on psychopathological conditions, and its natural model limited to biopsychosocial dimensions of human functioning. Excluded in this descriptive nosology is an existential perspective that emphasizes spiritual, moral, and historical dimensions of functioning. Only by incorporating the existential dimensions can a clinician achieve a complete multiaxial diagnosis, discern both the unity and uniqueness of individuals, and reach a comprehensive assessment of a client's condition and functioning.

This critique of secular psychiatric assessment is justifiable even though "religious or spiritual problems" have been subsumed under "other conditions" in DSM-IV. That classification marginalizes the spiritual dimension, though it also reflects a current consensus that spirituality is no longer considered pathological, defacto or dejure, contrary to the classical psychoanalytic critique of religion as neurotic illusion. Neither spiritual, moral, nor historical dimensions are fully appreciated in this secular nomenclature of mental disorders promulgated by the American Psychiatric Association.

The multidimensional approach of Christian humanism is both similar to, and different from, the multimodal approach to diagnosis and therapy advocated by Arnold Lazarus.[51] The acronym "BASIC-ID" suggests the modalities Lazarus stressed: behavioral, affective, sensory, imagery, cognitive, interpersonal, and drugs (biological). All of these natural dimensions that Lazarus notes should be included in a multidimensional diagnosis. The additional perspective that is needed relates to the existential realm expressed in the moral, spiritual, and historical dimensions.

Since the natural dimensions are covered thoroughly in clinical psychology, they will not be repeated here. Instead, the existential dimensions will be emphasized from the perspective of Christian humanism. The common condition evident in all three existential dimensions is *estrangement* experienced respectively in the spiritual, moral, and historical dimensions as unbelief, hubris, and ambiguity. Turning away from God toward oneself, one experiences an ambiguous life estranged from God, self, and others. Estrangement (alienation) is the consequence of the abuse of freedom, expressed as a repudiation of one's dependence upon God and manifest in selfish pride. This is the universal condition of human sin. The common effects are self-deception and human misery.

Are we to conclude that all suffering is caused by personal sin? No. Christian humanism acknowledges that good and innocent people suffer unjustly. The biblical stories of Job and Jesus are classic denials of the view that all suffering is caused by an individual's personal sins. One can argue from sin to suffering, but not from suffering back to sin. Bad things do happen to good people.[52] Nevertheless, one cannot comprehend human suffering from a Christian perspective apart from the concept of sin. The concept of sin functions as one explanation for human misery and evil, and helps to explain why the world is not the way it could be, and should be, nor the way God intends it. Consequently, the fundamental diagnosis of the human condition is not primarily ignorance; nor a misidentification of one's true self with the conscious ego;[53] nor is it desire or attachment per se; rather, the fundamental human problem is the pretense to divinity, expressed in one's turning away from God (unbelief) toward a life centered in self *(hubris)*,[54] and resulting in ambiguity and suffering.

Regardless of the particular theories about the etiology of sin and suffering, a general Christian consensus is that reconciliation involves liberation from alienation and from the oppressive power of sin and evil. The Christian mission and hope is to overcome alienation through liberating experiences of reconciliation. This religious purpose guides the experiential theory of psychotherapy informed by Christian humanism.

THEORY OF THERAPY

This section begins with discussion of the purpose of psychotherapy, followed by principles and processes of change occurring through several stages of therapy.

Purpose of Psychotherapy: A Reconciling Life

Proposition Six: *According to Christian humanism, the purpose of psychotherapy is to encourage a more reconciled life and reconciling relationships. This general goal involves helping clients to reduce their suffering, to solve their problems, and in the process, to help them become wiser, more compassionate and courageous, joyful and thankful, ethical and sanctified, and an agent of reconciliation with others.*[55]

Numerous goals have been advocated in teleological definitions of psychotherapy. Based upon his review of psychotherapy literature, Arthur Burton listed forty general goals with another thirty related to particular psychological concerns.[56] Various authors have advocated such ultimate purposes as self-actualization, self-acceptance, creativity, happiness, individuation, authenticity, self-integration, adjustment, autonomy, functioning fully, and being responsible.[57] As one example, the author of multimodal therapy, Arnold Lazarus advocated a twofold purpose of psychotherapy: "The aim is to reduce psychological suffering and to promote personal growth as rapidly and as durably as possible."[58]

The most generic goal of psychotherapy is to facilitate constructive change. Change is multidimensional, and just as the meaning of "cause" varies according to the dimension of life that is addressed, so the meaning of change varies. Three broad types of causes are those associated with the inorganic, organic, and spiritual realms. These three types of causes lead to three related types of changes. Respectively, they are quantitative, qualitative, and creative changes.[59] All three types of change occur in psychotherapy.

In the theological language of Christian humanism, the process of change is described as a movement from a condition of estrangement to reconciliation. In general, the change is from a condition of dis-ease, dis-integration, and dis-harmony to a condition of greater health, wholeness, and peace, or more succinctly, from an estranged life to a more reconciled life.

The Multidimensionality of Health

The word "psychotherapy" denotes psychological treatment. The goal of treatment is healing, which is the restoration of health. Health, disease, and healing must each be described in terms of the multidimensional unity of life. "All dimensions of life are included in each of them. Health and disease are states of the whole person; they are 'psychosomatic,' as a contemporary technical term incompletely indicates. Healing must be directed to the whole person."[60] Ultimately health is experienced as self-integration of the individual as a whole, symbolized as the reconciling life. This requires character formation and self-transformation in moral and spiritual dimensions through time. A healthy life is self-integrated, self-creative, and self-transcendent.[61]

In the natural realm of life, health occurs in biological, psychological, and social dimensions as physical health, mental health, and mutually satisfying relationships. In the existential realm of life, health occurs in spiritual, historical, and moral dimensions experienced as faith, hope, and love. Expressed in trinitarian terms, the goal is a person (body-mind-spirit) who is reconciled with God, who emulates the life of Christ, and whose spirit is guided and sustained by the Spirit.

The Goal Is a Reconciling Life

Multiple purposes have been advocated as the ultimate goal of the Christian life: life in Christ (Paul), a justified life (Luther), a sanctified life in the Spirit (Wesley), a redeemed life (Schleiermacher, Troeltsch), an unambiguous life (Tillich), an authentic life (Bultmann, Helminiak), a life according to the image of God (Howe), and a reconciling life (Olson). A Spirit-centered wholeness has been advocated as the goal of Christian counseling by Howard Clinebell.[62] Each of these goals could be applied to inform the purpose and practice of both psychotherapy and pastoral counseling.

According to the form of Christian humanism presented here, the central attribute of the *imago Dei* is the liberating potential to live a more reconciling life. Humans actualize the image of God within them insofar as they are liberated to reconcile one another. To facilitate actualization of this potential, the ultimate purpose of psychotherapy becomes a more reconciling life. The progressive tense ("reconciling") denotes two meanings: (1) that reconciliation is a lifelong process and a dynamic experience, and (2) the goal is not merely personal reconciliation, but to become an agent of reconciliation with and for others. Personal transformation is expressed in action leading to social reformation.

As the central concept of Christian humanistic therapy, reconciliation has been defined as follows: "Reconciliation is a multidimensional, unifying experience of resolving conflicts within and among alienated persons, whose being and relations are transformed through the power of forgiveness, and by the process of compassionate confrontation into a healing reunion of love, justice, and peace for the sake of which one decides to intentionally act."[63]

The Christian humanistic therapy presented here affirms that the general purpose of psychotherapy and counseling is to facilitate a liberating experience of reconciliation through the process of compassionate confrontation of client incongruities in the context of a Spirit-centered therapeutic relationship. Therapy may be construed as a process of dealing with some of the personal obstacles to living a reconciling life, including both self-deception and pride, as primary disorders of the intellect, and will.

A more reconciling life is indicated by a person who is becoming wiser, more compassionate and courageous, joyful and thankful, ethical and sanctified, and an active agent of reconciliation with others to reform political and economic institutions consistent with the vision of a reconciled society.[64] Living in a graced freedom, and being liberated from preoccupation with personal sin and guilt are further marks of the reconciling life. Unlike the apostle Paul, Jesus was never weighed down by a burdensome sense of sin.[65] His whole being was formed and suffused by his consciousness of God's merciful love. His embodiment of both human and theological virtues makes him an effective moral ideal to emulate.[66] He is the Christian paradigm of a reconciling life.

The reconciling life is a symbol for the Christian way of being and becoming. It refers to a life that is qualitatively different and of higher value as a result of being transformed by God's grace through one's encounter with Jesus of Nazareth, with his person and life, with his message of liberation and his ministry of reconciliation. In this experience of the unity of multiple dimensions, one senses the beatitude God intends for humankind. One becomes more whole and holy—a new being, a new creation, a new self.[67] In the psychological dimension of experience, the characteristics of a reconciling life include, but are not limited to, those attributed to a fully functioning person as described in client centered therapy.[68]

Principles of Therapeutic Change

Proposition Seven: *Christian humanism affirms a holistic, multidimensional, existential model of healing in spiritual, moral, and historical dimensions.*

Healing Is Holistic and Multidimensional

Most contemporary schools of psychotherapy minimize medical healing and eliminate the healing function of religious faith. The first is usually a matter of practice rather than of theory; the second is a matter of principle.[69] Christian humanism emphasizes the experience of holistic healing in all six dimensions of life, especially in the existential realm involving spiritual, moral, and historical dimensions.

Healing in one dimension can accelerate healing in another dimension, just as disease in one can create distress and dysfunction in another. Nevertheless, health may predominate in one dimension, but not in another. Examples are the healthy athlete with all the symptoms of neurosis, or the social activist whose involvement masks an existential despair.[70]

To say that all dimensions are interdependent is to affirm that they are both independent and dependent relative to one another. Their relative (not absolute) independence demands a comparatively independent way of healing, which means in some cases predominantly biological, psychological, or spiritual approaches to healing, and in other cases, combinations of approaches.

Spiritual Healing

Human experience and therapeutic change occur in the spiritual dimension of life as surely as they occur in other dimensions. The spiritual dimension of change involves *changes in felt meanings and ultimate concerns, in one's consciousness and way of being and relating.* All four concepts denote the experiential and existential nature of spiritual transformation. Spiritual meanings and ultimate concerns are not merely cognitive beliefs; they are convictions and commitments that are felt deeply, and known intuitively as well as rationally. Transformed by the Spirit, one develops a more sustained consciousness of God that is illustrated most clearly in the life of Jesus. One's way of being is transformed so that the apostle Paul can claim that a disciple of Jesus becomes a new creation as found in 2 Corinthians 5:17.

Although there are many similarities between healing within the psychological and spiritual dimensions of life, there are also important differences. These differences are sometimes expressed in contrasts between psychotherapy and spiritual direction, and particularly in terms of their focus, goals, and their respective interventions.

One illustration of differences in focus is the distinction between neurotic and existential anxiety. The independence of psychological and religious approaches to healing can be construed in terms of specializations with these different types of anxiety. Psychotherapy addresses neurotic anxiety, whereas religious healing addresses existential anxiety through prayer, sacrament, spiritual direction, and pastoral counseling.[71]

Just as the dimensions of life are not antagonistic to each other, so the various approaches to healing do not need to impede each other. The correlate of the multidimensional unity of life is the multidimensional unity of healing. No individual can exercise all the ways of healing with competence and authority, although more than one way may be used. But even if there is a union of different functions, for example, of the priestly and medical functions in one individual, the functions must be distinguished and neither confused with the other; nor may one be eliminated by the other.[72]

Healing of Character

Human experience is a moral experience just as it is biological, social, psychological, spiritual, and historical. It is particularly the moral and spiritual dimensions of human experience that distinguish life as uniquely and fully human. A moral life is a meaningful life, and a good life worthy of living. That being so, a religious theory of psychotherapy may look to *moral experience* as a further medium of knowledge relevant to understanding the reconciled life and to comprehending the experience of reconciliation that occurs through counseling and other human relationships.[73] "This involves a transformation of character as well as conduct, a change in conscience as well as cognitions, a reorientation of values in conformity with the will of God with the help of God's reconciling grace. This moral emphasis suggests a character-conduct therapy in contrast to cognitive-behavior therapy."[74]

A moral perspective on therapy is not the same as *moralism.* Therapy cannot be reduced to providing consultation about moral issues, but neither can therapy ignore moral issues and ethical dimensions of human problems in living.[75] The risk involved is that therapy becomes moral instruction or moralizing. Depth psychology has shown us that unconscious motives for personal decisions are not transformed by imposed moral commandments,[76] nor are unconscious defense mechanisms relinquished by rational argument or moral persuasion.

> An increase in awareness, freedom, relatedness, and transcendence does not imply a decrease in vital self-expression; on the contrary, spirit and life in the other dimensions are interdependent . . . directing one's life toward an integration of as many elements as possible is not identical with an acceptance of repressive practices as they are used in Roman asceticism as well as in Protestant moralism. The uncovering of the distorting consequences of such repression has been shown most convincingly by analytic psychotherapy and its application to the normal human being.[77]

Fragmentary Healing Through Time

It takes time to heal emotional wounds. Instantaneous insights resulting in immediate, complete change are rare occurrences in psychotherapy, just as immediate, emotional conversions in religion are rarely sustained in enduring behavior change. Psychotherapy is a gradual process of self-exploration and a new experience requiring time to assimilate.[78] An implication of the time required for clinically significant and sustained improvement is that the very brief forms of crisis intervention provided through health maintenance organizations is a flagrant form of health care rationing to the detriment of those who seek the benefits of medically necessary psychotherapy.[79]

Healing has a historical dimension and healing is often incomplete.

> Healing is fragmentary in all its forms. . . . Not even the healing power of the Spirit can change this situation. Under the condition of existence it remains fragmentary and stands under the "in spite of," of which the Cross of Christ is the symbol. No healing, not even healing under the impact of the Spiritual Presence, can liberate the individual from the necessity of physical death. Therefore, the question of healing, and this means the question of salvation, goes beyond the healing of the individual to the healing through history and beyond history; it leads us to the question of Eternal Life as symbolized by the Kingdom of God. Only universal healing is total healing—salvation beyond ambiguities and fragments.[80]

Processes of Therapeutic Change

Proposition Eight: *A central mechanism of therapeutic change is the experience of compassionate confrontation through the medium of a Spirit-centered therapeutic relationship.*

A generic statement of the ultimate goal of psychotherapy is "to facilitate constructive change in order to improve the client's quality of life." In Christian anthropology, constructive change is described as the process of *conversion*.[81] The stereotyped view of conversion as a singular, life-changing experience is much less common than an experience of gradual change through time. A developmental perspective seems more accurate and necessary to understanding faith formation, character formation, and spiritual growth. Moreover, a dimensional perspective helps one to comprehend that changes occur in biological, psychological, and social dimensions as well as spiritual, moral, and historical dimensions. The mutual interdependence of all dimensions suggests that change in one dimension of life impacts other dimensions and the person as a whole through the self-structure. Moreover, the holistic principle of Christian personalism points to the whole person as the agent of change. As with the process of psychotherapy, conversion is an experience of the person as a total unity in multiple dimensions through time. Conversion is an experience of transformation of the individual as a whole.

A fundamental principle of Christian humanism is that the experience of *compassionate confrontation* in a therapeutic relationship facilitates constructive change. In response to perceived genuineness, acceptance, and empathic understanding, individuals are liberated from the need to defend their sense of worth by clinging to the self-deceiving illusions they hold about themselves. Two terms expressing the significant role and transforming power of compassion are love and forgiveness. They are central concepts in the teachings of Jesus. Loving and being loved, forgiving and being forgiven, are also potent mechanisms of therapeutic change.[82]

Christian humanism is not a naïve or sentimental view of the human capacity to change. Rather, it recognizes the depth of human alienation and the need to confront individuals with their self-serving motives and rationalizations, and with the negative impact of their attitudes and behavior upon others in addition to their self-destructive consequences. Individuals who have been avoiding responsibility must be shown that even avoidance is a choice with consequences.

Individuals in therapy need encouragement in order to find the courage to accept their disowned past, to cope with their distressing present, and to anticipate an unwanted future or to envision a better one and make it happen. Reality is not easy to accept, and often painful to confront. But as with the pain after surgery, the stress of confronting reality holds the promise of potential healing. The experience of compassion is encouraging, and compassion enables and motivates one to be empathic toward self and others.

One cannot expect to facilitate an experience of compassionate confrontation with reality and self apart from a *therapeutic relationship*. The central role of the client-therapist relationship has been affirmed by most schools of psychotherapy, including integrative theories.[83] While there is disagreement whether a therapeutic relationship is sufficient for a positive outcome, based upon both their clinical experience and empirical research, most therapists affirm that it is necessary.[84]

The elements of a therapeutic relationship are well known: positive regard and empathic understanding by a therapist who is genuine and capable of communicating these attitudes and conditions concretely and effectively so the client experiences them. The current research on the *therapeutic alliance* adds the client's attachment to, and identification with the therapist, and patient-therapist agreement on both goals and strategies expressed in the form of a therapeutic contract.[85]

The therapeutic relationship and alliance facilitate the operation of mechanisms of psychological change. These include

> recognition that one has a problem, understanding it's origins and implications, feeling the emotions that surround it, honestly exposing one's soul to an empathic human being or in a group of supportive peers, suffering tragedy or loss, reenacting one's concerns in dramatic form—all these and other experiences trigger important shifts in the structure of psyche.[86]

A central mechanism is a change in one's *self-concept* through the self-explorations facilitated by a therapeutic relationship.

The empirically established elements of a therapeutic relationship and therapeutic alliance are affirmed by Christian humanistic therapy. However, by virtue of its existential model, additional therapeutic conditions are stressed for a therapeutic outcome with Christian clients. These are the experiences and development of faith in the spiritual dimension, love in the moral dimension, and hope in the historical dimension, including a sense of one's place in history and one's personal destiny. These existential dimensions are symbolized by emphasizing a Spirit-centered therapeutic relationship.

A *Spirit-centered* therapeutic relationship includes consciousness of the sacred, spiritual dimension of life as an essential condition in addition to empathic understanding, unconditional positive regard, and genuineness experienced by the client.[87] Christian humanistic theory construes the therapeutic relationship as a medium of the liberating experience of reconciliation. In this respect, the therapeutic relationship functions as an ordinary means of grace. Guided and sustained by the Spirit, it becomes both a sacramental and healing experience. A basic principle here is that an individual's potential to become a more reconciling person can be actualized only in those who have experienced the reality of a reconciling relationship, one form of which is the therapeutic relationship. People must be loved in order to become more loving toward themselves, others, and God. They must experience compassion in order to become more compassionate. A Spirit-centered therapeutic relationship is an experience of compassion.

A Spirit-centered therapeutic relationship is grounded in a *theonomous psychology,* which expresses in its creations an ultimate concern and a transcending meaning, not as something strange or foreign, but as its own spiritual ground and depth dimension.[88] By implication, theonomous psychotherapy is psychotherapy conducted under the impact of the Spiritual Presence. It is a Spirit-sustained and Spirit-guided therapy. It suggests that the direction toward which all potentialities shall be developed is a more reconciling life experienced presently within the realm of God's grace, and expressed symbolically in Jesus' religious vision of the kingdom of God. A reconciling life is the ultimate goal of Christian humanistic psychotherapy.[89] Christian humanism helps the therapist and client to discover, explore, and experience the spiritual dimension of healing as its depth dimension known in the therapeutic experience of reconciliation.

According to Christian humanism, the central source of healing is not the human therapeutic relationship. Rather, the therapeutic relationship is viewed as a medium of reconciliation whose ultimate source and power is not human but divine. Christians claim that the life and death, and the message and ministry of Jesus of Nazareth, revealed the power and love of God for all humankind. Therein lies the Christian foundation for human dignity, the cause of all Christian courage, and the source of all Christian hope: God's creating, redeeming, and sustaining love. The decisive revelation of this divine, healing love in Jesus of Nazareth, has been the basis for the claim of his uniqueness affirmed in the title, Jesus the Christ. The "Christ" is the Greek translation of the Hebrew term "Messiah." These terms connote the anointed one who saves.

To save is to heal. The root word *(salvus)* is the same for both terms. The Christian term of *salvation* is rendered appropriately as a therapeutic experience. The healing impact of one's encounter with the person and message of Jesus is that one experiences a changed awareness and feeling, a fundamentally different perception and purpose of life, a transformed orientation in thought, action, and relationships. According to the liberal Catholic theologian, Hans Küng, Christian humanism liberates and empowers people to experience their true humanity rather than creating for them something new and altogether different.[90] This is a qualitative and creative change.[91] The transformation of ordinary self-consciousness into God-consciousness is both liberating and healing.[92]

In more contemporary theological language, the central process of change highlighted by Christian humanistic therapy is the client's transition from a condition of estrangement to reconciliation. This is both a personal transformation and social reformation in which individuals and societies are reoriented to a renewed covenant with God, and consequently with one another and with themselves in a nurturing, communal life of love, justice, and peace.

The initial condition of estrangement is a multidimensional experience, which occurs in social, personal, and spiritual realms. Individuals are estranged from others, from their own true selves *(imago Dei),* and from God as the ground, power, and meaning of their being. "The central experience of the Christian faith may be described as the transformation of these three forms of estrangement by a new reconciliation with other persons, with ourselves, and with God . . . ."[93] These terms—estrangement and reconciliation—have an experiential reference, which for many people is no longer suggested by traditional concepts of sin and salvation.

Ian Barbour makes two additional points about this central transforming experience of reconciliation. The movement toward a more reconciled condition is both gradual and partial rather than sudden and total. "This reorientation must never be claimed as a completed accomplishment, but as a new possibility—the genuinely creative possibility for one's life, a pattern of existence of which one sees glimpses in one's own life and the life of others."[94] Life remains an ambiguous struggle requiring continued dependence upon God.

Stages of Therapy

Proposition Nine: *The process of psychotherapy may be construed in a teleological and voluntaristic theory of change that occurs in five stages of decision making and in seven stages of change from both the client's perspective and the therapist's functions.*

The teleological and voluntaristic nature of change highlight the relative freedom of the individual to pursue goals and to make deliberate choices as an agent of change. From this perspective, psychotherapy is defined as essentially a therapeutic relationship that facilitates a decision making process in which individuals deliberate about alternative ways of being and relating, and through which they eventually make a decision in favor of a particular alternative for the sake of which they subsequently and intentionally act. Consistent with this definition, an intermediate goal of psychotherapy is to help clients make wise decisions. Their decisions may be construed as telosponsive.[95]

Therapeutic change occurs through the *process of decision making.* The client makes a decision to resolve a dilemma or to solve a particular problem in a concrete life situation. Effective psychotherapy helps the client to make good decisions that ameliorate their suffering and enhance their quality of life. Accordingly, the stages of psychotherapy can be construed as stages of decision making.[96] One begins by appraising the challenge. This includes determining if the risks are serious if one does (or does not) change. Second, one surveys alternative, available solutions to assess which ones are acceptable means for coping with the challenge. In the third stage, one weighs the alternatives considered in terms of one's values and anticipated benefits and costs. In the fourth stage, one makes a commitment to implement the better alternative and to allow others to know of one's commitment. In the fifth stage one adheres to the decision based on the intended and experienced benefits, as well as the unintended effects.

The decision making process is not merely, or even primarily, an intellectual and detached weighing of alternative courses of action. Nor is making a decision a deliberate process of forcing oneself to choose. As in experiential psychotherapy, "choice is viewed as coming out of an open, patient, intuitive consideration of the range of one's current experiencing."[97] Decisions must be grounded in the felt meanings of one's actual experience.

Writing from the *subjective perspective* of the client's internal frame of reference, Carl Rogers suggested in his earliest formulation that the process of change in client-centered therapy occurred in twelve stages. About twenty years later, based on further research and clinical experience, he simplified these to seven stages of change.[98] These stages of change are construed in terms of the exploration of one's experience or perceptual field. "In general, the exploration of the perceptual field tends to move from others to self, from symptoms to self, from surface concerns to deeper concerns, from past to present, from negative to positive, and from experiences in awareness to experiences that have been denied to awareness."[99] Construed phenomenologically, therapy is described and understood more completely because the person is appreciated more fully as the one who learns to trust one's experience of meaningful feelings as a source of guiding values for liberating decisions and reconciling relationships.

Viewed in terms of the *therapist's functions,* the decision-making process occurs through seven generic stages of psychotherapy which can be summarized as follows:

1. establish rapport,
2. conduct a multidimensional assessment,
3. encourage the client's commitment to the treatment goals and strategies derived with the client,
4. implement the treatment plan,
5. evaluate progress,
6. continue or modify the plan as indicated, and
7. terminate therapy.

PRACTICE OF THERAPY

Christian humanism leads to a form of integrative psychotherapy guided by the purpose of encouraging change in the direction of a more reconciling life. This theory does not prescribe a restricted set of techniques. A variety of therapeutic strategies that focus on one or more of the six dimensions of experience are employed in a flexible approach tailored to each individual client.

Establish Rapport

The goal of the first stage is to establish rapport by being fully present to the client's experiencing. Rapport is facilitated by the therapeutic *attitudes* of empathy, genuineness, and positive regard, all of which are communicated through the standard listening *skills* of reflection, paraphrasing, and amplifying of the client's felt-meanings. These attitudes and skills encourage the client to experience, express, and explore the meaning of their experience, their perceptions and thoughts, intentions and goals, decisions and actions, and their past and present relationships. In this human encounter between authentic persons, trust and hope are instilled as relevant information is disclosed and processed through reflective dialogue.[100]

Conduct a Multidimensional Assessment

Assessment of both natural and existential realms of experience is essential in order to describe and understand the client, to ameliorate their suffering, and to help them experience an improved quality of life. The natural realm of biopsychosocial dimensions can be summarized in a DSM diagnosis or as an International Clinical Diagnosis (ICD). Assessment of the existential realm of spiritual, moral, and historical dimensions requires additional evaluation.

The biopsychosocial assessment includes the biological dimension. This dimension is assessed through medical examination and neuropsychological testing to rule out physical causes. An example from clinical health psychology is to rule out a tumor as a cause of headaches before proceeding on the assumption they are tension headaches. Another illustration is to rule out hypothyroidism as a cause for clinical depression. In the psychological dimension, all four domains are assessed: cognitive, affective, conative, and behavioral. The person's readiness to change, and degree of self-awareness, their self-concept, and self-esteem are important elements to explore, along with cyclical patterns of maladaptive expectations and experiences. In the social dimension, past and present interpersonal relationships are explored to assess core conflictual relationships. Interviews with significant others usually provide helpful information, and may indicate marital or family therapy as the treatment of choice. Analysis of the interpersonal dynamics of transference and countertransference is also relevant, though less central than in psychoanalytic therapy.

Assessment in the spiritual dimension focuses on the person's

- religious life history
- present identification with a particular faith tradition
- attitudes toward faith tradition
- degree of present involvement in a faith community
- perceived faith resources and religious barriers to growth and health
- stage of faith development,[101]
- current practice of spiritual disciplines
- ultimate concerns and spiritual strivings[102]

Inventories can be useful to assess levels of spiritual development, including the capacity to forgive self and others.[103]

In the moral dimension, the stories clients relate in therapy, their attitudes, and actions are sources for identifying their dominant values. Kohlberg's stages of moral development can provide a framework for assessing a client's status in this dimension. Explicit dialogue about implicit duties, virtues, and values raise ethical questions concerning the good life, what one ought to do, and who one should become. What are the relevant moral issues? What are the client's hierarchy of values, ultimate loyalties, characteristic virtues, and felt obligations? Is the client competent in moral reasoning to resolve ethical dilemmas?

Whether clients are oriented primarily toward the past, present, or future can be inferred from interviews to assess their state in the historical dimension. It is also desirable to assess which factors in the past or present seem salient as predisposing, precipitating, reinforcing, or primary causes. It is especially important to assess the individual's intentions and goals in a teleological approach such as Christian humanism. Present experience is bracketed by both memories of the past and strivings toward the future. Personal strivings are likely to express one's spirituality, which is characterized by ultimate concerns and goals.

Encourage the Client's Commitment to the Treatment Plan

One of the causes of premature terminations of therapy is that the client is neither ready to change nor prepared to change. An assessment of the client's readiness is essential. Even if the client wants to change, another reason for therapy drop outs is that the client has insufficient commitment to a relevant treatment plan developed collaboratively. The individualized treatment plan addresses the client's problems and needs, and it takes into account realistic limitations as well as available resources. Time needs to be spent showing clients the connections between their symptoms, distress, and its causes as they relate to the treatment goals and strategies.

Collaborative goal-setting is also vital to developing a therapeutic alliance and contract. Moreover, treatment goals must be clear, attainable, and sufficiently "measurable" so both the client and therapist can determine if and when the goals are achieved. Consistent with the principle of shaping behavior by successive approximations to the desired goal, it is usually helpful to begin with realistic goals that are likely to yield success early. A therapy-by-objectives approach seems an appropriate model for case-management purposes,[104] consistent with the teleological model of Christian humanistic therapy, so long as objectives are defined in all six dimensions of experience.

Although the course of therapy is a deliberate and goal-oriented process, change is not limited to, nor does it occur primarily in, cognitive or behavioral domains. As noted previously, a client's experience of compassionate confrontation in a therapeutic relationship is postulated as a central mechanism of change. This principle expresses the experiential emphasis of Christian humanistic therapy, and its appreciation for the client's emotional experience and its facilitation. Much of the focus of therapeutic work is upon the emotional meanings of the client's experiences. The therapeutic relationship is a medium for a corrective emotional experience,[105] not merely a means for effecting insight, cognitive restructuring, or behavioral change. Emotions are often the core of a complex of ideas, as Carl Jung suggested. Emotions are motivating, often problematic, but also function as indicators of an individual's needs, values, and the quality of their encounters with others.

Implement the Plan

A variety of strategies can be applied to implement the treatment plan. A generic approach is to construe the course of treatment as a problem-solving and decision-making process.[106] Both direct and indirect approaches can be used to help clarify what the client wants and needs relative to what is achievable. After defining the problem and evaluating alternative solutions, clients are encouraged to make a decision in favor of a particular alternative, for the sake of which they are encouraged to intentionally act. They are supported as they take action and helped to evaluate the outcomes of their action. Much of the work of therapy is helping clients persist in their efforts to change despite their fears and ambivalence, and the obstacles or set backs. Presented graphically, therapeutic progress is more of a gradually ascending, saw-toothed curve than a continuously ascending, straight line.

Both in the formulation and implementation of the treatment plan, therapists and clients can draw upon their respective "spiritual intelligence." Core components of spiritual intelligence include

1. Transcending the physical and material realm
2. Experiencing heightened states of consciousness
3. Sanctifying everyday experience
4. Utilizing spiritual resources to solve problems
5. Being virtuous[107]

Evaluate Progress

The process of assessment is continuous in psychotherapy. As alternative solutions are attempted, the client's feelings and attitudes are explored to help process the change taking place. The progress can be evaluated in terms of the level of goal attainment relative to the treatment goals previously set. Goal Attainment Scaling is a practical instrument for measuring both qualitative and quantitative goals set in all dimensions with a wide range of clients with different problems in a variety of settings.[108] Repeated measures of the frequency, intensity, and duration of symptoms such as anxiety and depression help to assess therapeutic progress.

Evaluation of therapeutic progress requires clear evaluation criteria. Insofar as the general goal of Christian humanistic psychotherapy is a client who experiences a more reconciling life, the indicators of the latter become relevant outcome criteria. Thus one looks for an increase in wisdom, compassion and courage, joy and gratitude, rational decision-making, ethical conduct, and caring about others. Insofar as the goal of therapy is to assist the client to make a good decision, the criteria for an effective decision-making process are germane.[109]

Continue or Modify the Plan and Strategies As Indicated

The purpose of continuous assessment of progress is to help the client and therapist make necessary modifications in the treatment plan and strategies. The initial treatment goals may have been too high or too low, or the strategies too difficult for the client to apply and perform. Skills-training may be prerequisite to attainment of some treatment goals. Realistic expectations help to prevent premature discontinuation of efforts required in a particular strategy of change. The standard procedure of goal-attainment scaling includes estimation of five levels of expected outcome for each treatment goal ranging from "much less than expected" to "much more than the expected level of outcome."

Taper and Terminate Therapy

Although the client is presumably improved at the time of termination, ending a therapeutic relationship is usually a cause of ambivalent feelings. The therapist has become a confidant and source of significant support for the client. Ending this relationship may involve both anticipatory grieving and anxiety. Gradually increasing the length of intervals between sessions (tapering) is one practical solution, and scheduling follow-up sessions is usually advisable. It is important that the client knows he or she may return if needed.

An important part of preparation for the ending of therapy is to apply strategies that facilitate transfer of training and relapse prevention, so that what the client has learned, experienced, and practiced throughout the course of therapy can be applied and maintained in their own life. The client's practice of decision making and other skills should contribute to his or her confidence to "go it alone."

Techniques

Christian humanistic therapy does not limit interventions to a particular set of strategies. A variety of therapeutic techniques can be applied to assist clients to explore and express their thoughts, feelings, and intentions, to make decisions, and to take action in order to solve their problems, and to reduce or cope with their suffering. Most of the empirically established, efficacious techniques used by psychotherapists can be applied selectively to address clients' problems. The variety of techniques derived from the standard biopsychosocial model and psychotherapy research can be incorporated, and need not be repeated here. Rather, some techniques will be suggested that address the existential realm involving the spiritual, moral, and historical dimensions of life. The approach taken is eclectic, but not an a-theoretical, technical eclecticism. Christian humanistic therapy is a form of integrative psychotherapy of an interdisciplinary nature.

In the *spiritual dimension,* the client can be encouraged to seek spiritual direction to acquire and develop spiritual disciplines that foster spiritual healing and growth.[110] The classical spiritual disciplines are prayer, meditation, study, service, worship, celebration, confession, guidance, solitude, and simplicity.[111] All of these may help to create, sustain, and strengthen faith, which is the primary domain of the spiritual dimension and a medium of healing. Therapeutic effects can be expected in the psychological dimension.

Prayer and meditation were central spiritual disciplines practiced by Jesus (e.g., Luke 3:21; 5:16; 6:12; 9:18; 11:1). As a devout Jew, Jesus is likely to have recited the Shema as a daily devotional expression of his monotheistic faith: "Hear, O Israel, the Lord our God is one Lord; and you shall love the Lord your God with all your heart and with all your soul, and with all your might" (Deuteronomy 6:4-5). In fact, Jesus cited this prayer as the first great commandment.[112]

The practice of meditation has been preserved and nurtured in the Catholic tradition in a variety of forms such as meditative reading of scripture *(Lectio Divina)* and contemplative or centering prayer.[113] Another variation of meditation is the use of "pneumogenic phrases."[114] (The Greek word *pneuma* signifies both spirit and breath.) Analogous to autogenic phrases,[115] which are physiologically directed suggestions (e.g., "my hands and arms are heavy and warm"), pneumogenic phrases are spiritually directed, but also yield a deeply relaxed body and a calm, quiet mind. The client is encouraged to repeat various biblically based phrases in a slow, silent manner. Examples of such phrases include: "to set my mind on the Spirit of God is life and joy and peace"; "the breath I breathe is the Breath of God"; "the Lord reigns, my heart is calm"; or "the love of Christ holds my life together." A variety of phrases may be taken from biblical passages, spiritual writings, and hymns, each selected according to the client's needs and preferences. One or more phrases may be repeated during a particular meditation. The phrases are repeated slowly and silently in a quiet place, sitting comfortably with eyes closed to facilitate focused attention and concentration. In addition, these phrases may be applied singularly and quickly in stressful situations to maintain self-control, to cope with anticipatory anxieties, and to inhibit negative self-talk and expectancies.

The use of scripture in psychotherapy and counseling has been debated for some time among Christian counselors. Some consider it inappropriate, and never to be used; others suggest it should be used with all clients; still others (including this author) recommend its judicious application.[116] Donald Capps has shown how to use proverbs in premarital counseling, the psalms in grief counseling, and Jesus' parables in marriage counseling. The parables are particularly effective for reframing perceptions through an indirective approach to counseling, which is distinct from both directive and nondirective approaches.[117] A thematic approach to the use of scripture in therapy has been presented by William Oglesby.[118]

In the moral dimension, techniques of value clarification and value modification are appropriate strategies. Helping clients experience themselves as responsible agents of their actions is facilitated by working through the steps involved in making a good decision. Since conduct discloses character and conscience, dialogue about the relationship among all three may be helpful. The Adlerian concept of a lifestyle analysis is relevant here, with special reference to the client's values and the ethical principles implicit in one's actions. Allowing clients to confess their "sins of omission and commission" is usually therapeutic, but may be done more meaningfully through religious rites or sacraments of reconciliation by referring them to competent clergy.

The concept of the will is central to both the moral dimension and personality dynamics. Strengthening and redirecting the will is an important part of therapy. Roberto Assagioli's techniques are germane here.[119] As the primary domain in the moral dimension is love, experiences which foster a more loving orientation are to be encouraged. These include social involvement in a religious community for worship, study groups, and social action to practice becoming a liberating agent of reconciliation for others. The experience of being loved by God, which occurs through faithful contemplative prayer, is a healing experience in part because it effects a union of the human will with the divine will of actualizing the liberating realm of reconciling love.

In the historical dimension, the relevant domain is hope as the antidote to despair. The development of hope is no quick and easy task. It takes both time and effort, faith and love. Andrew Lester has shown how clients project themselves into the future by creating "future stories." He presents a variety of specific strategies to generate and strengthen hope such as inviting the client to imagine what is coming in the future, using dreams and daydreams, free associations, guided imagery, and relating their future stories to the sacred story told in their faith tradition.[120] The principles and practices of narrative therapy are relevant to change in this historical dimension.

EVALUATION

Proposition Ten: *The efficacy of therapy guided by a Christian perspective has been documented in a few controlled, empirical studies.*

An assessment of any theory of therapy requires discussion of evaluation criteria as well as actual outcomes documented in empirical research.

Evaluation Criteria

Kurt Lewin once stated that there is nothing so practical as a good theory. But what constitutes a good theory? Several criteria have been offered. A *good theory* is important, precise and clear, parsimonious, comprehensive, integrative, operational, empirically verifiable, heuristic, and practical. By these criteria, Christian humanism can be judged as a potentially viable theory to inform the practice of psychotherapy. The central construct of reconciliation has been defined theoretically, and its existential dimensions have been described phenomenologically and grounded biblically.[121] However, to become a scientific theory it must provide operational definitions and empirically verifiable hypotheses. Operational definitions are being developed to allow measurement of changes in the direction of a more reconciling life. This research is prerequisite to achieving the goal of determining the antecedents and consequences of the therapeutic experience of reconciliation.

David Wells provided five criteria of a *satisfactory Christian anthropology*. These criteria are relevant to evaluating psychotherapy, which is guided by a Christian theory of personality. The criteria are:

1. It appreciates the uniqueness of the person as one made for relationship with God.
2. It preserves human worth and dignity.
3. It appreciates both the depths and heights of human potential (hence it is realistic, not pessimistic nor optimistic).
4. It relates persons to the created order in such a way that the realization of our full humanity is given high priority by affirming both the reality and the meaning of the self as related.
5. The view of human nature must be compatible with the understanding of divine nature, that is, with God's purposes, ways, and mode of communication in the world, as well as with the means of salvation God has provided for our sin and guilt.[122]

Since one of the intermediate goals of psychotherapy is to help clients make high quality decisions, the process criteria that define the latter may be used to evaluate the former. A good therapeutic outcome is a *high-quality decision* defined as a process involving seven steps:

1. Thoroughly canvass a wide range of alternative courses of action.
2. Survey the full range of objectives to be achieved and the values implicated by the choice.
3. Carefully weigh whatever you know about the costs and risks of negative consequences, as well as the positive consequences which could flow from each alternative.
4. Search intensively for new information relevant to further evaluation of each alternative.
5. Assimilate accurately, and take account of any new information or expert judgment to which you are exposed, even when the information or judgment does not support the course of action you initially prefer.
6. Reexamine the positive and negative consequences of all known alternatives, including those originally regarded as unacceptable, before making a final decision.
7. Make detailed plans and provisions for implementing or executing the chosen course of action with special attention to contingency plans which might be required if various known risks were to materialize.[123]

It is important to note that these criteria address the process of decision making. The outcome is not always under the decision maker's control.

Insofar as the general purpose of psychotherapy is to encourage a more reconciled life and reconciling relationships, the criteria defining the *traits of a more reconciled person* can be applied to evaluate outcome. Through the experience of solving their problems and reducing their distress, clients can become wiser, more compassionate and courageous, joyful and thankful, ethical and sanctified, and an agent of reconciliation with others. Presently these attributes or elements of the experience of reconciliation are theoretical. Research is being conducted using the Semantic Differential to determine the factors that individuals apply in their determination of the meaning of reconciliation. Factor analyses will serve as the basis for development of an empirical measure to assess change on this dimension from a state of being less reconciled to being more reconciled, and for the development of a reconciled personality inventory.

Construing reconciliation as a tripartite *attitude* involving cognitive, affective, and behavioral dimensions may be helpful both conceptually and empirically, since it invites an application of research on attitude change to therapeutic practice. Perhaps a *state/trait inventory* would distinguish temporary experiences of reconciliation from a more enduring disposition to be reconciling across situations with a variety of individuals. The eventual goal is to be able to evaluate outcomes of psychotherapy guided by this general purpose of attaining a more reconciling life.

Results

Controlled-therapy outcome studies have been conducted to evaluate the efficacy of Christian-based forms of cognitive-behavioral therapy[124] and pastoral counseling,[125] but the studies are few in number. Positive results have been reported relative to both no treatment and to standard forms of psychotherapy. It is not necessary to demonstrate that "Christian therapy" is superior to other established approaches. It is sufficient to show comparable results, and also reasonable to predict efficacious outcomes in light of the repeated findings of no significant differences among standard approaches to therapy.[126] The form of Christian therapy must be described in such studies to be clear about its goals, processes, and strategies.

The Christian humanistic theory of psychotherapy presented here awaits empirical testing.[127] Only indirect support exists as noted previously. Christian humanistic therapy is a form of integrative psychotherapy. To put this in perspective, most new approaches to integrative psychotherapy lack controlled research to support either their efficacy, their hypothesized mechanisms of change, or the specific constructs and combinations of techniques utilized.[128]

Insofar as reconciliation therapy includes already established elements, then extant research showing the efficacy of these elements provides indirect support for this theory. For example, as the experience of forgiveness is a salient mechanism of personal transformation from an alienated to a more reconciled state, the current empirical research on the therapeutic efficacy of forgiveness is relevant.[129] Additional research from which to derive empirically validated processes and techniques applied in a variety of therapeutic approaches has been summarized by Allen Bergin and Sol Garfield.[130] A practical discussion of common factors contributing to positive therapeutic outcome was provided by Garfield.[131]

Future Research

An interdisciplinary research agenda has been outlined to advance this theory philosophically, theologically, psychologically, and scientifically.[132] *Outcome evaluation* should be conducted with heterogeneous populations, and in a manner consistent with the teleological nature of both Christian psychotherapy and human behavior. An appropriate measure for psychotherapy outcome research is goal attainment scaling,[133] in addition to pre-post measures of psychological and spiritual well-being.[134]

Process research is equally relevant to assess actual stages of therapy and to identify the salient mechanisms and episodes of change. The discovery-oriented method,[135] which employs a "process diagnosis" of various types of potential change events, seems to be a fruitful approach for describing and understanding the client's experience in Christian humanistic therapy. An area for future research is to identify the various types of change events and their markers in all six dimensions of experience: biopsychosocial (natural) and moral-spiritual-historical (existential).

The research approaches to the discovery of process patterns and change mechanisms, which seem particularly promising and consistent with the experiential emphasis of Christian humanistic therapy, include task analysis and the use of patient and therapist experiencing scales. Task analysis is relevant because among the change episodes studied in this approach to psychotherapy research are resolutions of problematic emotional responses and problem-solving processes. Both types of episodes in therapy could be subsumed as "reconciling episodes," which are change events leading to personal transformation and improved relationships. Intensive and rigorous observations of clinically significant episodes of change in psychotherapy provide the basis for development of a science of psychotherapy characterized as a process of experiential change facilitated by a therapeutic relationship.[136]

POINTS OF DIALOGUE

With Other Religions

Various positions have been taken by Christians toward those of other religions. These range from an imperialist exclusivism to a more inclusive pluralism. Beyond these positions within Christianity are religious and cultural relativism. Christian humanism is pluralistic, humanistic, existential, postmodern, and ecumenical.

Christian humanism adopts a *pluralist perspective* on other world religions. It affirms that the Spirit of God was present in Jesus of Nazareth as the power of life bringing new being and meaning, and that this same Spirit is present among peoples and in religious groups not consciously Christian.[137] This does not make Christian humanism relativistic. Quite the contrary, it denies the relativist's claim that there is neither a universal human condition nor human essence, nor any unconditional human norms or ultimate religious truths. For the Christian humanist, the divine revelation and saving grace in Jesus as the Christ is decisive but not absolute, normative but not dogmatic, unique though not singular, an authoritative source of truth and grace which cannot be claimed in an authoritarian manner nor proclaimed in an intolerant tone.[138]

The term "Christian humanism" suggests both Christian and *humanistic criteria* for judging the value of religious beliefs and practices. An existential analysis of the human condition reveals fundamental needs and dimensions, anthropological constants, and existential questions as humanistic criteria. To be relevant, religious systems must address these human needs in all dimensions and provide relevant answers to the associated existential questions. As the essence of being human is expressed in the phrase "finite freedom," a religion that fosters human liberty and liberation is more worthy than one that rationalizes economic inequality or condones political oppression and religious intolerance.

Christian humanism adopts an *existential interpretation* of Jesus' message. An existential interpretation presents his message as an answer to existential questions. These questions address the nature of existence, the meaning of persons and their human potentials, the nature and purpose of healing, determining values, and the purpose of life in the face of human suffering associated with natural disasters, diseases, and social injustice. These are spiritual questions, for the spiritual dimension of life addresses the realms of both meaning and being, including ultimate concerns and values commanding loyalty and trust. Religions can be compared in terms of their respective answers to these existential questions.

In addition to being existential, humanistic, and pluralistic, Christian humanism is postmodern in its approach to both anthropology and other religions in ways analogous to a post-modern Christology:

a. in awareness that different periods and places will give rise to different anthropologies
b. in recognizing that complete rational proof or unambiguous revelation of true human nature is not possible, only probable
c. in rejecting intemperate and insistent claims for any Christian form of humanism that would reject the truths of other anthropologies in demeaning and exclusive claims, all in the name of a man named Jesus, who excluded no one.[139]

Christian humanism is also an *ecumenical* theology and anthropology. An ecumenical theme of reconciliation was affirmed by the Second Vatican Council in one of the sixteen documents produced, titled the *Decree on Ecumenism.* That document suggested that Protestant churches can engender a life of grace, and can be rightly described as capable of providing access to the community of salvation. Salvation is not limited to those who belong to the Roman Catholic Church.[140] This is a radical change from previous dogmatic views that declared no salvation outside the one true, holy Catholic Church. But what of the salvific nature of non-Christian religions? A more inclusive position is warranted, based on Jesus' good news about the liberating realm of God's reconciling love as a universal, inclusive reality expressed in his religious symbol of the kingdom of God,[141] and in his practice of open-table fellowship.

The multidimensional unity of life is another foundation for a more unifying world of theological diversity. The multidimensional unity of life leads to a multidimensional unity of religion as a realm of life. Nevertheless, unity is affirmed with diversity, not in spite of or instead of it.[142] The many exist with the One, and the One with the many.

A Christian humanist affirms that the Spirit of God is revealed through one's encounter with the Gospel of Jesus in the experience of faith, hope, and love nurtured by regular meditation on scripture, and by sustained worship, study, service, and prayer in the community of faith called the Church. The Christian faith affirms that Jesus Christ is the way, the truth, and the life (John 14:6). This faith may be confessed, however, without denying that the Spirit of God is revealed through the world's magnificent religions. The Spirit moves where it will, and the kingdom of God is present and manifest wherever humanity becomes more liberated and reconciled in a life of love, justice, and peace. The kingdom of God cannot be identified with the Christian Church, whose sign and servant it is called to become. Jesus' vision of the kingdom of God requires and maintains a prophetic witness and an appropriate humility in Christians' relations with those of other faiths.

With Judaism

Christianity has the closest affinity with Judaism by virtue of its historical origins within Judaism. Jesus of Nazareth was a Palestinian Jew. The present resurgence of interest in the historical Jesus (known as the Third Quest) has accentuated his Jewish identity. "If he belongs anywhere in history, it is within the history of first-century Judaism."[143] Moreover, the apostle Paul was a Hellenistic Jew prior to becoming the most noteworthy Christian missionary of the first century.

Aside from a common historical heritage, Christianity and Judaism share sacred scripture, a common monotheism, and a history of God's irrevocable covenants with Adam, Noah, Abraham, and Moses.[144] Christian humanists affirm with Jews that the Tanakh ("Old Testament") is the record of God's covenant with the people of Israel, revealing both what God is like and how people ought to live. Both religions emphasize the reconciling experiences of repentance and forgiveness, and a common striving for the sovereignty of God's redeeming love on earth. Moreover, both are grounded in a theology of hope. Christians share with Jews a vision of a society characterized by justice *(mishpat)*, compassion *(hessed)*, and peace *(shalom)*.[145] Liberation and reconciliation are central themes in both religious traditions. Moreover, both faith traditions depict human beings in search of an ultimate meaning for life, and both affirm that partial meanings (in terms of one's function or one's place in society) are not ultimately fulfilling, for these meanings are themselves open to question.[146]

Although there are fundamental similarities between Judaism and Christianity, there are also decisive differences, not the least of which is the Christian affirmation of God's covenant with humankind through Jesus as the Messiah, denied by those in the Jewish tradition. Moreover, the kingdom of God envisioned by both traditions was given a unique emphasis by Jesus of Nazareth.[147] Further differences between the two religions have been characterized (and caricatured) as contrasts between old and new covenants, Old and New Testaments, law and Gospel, letter and spirit, obedience and trust, works and faith. Their discontinuity has been emphasized over their continuity.

Tragically, their religious differences have been exploited as a cause of alienation between Christians and Jews, and the Holocaust of World War II forever changed Judeo-Christian relations. The Holocaust has had the redemptive effect of leading more Christians away from intolerant, exclusivist claims to a more inclusive position that sees Jews and Christians united in the kingdom of God.[148] Christian humanism honors the Jewish faith tradition as both its historical home and as a present pathway to reconciliation with God. It honors Islam and Eastern religions as additional authentic paths.

With Islam

Islam shares a monotheistic faith with Judaism and Christianity. The God of Moses and Israel, and the Abba of Jesus is the One called Allah by the prophet Muhammad. The Sufi tradition within Islam finds a parallel in the Christian contemplative tradition. Moreover, while the content of the moral law varies, Islam teaches the importance of living an ethical life. There are also shared images of the person as a body-mind-spirit unity.

There are differences of course. The Quran is sacred scripture unique to Islam. Islam agrees with Judaism that Jesus was a prophet. Christians acknowledge Jesus' prophetic role, but add more in their concept of Jesus as the Christ. Most Christians would not agree with Muslims that Muhammad is the seal of the prophets, although his prophetic teachings may be honored. Moreover, the Muslim's emphasis upon salvation via good works is a secondary theme in Christian thought. As expressions of sanctification, acts of love are presumed to be the consequence of the prior human act of faith, which in turn, is a response to God's decisive act of grace in the person of Jesus Christ.

With Hinduism, Buddhism, and Taoism

Christian monotheism distinguishes God as Creator from humans who are created. Christians are also likely to emphasize the concept of a reconciling relationship between human individuals and a personal God through a union of love between the human will with the divine will. This personal and interpersonal view of the relation between the human and the divine has been characterized as "dialogical personalism."[149] It differs from the Eastern idea of absorbing all individual beings into the totality of Being. The latter view is found in the pantheistic-monistic religions such as Vedanta Hinduism, in which individuality is an illusion submerged in the All, or essentially a part of the One, hence not a separate reality.[150] Nevertheless, the Reformed theologian, David Wells, finds the latter monistic theme evident in Christian theology and anthropology illustrated by Schleiermacher, Hegel, and Tillich; by process theologians such as Ogden, Williams, and Cobb; and in Pannenberg and Moltmann who view God immersed in social reality and moving the world toward a future which is qualitatively different from the present. Wells suggests these anthropologies lead to a loss of individuality of the human self.[151]

The Christian concept of God is both personal and theistic, expressed in concepts of being and person, purpose and will, and the "acts of God," which affirm an active, divine agency and the dynamic presence of God in human history. Nevertheless, this view cannot be rationalized simply by a personal, teleological anthropology or theology.[152] The question of human being is the question of being itself, which is the question of God. Thus, theology is grounded in ontology as well as historical revelation and religious experience. Moreover, both Catholic and Protestant theologies have affirmed the concept of God as the supreme being, being itself, or the ground, power, and meaning of being. Christian humanism is a psychology of being, consciousness, and meaning, so there is a basis for dialogue with the anthropologies of Eastern religions rooted in similar ontological assertions.[153] Moreover, the chief attributes of ultimate reality in Hinduism—infinite being, infinite consciousness, and infinite bliss *(sat, chit, ananda)*[154] are found in various Christian concepts of God. Thus in both religions the deepest human wants for eternal life, infinite knowledge, and endless joy are affirmed as attainable blessings. Whereas Christianity affirms justification by Grace through faith in love as necessary for people to experience these beatitudes, Hinduism claims people possess them naturally.

The principle of "inculturation" was accepted by the Roman Catholic Church in Vatican II, namely, the view that as a consequence of the incarnation itself, Christianity should accommodate itself to the cultural forms of different peoples. The Roman Catholic theologian, Raimundo Pannikar, expressed this principle in his book titled, *The Unknown Christ of Hinduism.*

The "Christ" who is unknown in all religions is the universal word or *Logos,* affirmed as the universal Absolute in Hindu philosophy. This ultimate reality incarnate in Jesus is incarnate in diverse forms and in other faiths; it is also the goal of every religion, though always beyond what is said or thought.

Moreover, corresponding to the personal theism of Christianity is *Isvara* as the portrait of ultimate reality in the Hindu religion, the personal aspect of Brahman, and the mediating reality between the transcendent ultimate and the world. The personalistic conception of ultimate reality as the One Self *(Atman),* who is incarnate as Krishna in the *Bhagavad Gita,* seems more compatible with Christian humanism than impersonal monistic views expressed in the Vedanta. Moreover, in personal terms, the Hindu and Christian God stands in relation to the world as an artist to one's handiwork. And in both religions, a triune conception of ultimate reality is expressed. In Hinduism, God is creator (brahma), preserver (vishnu), and destroyer (shiva); in the Christian tradition, God is creator (father), reconciler (son), and sustainer (Holy Spirit).

With its emphasis upon reconciling love, Christianity has been viewed as closer to the Hindu path of devotion *(bhakti-yoga)* than to the way of service *(karma-yoga),* the way of knowledge *(jnana-yoga),*[155] or to the way of meditation *(raja-yoga);* however, this comparison fails to appreciate the Christian emphasis upon good works and on social justice, as well as its rich tradition of contemplative prayer. Pannikar described three forms of Hindu spirituality as the way of obedient action *(karma-marga),* the way of devotion to a personal deity *(bhakti-marga),* and the way of contemplative knowledge or mystical communion through meditation *(jnana-marga).* He suggested that all three types of spirituality are incorporated into Christianity and reconciled in its trinitarian view of God.[156]

The Anglican theologian and religious relativist, Don Cupitt, finds in the Christian idea of incarnation an expression of the notion of the universal in the particular. In this respect, his view seems analogous in a formal sense to the Zen vision of finding nirvana in the midst of *samsara.* As with Zen, he also denies a substantial, individual self.[157] By contrast, Christian humanism is a form of personal realism.[158] The human self is not an illusion as suggested in Zen Buddhism. A unique personality as an individual reality in relation to others is a central construct in Christian anthropology. Nor can the Christian experience of reconciliation be comprehended as an enlightened detachment.

Like Gautama the Buddha, Jesus the Christ founded a movement for renewal and revitalization. Both Buddha and Jesus had a prophetic vision of reality that was contrary to the conventional wisdom of his time, though neither one sought to establish a new or separate religion. Both of these movements originated in the intense religious experience of their founders. These were also peace movements—promoting a way of peace with wisdom, compassion, and justice.[159] Neither one was engaged in a violent revolution to overthrow their governing authorities. The Christian and Buddhist movements were both nonviolent forms of resistance, reform, and renewal.

The Buddhist principle that suffering is an ontological reality was applied to the Christian concept of God by the Japanese theologian, Kazo Kitamori. In his view, suffering belongs to the essence of God, and the heart of the Christian gospel is the Cross, not the incarnation. Kitamori relates Lutheran Christianity with the Kyoto school of Japanese philosophy. The latter originated in the 1920s. It has its roots in Zen Buddhism and in modern European philosophies, especially existentialism.[160]

Insofar as the "Tao" is translated as the "Way," we may speak of the Tao of Christ. Indeed, as in Taoism, the earliest name for the Christian movement was the "Way" (Acts 9:2), and Christ is affirmed as the way, the truth, and the life (John 14:6). Jesus taught about a way of life, a path of inner transformation of the heart centered in God and expressed in acts of healing love and liberating justice. The Tao of Christ is a path of renunciation of a self-centered and materialistic existence. One must let go of selfish concerns for fame and fortune to become concerned ultimately with God's purposes in a Spirit-centered life.[161]

Insofar as the Tao is a metaphor for nature as ultimate reality, Christian humanism agrees that the natural world is real, but not the only, or ultimate reality. Nevertheless, the Taoist notion of balance between *yin* and *yang* is analogous in a formal sense to the Christian idea of reconciliation. Both concepts serve a synthesizing function, and they are symbols of the multidimensional unity of life and its dialectical dynamics.

This discussion suggests both similarities and differences between Christian humanism and the anthropologies of other religions of the world. Implicit in this discussion is the principle that although a spiritual life may be expressed and nurtured in a particular organized religion, it is restricted to none. In fact, a number of people have sought spiritual pathways outside an institutionalized religion. The so-called "New Age" spirituality is an example.

Since Dietrich Bonheoffer's call for a "religionless Christianity," there has been a growing recognition that many are unable to be "religious," that is, dependent upon a God of the gaps to fill the holes not yet claimed by science, or on a *deus ex machina* called upon to solve insoluble problems or to provide support in times of human failure. A religionless Christianity will be freed from individualistic piety and a supernatural metaphysic in favor of a this-worldly transcendence expressed in a new life for others. Only as a suffering servant to the secular world can Christians come of age and remain grounded and centered in the Being of God.[162] At a minimum, this is a call to dialogue with those of other faiths in a genuine ecumenical spirit of faith, hope, and love to bring forth mutual understanding, justice, and peace.

With Other Theories of Personality/Psychotherapy

The dominant approach in contemporary psychology is based on the tripartite biopsychosocial model. This model of human behavior is unsatisfactory insofar as it claims to represent either the whole person or the essence of human experience. While it envisions the person as a mind-body unity in relationships, secular psychology ignores or minimizes the dimensions of spirit, conscience, and time. In place of psychology's partial image of the person, a more inclusive and complete image is needed to describe and understand both the individual personality and human transformation, including the human predicament of estrangement and its essential need for the healing experience of reconciliation. The spiritual, moral, and historical dimensions of human experience must be included to understand what it means to be a person and what it means to be healed and whole.

Clinical psychology has fallen short of providing a description of authentic human experience and what it means to be. It has replaced reverence for the human spirit with a science of human behavior. Sustained care of the soul *(seelsorge)* has been reduced to modification of behavior; reconciliation has been rendered as adaptation; sanctification has been replaced by mental health. The *imago Dei* that defines human nature as including an essential spiritual dimension has been replaced by a psyche without spirit. Its secularized image of the self and ultimate goal of self-actualization make psychology a discipline lacking both spirit and character. Its miniature theories and parochial specialties have fragmented and demeaned human beings, and limited human potential by espousing psychological egoism and hedonism, expressed in the goal of the fulfillment of personal needs. To paraphrase Hamlet, there are more things in human nature than are dreamt of in secular psychology.

Similar to the hedonistic paradox, the autonomous quest for self-actualization will forever elude human hope. It is a Christian principle that those who seek to gain their life will lose it; those who lose their life for the sake of another find it. To paraphrase Reinhold Niebuhr,[163] the Christian truth is that egoism is self-defeating, and to give selfishness the appearance of normality or to claim it as a virtue[164] betrays a desperate and destructive illusion to which one can cling only with an uneasy conscience. Religious theories of human nature are needed to lift human aspirations to self-transcendence beyond self-actualization, to duty beyond desire, to purpose greater than pleasure, to virtue beyond need, to an open future over a confining past, to growth beyond adjustment, and to justice beyond accommodation.

The tri-dimensional (biopsychosocial) framework of clinical psychology provides a viable skeleton, but it lacks muscle and nerve, inspiration and transcendence. Vitality and values, meaning and purpose, will and spirit, conscience, character, and time are all concepts necessary to an accurate description and understanding of the person. Religious theories of personality may help scientific psychology recover the person. A basic premise of Christian humanistic theory is that psychotherapy must be grounded in a Christian understanding of human existence, about what it means to be human in a God-given world infused with grace. A theological anthropology is needed to restore the person to a rightful place in psychological theory and to a harmonious self-world relation.

A personalistic definition of psychology (e.g., Murray, Stern, Allport, Rogers, Maslow) varies considerably from the dominant view of psychology as "the science of behavior." A more appropriate definition of psychology as a truly human science is "the science of the person considered as having experience or as capable of having experience."[165] Stated more simply, psychology is the science of personal experience. Existential and phenomenological psychology make comparable efforts to reclaim both the unity and uniqueness of the individual as one who experiences life concretely and personally.

Personal experience is, however, only one aspect of human existence, hence more than a psychology of experience is needed. The person is complete and enduring, whereas experiences are fragmentary and transitory. The person is capable of having experience, but the person cannot be reduced to experience.[166] The latter reduction is the error of empiricism. A helpful correction is to define experience itself as a multidimensional unity with biopsychosocial and spiritual-moral-historical dimensions. Another correction is to strive to recover the person in psychological theory.[167] Affirming concepts such as a self-structure, self-concept, or identity helps to recover the person as a whole. An emphasis upon human agency and personal strivings that include spiritual aspirations are additional viable approaches.[168]

A Christian humanistic theory of personality and psychotherapy needs to be guided by the compassionate wisdom expressed in the liberating gospel of reconciliation taught by Jesus of Nazareth, as recorded and interpreted in the Synoptic Gospels. A *liberating psychology of reconciliation* is needed, informed by the liberating covenant of reconciliation expressed religiously and symbolically by Jesus in his teachings about life in the kingdom of God. The underlying norm for this theological anthropology called Christian humanism is the liberating covenant of reconciliation with God in Christ as our ultimate trust, loyalty, and concern. This theological norm is vital to transform secular psychology. Theology is not anthropology, but theology provides answers to anthropological questions, such as the purpose of life, the meaning of personhood, and the problem of human estrangement associated with finite freedom.[169]

To paraphrase the Catholic existentialist, Jacques Maritain, (using gender-neutral language), Christian humanism would (a) consider humans in all their natural grandeur and weakness, in the entirety of their wounded being inhabited by God, in the full reality of nature, sin and saint-hood. Such a humanism would (b) recognize all that is irrational in persons in order to tame it to reason, and (c) all that is suprarational, in order to have reason vivified by it and to open individuals to the descent of the divine into their personal lives. Its main work would be (d) to cause the Gospel leaven and inspiration to penetrate the secular structures of life—a work of sancti-fication of the temporal order.[170] This is a call for renewal of the social order based on a theistic and Christocentric vision. Christian humanism is also a vision for psychology as a truly human science of personal life understood as a multidimensional unity embedded in reconciling relationships trans-formed by the grace of God.

CASE STUDY*

The discourse analysis of the selected case is an example of the natural model of both personality and the process of therapeutic change. However, the psychological and social dimensions of experience are emphasized and the biological dimension is neglected. Moreover, within the psychological dimension, the cognitive domain of meaning is emphasized by discourse analysis over the affective and conative domains. Moral experience is par-tially recognized, but not the spiritual or historical dimensions. The absence of the latter two dimensions make the discourse analysis a less comprehen-sive interpretation than Christian Humanistic Therapy (CHT), which inte-grates both natural and existential models in a multidimensional view of change.

Alternative case formulations and intervention strategies are presented here in the multidimensional model of CHT. For the purposes of this discus-sion, it will be assumed this woman identifies with the Christian tradition.

Biological Dimension

Although the diagnosis was a major depressive episode, there were sug-gestions that this was not the first episode. Repeated episodes suggest a bio-logical component to the etiology of this mood disorder. CHT includes at-tention to the biological dimensions of symptomatology, etiology, diagnosis, and treatment. In terms of etiology, it is important to rule out a family his-tory of depression, hypothyroidism, and menstrual irregularities as potential biological factors. Treatment would include attention to this woman's sleep,

---

*The case selected is the analysis of a forty-two-year-old, married, employed, Caucasian woman suffering from a major depressive episode. Madill and Barkham (1997). From "Discourse analysis of a theme in one successful case of brief psychodynamic-interpersonal psychotherapy," *Journal of Counseling Psychology, 44* (2), 232-244.

eating, and exercise habits; monitoring her energy level, weight changes, menstrual cycle, and sexual desire and satisfaction; and compliance with medication prescribed at a therapeutic dosage. Her response to particular psychotropic medications taken during previous depressive episodes should be explored as a basis for psychiatric referral. CHT supports a combination of medication and psychotherapy for major depression.

Psychological Dimension

Although discourse analysis was presented as a case formulation devoid of "mechanisms of change hidden within the client's head" (p. 243),[171] in fact the analysis focused upon the client's expressions of her own internal attitudes toward herself and her mother. In this respect, the psychological dimension was addressed and internal constructs were actually employed.

In the case study, the psychological domain emphasized was primarily cognitive. The process of change was construed in terms of the client's use of language, and the cultural meanings expressed in the expectations and role obligations associated with her "subject position" as both a woman and a daughter (but not as a wife). There was little appreciation for the "common feeling language" that was utilized as one of the conversational strategies in the therapeutic protocol.[172]

Within the cognitive domain, CHT includes the concept of "meaning" as a basic personality structure, and perceiving and understanding are among the basic cognitive functions affirmed; however, CHT also includes in case formulations the affective, conative, and behavioral domains. All of these domains are relevant to the client's self-concept.

Within the humanistic tradition, the client's attitudes toward oneself are considered central to both the etiology and treatment of various forms of maladjustment.[173] From this perspective, this woman's mood improved primarily as a function of her changing self-concept. However, this change is not merely cognitive. Changes in self-concept are influenced by one's actual experience of self. This experiential dimension seems neglected in the discourse analysis due in part to the cultural linguistic definition of the self in terms of "subject position."

The experience of self is much deeper and richer than a functional-linguistic analysis could reveal, even if all ten presenting problems were subjected to discourse analysis. In other words, the psychological change that occurred in this case, occurred in multiple domains: that the client experienced a reorganizing of herself-structure, which entailed new perceptions about herself in terms of values and personal meanings, with related changes in her feelings, intentions, and actions. In terms of the central construct of CHT, the woman who was vulnerable to distress because of the estrangement in the psychological dimension between her self-concept and her felt experience (and her self-ideal) was restored to health through a greater reconciliation between her self-concept, her experience, and her self-ideal. She began to live as a more integrated, whole human being with greater self-acceptance as a responsible, decision-making agent of action.

This latter point reflects the emphasis of CHT upon the *unity of the personality* which appears absent in discourse analysis. The personhood of the client was not transparent in the abstract discourse analysis in part because of its focus on a particular thematic problem. A person cannot be defined by social positions, nor reduced to a particular problem, not even to a listing of ten presenting problems that this client was asked to provide in the pretherapy intake assessment. CHT is primarily person-centered rather than problem-centered. Who is the person that is changing? How is she experiencing the changes? Is she experiencing them passively or actively as a free and responsible agent of change?

Related to this discussion of the change in the client's self-concept is the authors' definition of the self as a particular manifestation of the acceptable descriptions available at a particular time and in a given culture. Although this reflects the role of culture as a limiting factor, Madill and Barkham's analysis approaches a form of *cultural determinism* that does not appreciate the capacity for creative transcendence and personal transformation possible in individuals who are liberated from the conventional wisdom of their time and culture, including socially prescribed roles. CHT affirms *conditional freedom* in lieu of any form of determinism. This notion is central to a voluntaristic theory of change, which affirms that human choices and decisions function as significant "causes" of change. The client in this case seems to be increasingly aware that she must make a choice between caring for her mother at home and her own mental health. She is experiencing the stress of making this decision and the burden of responsibility for making it.

This voluntaristic principle in CHT is expressed in its preference for the "telosponse" over "response" to highlight the whole individual as the agent of action and change. The favorable change this woman experienced may be construed as a function of the therapy that helped her transcend the culturally bound definitions of a "dutiful daughter" in favor of a more internal focus of her own self-definition. She made intentional decisions about those obligations she felt she should fulfill and how she should meet them. Her decision-making process was telosponsive: deliberative, intentional, and self-directed.

The reluctance of Madill and Barkham to consider hidden mechanisms of change within the individual results in an interpretation that is *lean on motivational constructs,* and especially those terms that express a voluntaristic-teleological theory of action, change, and human agency, such as the concept of "will." Although the client's decision to place her senile mother in a nursing home was mentioned, it was not explored dynamically in terms of the client's motivations for making her decision. The article mentioned reasons for the client's actions, but these were construed cognitively as expectations and role obligations. There was little or no analysis of any therapeutic dialogue that may have occurred about the client's needs and desires, about what she wanted to occur and willed to happen.

A Christian humanistic therapist would explore the client's needs in all six dimensions. The therapist could note the universal and innate nature of these needs, including the God-given need to be healthy, whole, and happy, and the deepest need for a reconciling life with God, others, and self. Therapeutic conversation could confront the client (compassionately) with the manner in which her goal of caring for her mother at home was frustrating her own needs; that her mother's need for care could be fulfilled in a nursing home; that the client's own need for positive regard from her mother, which was not fulfilled in the past, would not be fulfilled by her continued caring for her mother at home; that fulfillment of her need for self-esteem was overly dependent upon her performance in her role as caretaker (or "dutiful daughter"); or that she may have repressed her resentment associated with her frustrated needs, and experienced it as guilt and self-blame.[174]

In addition to discussion of her needs, a change in this woman's self-concept could be facilitated by teaching her the insights from psychological theories of stress. Construing her depression as a stress response could prove therapeutic. An understanding of the alarm-adaptation-exhaustion phases of the human stress response could help the client understand her depression not as the consequence of a moral failure to fulfill her obligations as a daughter, but as a natural (acceptable) response to an inordinate amount of sustained stress. We are, after all, not gods but mortals with limitations. Each of us has a unique threshold of stress, which the client has exceeded as the result of several years of caring for her mother at home, in addition to her full-time job, and her household responsibilities as a wife. For years she has carried an excessive workload, and the cumulative pressure has led to an understandable exhaustion expressed and experienced as depression. Each of us has a finite supply of adaptation energy.[175] Just as the banks of a river, which give it structure and direction, can erode from continuously flowing and turbulent waters, so too can our personality structure and our ability to cope erode from sustained exposure to pressure, frustration, and conflict. The psychophysiology of the stress response suggests its effects are cumulative and long term, as well as immediate. The long-term effects of protracted stress lead to the prediction that placement of her mother in a nursing home may not result in immediate reduction in the client's distress. This client's reduced depression occurred after about eight weeks. During some of this period her mother was apparently hospitalized.

The client in CHT would be encouraged to explore her decision according to the stages and criteria of decision making that lead to a good quality decision. She would be invited to determine the potential and probable risks, costs, and gains of continuing to care for her mother at home versus placing her in a nursing home. Moreover, she would be encouraged to consider other alternatives. For example, what about home health care provided by a visiting nurse or nursing assistant to feed and bathe her mother? Are there other relatives who might care for her mother for a period of time, either in their own home, or in the client's home to provide the client and her husband periodic relief and vacations? In terms of the spiritual dimension of CHT, the client would be encouraged to weigh her decision in light of the life God calls her to live, the paradigm for which is the life of Jesus of Nazareth. In her struggle to decide, she would be encouraged by the knowledge that one indicator of the image of God within her own life is her God-given capacity for weighing possibilities and deliberating about alternatives.

Social Dimension

The form of therapy reported in this case was a variant of psychodynamic-interpersonal therapy based on Hobson's conversational model. Three key features of this therapeutic approach are its emphases upon (1) the interpersonal origin of client problems, (2) the therapeutic relationship as the medium for modification of such problems, and (3) conversational strategies as interventions: posing hypotheses, use of negotiation, and metaphor, and development of a common feeling language. The therapeutic approach seems appropriate in light of the identified problem as a relational theme and the client's mood disorder. Implicit in the problem was the theme of alienation between the client and her mother. Absent from the discourse analysis was any consideration about potential alienation between the client and her husband.

The discourse analysis seemed to minimize the significance of the therapeutic relationship as the medium of change, and particularly the client's expression of affect as a mechanism of change. This relative neglect was evident in the analysis of mostly client statements rather than client-therapist-client triads. The extracts reported give the impression of a monologue going on inside the client's head more than a therapeutic dialogue. Moreover, the definition of dyads as a therapist comment followed by a client comment discouraged an analysis of the impact of the therapist's responses occurring after client statements. The definition and procedure for selecting therapeutic extracts in discourse analysis, in turn, limited the reader's ability to assess both the degree to which the client validated the therapist's reflections and interpretations, and any change episodes as a function of therapist statements.

The authors presented their discourse analysis as an alternative to case formulations based on hypothesized internal mechanisms of change. They also contrasted their approach with the developmental model of therapeutic change occurring through stages of assimilation. They did not contrast their own case formulation with the one that seems most consistent with the clinical approach taken in this case. In other words, their analysis neglects the salient conditions within the therapeutic relationship itself as a visible and interpersonal mechanism of change.

From the few therapist responses reported in the article, others discussed, and from the therapist's psychodynamic-interpersonal approach, it seems reasonable to hypothesize that the therapist was genuine, regarded the client positively, understood her empathically, and communicated these facilitative conditions concretely so the client perceived and experienced them. These defining elements of the therapeutic relationship have been affirmed consistently across theoretical orientations to psychotherapy as necessary to constructive personality change, and within the client-centered tradition, as generally sufficient.[176] The presence and effects of these facilitative conditions provide an alternative explanation of the client's change, which seems more compatible with an interpersonal approach than the explanation provided by discourse analysis; it is equally coherent, parsimonious, experiential, and relational.

To be more specific, the client may have cared for her mother with conscious or unconscious hopes that she might finally gain and maintain positive regard from her mother. The absence of this feeling of acceptance and love from her mother made her vulnerable, and ironically, dependent upon caring for her mother for the sake of the client's own self-esteem. Her childhood experience of being molested predisposed her to low self-esteem. Being vulnerable, the client tends to perceive her mother's actions as potentially threatening of even more rejection, failing to appreciate the limitations that her mother's dementia placed upon her ability to reciprocate. It is likely that the client did not feel either loved or understood by her mother.[177]

A loss of self-esteem has been implicated as a causal factor of depression, and in some cases, due to the person's felt inability to live up to personal aspirations or obligations. Depression is the emotional correlate or consequence of the loss of self-esteem. Moreover, a recovery or rise in self-esteem is considered a mechanism of therapeutic improvement.[178] These observations are offered to support another interpersonal explanation for the client's improvement, namely, that the therapist provided the client with the facilitative conditions characteristic of a therapeutic relationship, which helped her to experience an acceptance of self she had not experienced from her mother. This experience enabled the client to accept her own needs for well-being, and to make a decision that valued herself as well as her mother. The experience of being accepted in therapy enabled her to grow in her self-acceptance.

The facilitative conditions provided in a therapeutic relationship are summarized in CHT as "compassionate confrontation." This is an interpersonal construct which suggests that a major mechanism of change is the client's experience of a therapist who genuinely cares about her in a more unconditional manner than the client has experienced in other relationships. Simultaneously. the client is confronted with the estrangement she is experiencing both intrapsychically and in relationships with significant others.

The strength of discourse analysis is the way in which it highlights cognitive changes in the client's meanings associated with her social role as culturally defined. However, it does not seem to appreciate two salient interpersonal dimensions: the role of the client's relationship with the therapist in the process of change, and the client's relationship with her husband. Both are legitimate agenda for therapeutic conversation in CHT, since both are potential realms for change, and both fall under the rubric of interpersonal-psychodynamic theory.

The social dimension included in a case formulation according to CHT would alert the therapist to explore this client's relationship with her husband. Given the stress upon her from her full-time job, household responsibilities, and caring for her mother, another avenue of potential change is the role her husband plays. What household responsibilities does he assume? Does he help care for the client's mother? Does he resent his mother-in-law being in their home, and express that in his demands upon his wife? Is he jealous of the care and attention his wife gives to her mother? CHT would explore these and other aspects of his experience, and other family roles, rules, and communication patterns as potential factors contributing to the client's depression or its resolution. CHT emphasizes the person-in-relationships, which seems more compatible with an interpersonal-psychodynamic approach than discourse analysis. CHT may lead to individual sessions with the client's husband or conjoint sessions with this couple.

Moral Dimension

One of the reasons the authors seem to favor discourse analysis is that it appreciates the moral dimension. The client's depression was construed as a function of an ideological (ethical) dilemma of "duty to other" versus "duty to self. " Her condition was interpreted in terms of the cultural definition of a woman who should be selfless and live for others. This set of moral standards was presumed to be delimited by social convention and expressed in role expectations and normative obligations of daughters in relation to their mothers.

This appreciation for the moral dimension of the client's change is commendable, particularly in light of the way many theories of psychotherapy seem to ignore the moral dimension of change. Were the client a Christian, one could appeal to the mutuality affirmed in the second sacred commandment: Love your neighbor as yourself. The Christian humanistic therapist could point out that the commandment is not "love your neighbor [mother] more or less than yourself." The client's decision to place her mother in a nursing home could become morally defensible to her by construing it as fulfillment of the second commandment rightly understood as affirming equality and mutuality. In other words, the moral principle of altruism was dominant in this case, and as the woman began to accept an alternative principle of mutuality, she became less depressed. In transactional analysis terms, she moved from a "you count-I do not" position to "you count-I count."

The moral dimension appears to be more salient in this case than the discourse analysis discloses. Diagnostically, it appears that the client suffers from a form of existential anxiety called moral anxiety involving guilt and self-condemnation.[179] This form of anxiety results in despair as the primary symptom, manifested clinically as depression in this case. The fact that the client kept secret her childhood experience of molestation suggests unresolved guilt. In addition, the client feels guilty about her decision to place her senile mother in a nursing home. Her depression may function as self-inflicted punishment, the need for which is created by her sense of violating her own conscience. More specifically, she feels she has failed to fulfill her ideal image of what a good daughter is, and should be. From the perspective of CHT, her distress may be construed accurately as a conflict between her conscience and conduct, between what she believed she ought to do and what she was actually able to do, and decided to do. This is less a conflict with her culturally determined superego (as in discourse analysis), and more a conflict between her own internal values (conscience, self-ideal) and her decision.

Particularly missed in the discourse analysis is an understanding of the client's moralism and her attempts at self-justification by being a dutiful daughter. In CHT, the client's condition may be construed as a legalistic attempt to establish her worth through her own efforts to achieve her standards defining a good person. In theological language, her problem is "works-righteousness," as a form of self-salvation. By contrast, in her relationship with her therapist, she experiences a more unconditional acceptance, which may be construed in theological language as the experience of forgiveness or grace. She experiences less need for positive regard from either her mother or others because she has experienced grace in her relationship with her therapist.

The process of change in this case can be construed as a movement from guilt through grace to gratitude. Of course, in Christian terms the therapeutic experience would be construed as a medium of divine grace. Because of the acceptance she experienced in therapy, she was enabled to forgive her mother and she forgave herself for not being able to continue to care for her mother. Stated in terms of self-theory, the client became less depressed because her moralistic self-ideal became less rigid and legalistic; and her self-concept became more realistic, which enabled the client to accept her limitations and actual experience. She became more compassionate with herself as a consequence of her experience of compassion in the therapeutic relationship.

Another viable interpretation of the client's conflict in CHT terms is to construe it as a value conflict, that is, a matter of conscience. The reduction in her depression occurred because of a value modification, or a reconciliation between the moral obligation she accepted to care for her mother, and the value she placed on her own well-being. However, her difficulty was not merely an ideological dilemma between her action and a cultural norm; rather, to the degree her depression was not biological, it may be interpreted as an incongruity between her own self-ideal and her experience. Her guilt is symptomatic of conflict within her own conscience, which obligates her to care for her mother on the one hand, but which, on the other hand, does not appreciate her own worth as one deserving to be liberated from depression.

Another dynamic interpretation, which could be applied in CHT, is that this woman may have unconsciously wished her mother would die, repressed that desire, but experienced its associated guilt, hence the need for punishment, which she experienced in the form of a depression and in her self-inflicted servitude to her mother. This interpretation requires more clinical evidence and should be offered to the client very tentatively and only if further clinical data suggest it is appropriate. One clue leading to this hypothesis was the client's statement that to whatever nursing home her mother goes, that is where she would die. The client's guilt might be eased by helping her to understand that such wishes for relief are normal (rather than evil) for someone who is overwhelmed and exhausted by the burden of so many years of caretaking. Confession and forgiveness may serve as salient mechanisms of change in this case.

Historical Dimension

One of the strengths claimed for discourse analysis is that it links the process of psychotherapy to a socio-historical context in terms of culturally conditioned identities and roles ("subject positions"). Contrary to this theoretical assumption, the analysis suggested that the client improved precisely because she became more reconciled with her own personal past. From the perspective of CHT, discussion of this case would be enriched by further analysis of the client's experiences in her family of origin. Does the client believe that her sister-in-law's story is true, namely, that the client was an unwanted child whom her mother attempted to abort? What were the messages of conditional worth communicated by her mother? Did the client develop a negative self-concept and low self-esteem from her mother's criticisms and expressed expectations that her daughter was a failure, hence that she would fail at marriage if not at life? Past experiences are relevant to present therapeutic intervention, though not always determinative. Life stories have historical dimensions.

Another potential interpretation of the process of change suggested by CHT is a change in the client's orientation in time. Depression associated with guilt reflects one who is tied to the past. The client's final statements about letting go of everything that was ever bad when she was young, and how her mother's presence in her home had reminded her of all that, suggests her depression was a function of her predominant orientation toward the past. The struggle of deciding to place her mother in a nursing home was more of a present focus. The process of change can be described as a shift in time orientation from a focus on the past to the present and eventually toward the future. In other words, the process of change salient in this case could be construed in terms of the client's experience of hope.

The loss of hope has been identified as a precursor of depression.[180] Its indicators include a negative view of the future, anticipated helplessness, or feeling thwarted.[181] Hopelessness is expressed by clients who have given up, who feel there is no sense in doing anything, and it is useless to try because nothing works, and their situation will never change. "What's the use? What's the difference? Nothing seems worth the effort." The tone of despair is implicit in such statements.

The antidote to despair is hope. The client began to feel hope that she could take effective action to resolve her conflict, and anticipated that she would experience relief from her suffering and from her burden as a caregiver. From the perspective of CHT, hope is motivating and it helps to restore health. The experience of hope is an active ingredient of change, and eliciting hope in clients is recommended as an important therapeutic strategy in CHT. Hope is good medicine. It is also a category related to the spiritual dimension of experience.

Spiritual Dimension

The positive change in self-concept alluded to in the psychological dimension could be both construed and encouraged in the spiritual dimension by helping this Christian client to assume her true spiritual identity as one who has been created in the image of God. The *imago Dei* provides content to the Christian's self-concept through identification with the model life of Jesus of Nazareth. To be created in the image of God is to possess freedom, intellect, and will, and to act purposefully as a personal and responsible being in relationship with others. To be made in the image of God, however, is not the same as being God. The human limitations implied by finite freedom must be accepted to avoid a pretense to divinity *(hubris)*. In this manner, the client may be helped to accept her limitations as a human being, and to make placing her mother in a nursing home morally acceptable.

The client's self-esteem may be enhanced by construing her own compassion for her mother as a cardinal virtue, an expression of the *imago Dei* in the client, and the work of the Spirit in her life. She has shown the gracious love of God faithfully and effectively through her love for her mother, despite her mother's apparent failure to communicate love for the client and to protect her from childhood molestation. The client's loving care for her mother may be construed as the work of the Spirit within her soul, prompting the client to forgive her mother and to persevere in love without reciprocity from her mother. But the client must also understand that the Spirit seeks the healing of her own soul, which means liberation from the oppression of her own mental illness, and in order for that to occur, the client must allow God to continue to care for her mother through the staff of the nursing home. It is their calling (and paid job) to provide such service to those in need of more intensive nursing care.

It may help to enhance this Christian woman's self-esteem further by indicating that both her previous decision to provide long-term care for her mother in her home, and her decision to place her in a nursing home reflect her fortitude (courage), which is a spiritual gift. Moreover, her inordinate patience, goodness, gentleness, and charity toward her mother all these years are fruits of the Spirit as a blessing of God. She may be encouraged to pray for these and other spiritual gifts and fruits, including understanding, wisdom, self-control, peace, and reverence for God. All are intended as blessings in her own life, and as sources of guidance for her decisions and actions. It is helpful for depressed individuals to appreciate the virtue and nobility of their own life, and that they have been blessed to be a blessing for others and for themselves.

Psychotherapy is not the same as spiritual direction. The contrast with psychotherapy is suggested by the following definition of spiritual direction as (a) a professional helping relationship in which (b) one person provides spiritual guidance (c) to enhance and encourage the spiritual healing and spiritual formation (growth) of another, (d) through the experiential learning process of spiritual discernment of ultimate concerns, and (e) through the practice of spiritual disciplines (acts), (f) which lead to a more reconciled life with self, others, and God (ultimate reality) experienced and expressed in wisdom, courage, compassion and gratitude.[182] Despite these differences between psychotherapy and spiritual direction, in CHT a Christian client may be encouraged to seek spiritual direction to nurture spiritual gifts and to experience the fruits of the Spirit that enable believers to express the requisite virtues, and thereby to empower them to fulfill their divinely ordained duties such as honoring one's parents. Prayer and meditation are two examples of spiritual disciplines practiced by Jesus, whom Christians strive to follow (e.g., Luke 3:21; 5:16; 6:12; 9:18; 11:1). They are practices endorsed by CHT.

Healing within the spiritual dimension of life involves a growing consciousness of God's love, and consequent changes in one's way of being and relating. Spiritual healing also involves changes in felt-meanings, especially ultimate meanings concerning the nature and purpose of life, and the meaning of suffering. The absence of any reference to the spiritual dimension in the discourse analysis is remarkable in light of (a) the authors' emphasis upon the role of constructed versions of reality, and (b) the visions of reality found in religious constructions. The spiritual dimension is implicit within this case, but not addressed explicitly by the discourse analysis. There was no mention in the analysis of this woman's religious orientation, as if her religion were not a part of her culture or the socio-historical context, both of which are salient in discourse analysis.

The worldview implicit in discourse analysis depicts a one-dimensional, visible reality in time and space. This modern worldview is a secular vision grounded in the scientific and technological revolution antedated by the period in Western intellectual history known as the Enlightenment. It is a nonreligious vision of reality based on autonomous reason, and which some have termed as naturalistic humanism. Discourse analysis relies solely upon human uses of language and human culture as its frame of reference.

Jesus' vision of reality was spiritual, not exclusively natural. His teachings were grounded in his own spiritual experience, and his ministry was Spirit-centered. He affirmed the Spirit of God as an experienced reality, experienced within present personal-social-historical life. He called individuals to be reconciled with God and to be liberated by divine compassion in order to become reconciling agents with one another in a life of love, justice, and peace. Jesus was a charismatic Sage as well as a prophetic social reformer. His life and mission were marked by an intense experiential relationship with the Spirit (Lk. 4:20-21). Indeed, his relationship to the spiritual dimension of life is the key to understanding his ministry as healer, sage, prophet, and as the founder of a revitalization movement.[183]

A more comprehensive, cultural perspective than discourse analysis would be cross-cultural, and it would disclose the worldview or picture of reality as it impacts both clients and therapists. Virtually every human culture seems to have affirmed a spiritual dimension of reality, a "world of Spirit." This primordial tradition[184] seems to be a universal perspective that affirms a spiritual dimension of reality that is charged with transforming energy and power, and which is known experientially by persons attuned to it. This spiritual vision of reality Jesus of Nazareth taught in his parables and sayings about the realm of God, and he invited people to experience this healing reality, whose ultimate quality is compassion. CHT is based on an understanding of this spiritual reality as a liberating experience of reconciliation. The ultimate concern of a disciple of Jesus is to experience and to advance this spiritual realm, symbolized by the kingdom of God, and thereby to transform human culture in all other realms—political, economic, social, and religious.

This spiritual world is known historically in such events as the Exodus and the return from exile of the Jews, and in the lives and teachings of Moses, Jesus of Nazareth, Lao-tzu, Buddha, Confucius, Krishna, Muhammad, and Red Elk. It is experienced cultically in communal worship in temple, synagogue, and church, and personally in devotional and spiritual experiences of ordinary people and especially in charismatic prophets as Spirit-filled mediators.[185] What is added and emphasized in CHT is that this spiritual dimension of reality is known also in concrete interpersonal relationships in which people have liberating experiences of reconciliation. These experiences are mediating ciphers of a Spiritual Presence revealed in human life and human history. This cross-cultural and spiritual context might encourage the client to explore how God has been present in her life, and what God is doing now to lead her to a good and blessed life. It may help her to see the Spirit at work in the reconciling episode occurring in therapy as she comes to terms with her situation and makes a decision to resolve the conflict. In such ordinary experiences of life one witnesses the extraordinary acts of God.

Attention to the spiritual dimension in CHT could lead further to an exploration of the client's meaning of her own suffering with depression in terms of her Christian faith. Given the guilt she is feeling, it seems probable that she may have a negative image of God. She might interpret her depression as God's punishment for her sin. She may endure her suffering in order that God would be lenient with her, as if she must earn God's forgiveness via penance instead of receiving it as a gift. Her image of God needs to be explored in light of Jesus' message of God's mercy and forgiveness, and the second commandment which counsels mutuality over either altruism or egoism. The client needs to hear that God loves her and seeks to liberate her from her depression by inspiring greater self-care as well as nursing home care for her mother. Even if her biological mother never wanted her, the client is the wanted child of God.

Assuming this woman was striving to do the will of God, perhaps if she were to come to believe it is God's will for her mother to be in a nursing home she could be more settled with the decision, and liberated from her guilt. The client might be encouraged to meditate upon Jesus' second commandment and to pray for divine guidance as to what following this commandment means in her concrete situation, here and now, as it relates to her decision about placing her mother in a nursing home.

In general, unconscious needs or motives for personal decisions are not transformed by moral commandments, but the "law of love" may help to liberate this woman from her self-condemnation and chronic low self-esteem, when discussed in the context of a therapeutic relationship in which she actually experiences genuine understanding and caring. A Christian humanistic therapist seeks to provide this kind of hospitality of soul, and as a soul friend, helps the client experience the healing that comes in one who does not merely believe, but knows "God loves me." This is a heart-felt knowing, not merely an intellectual belief. One knows because one has experienced God's love through the medium of a therapeutic relationship. The client would know herself to be of infinite worth, not merely as a dutiful daughter, but as a child of God, loved eternally. Through the experience of real acceptance in CHT, she may be enabled to accept the divine love for her, incarnate in the Spirit-centered therapeutic relationship implicitly, and explicitly and decisively in the life and teachings of Jesus. As she experiences reconciliation through the therapeutic relationship, she becomes more open to further growth toward an even more reconciling life in communion with God as modeled by Jesus of Nazareth. As she embraces the God-consciousness of Jesus, lives in it and by it, thus is she redeemed and healed.

Because the spiritual dimension is included in CHT, it is legitimate to raise questions with a Christian client such as "What does your faith lead you to do?" "What do you think God is calling you to do?" "How do the actions and teachings of Jesus inform your decision?" "Do you accept God's acceptance of you?"

CHT describes the Christian experience of personal transformation as the movement from a condition of estrangement to reconciliation. Construing this woman's change in psychotherapy as an experience of reconciliation is supported by the various connotations of this term, which can be illustrated in this case.

As a transitive verb, "to reconcile" means to make consistent, congruous, harmonious and compatible. An example is to reconcile one's ideals with practical reality. One interpretation of the successful psychotherapy for the depressed woman in this case was that her therapist helped her to reconcile her ideal self as a dutiful daughter with the practical realities of her workload and her own illness. She was enabled to develop a more realistic (and forgiving) self-ideal, which was also more congruent with her experience, and more compatible with both her own, and her mother's human needs.

Another meaning of the verb "to reconcile" is to adapt, to adjust, or to cause one to accept a condition (e.g., one becomes reconciled to hardship). These connotations would lead to an interpretation that the client became reconciled to (accepted) the need for her mother to receive care in a nursing home. However much the client felt consciously that she ought to/wanted to care for her at home, both she and her mother needed the alternative solution. The client became reconciled to that reality. She adjusted to this needed change and her level of functioning became more adaptive as her depression lifted.

Finally, synonyms of the verb "to reconcile" include: to settle something, and to change from an agitated, disturbed state of alienation to a more calm state of harmony and peace. The woman in this case changed from an agitated state of major depression to a condition of greater calm, which she described as letting go of everything that was ever bad when she was young. Through this reconciling experience, the issue was settled by working through the felt-meanings of her experience to reach her decision, and she achieved a greater sense of peace.

By way of summary, CHT provides a practical, comprehensive, coherent, experiential, and interpersonal explanation for therapy change with a Christian client. This approach appreciates human motivations and emotions associated with relationships, which a more cognitive case formulation neglects. Moreover, CHT affirms the existential dimensions of human experience—moral, historical, and spiritual—in addition to the natural dimensions—biological, psychological, and social.

Finally, CHT meets the criteria for a satisfactory case formulation:[186]

1. It helps organize often complex and contradictory information about a person.
2. It provides a frame of reference enabling the therapist to understand the client better.
3. It provides hypotheses about the causes and influences maintaining a person's psychological and interpersonal problems.
4. It serves as a blueprint guiding treatment planning and as a marker for change.
5. It helps the therapist to experience greater empathy for the client.
6. It helps to anticipate therapy-interfering events.
7. It organizes descriptive information coherently and comprehensively while leading to prescriptive recommendations tailored to the unique needs of the client.

NOTES

1. "Common Era" means the dating accepted by all, including non-Christians. Jesus was born about 4 B.C.E. ("before the Common Era"), near the time of the death of Herod the Great. Sanders, E. P. (1993). *The historical figure of Jesus.* New York: Penguin Books, p. 11.

2. This date of Jesus' crucifixion is the estimate of contemporary New Testament scholars. Funk, R., Hoover, R., and The Jesus Seminar (1993). *The five Gospels: The search for the authentic words of Jesus.* New York: Macmillan, p. 128.

3. Sanders, *The historical figure of Jesus,* pp. xi, 1.

4. Liberal Christians have generally favored historical theology over dogmatic theology since the latter has been shaped by ancient metaphysical ideas. Liberals may

actually deny the orthodox image of Jesus in the creeds as a divine or semi-divine being who allegedly saw himself as the savior whose purpose was to die for the sins of the world, and whose message consisted of proclaiming that. This is an image written into the New Testament and imposed upon the historical Jesus by the early Church, which many contemporary New Testament scholars claim is not a historically accurate portrayal of who Jesus was and what he taught. See Borg, M. (1987). *Jesus—a new vision: Spirit, culture, and the life of discipleship.* New York: HarperSanFrancisco, p. 7.

5. Among titles ascribed to Jesus, "Christ" appears multiple times, especially in Paul's letters (Synoptics, 37; John, 19; Paul, 374). The English equivalent title "Messiah" appears only twice (in the gospel of John). By contrast, the title "Savior" appears only twenty-three times, primarily in Paul's letters (Synoptics, 10; John, 1; Paul, 12). Other titles appearing in the New Testament as a whole include Lord, Son of Man, Son of God, Lamb of God, Mediator, Redeemer, Master, Rabbi, Teacher, and he who comes in the name of the Lord (Matthew 23:39). For a review of the titles ascribed to Jesus, see Barclay, W. (1962). *Jesus as they saw him.* Grand Rapids, MI: William B. Eerdmans. The title ascribed to Jesus most frequently in the Synoptic Gospels (Matthew, Mark, and Luke) is "Rabbi." The oral teachings *(mishnah)* of this "local Sage" centered on his vision of the kingdom of God. Chilton, B. (1996). *Pure kingdom: Jesus' vision of God.* Grand Rapids, MI: William B. Eerdmans, pp. 46-47, 103-106.

6. For a thorough history of the Christian religion, see Latourette, K. S. (1953/1975). *A history of Christianity,* Vol. I and II. New York: HarperCollins.

7. Illustrative contemporary research yielding various conclusions about Jesus' context, life, and teachings are Borg, M. (1994). *Jesus in contemporary scholarship.* Valley Forge, PA: Trinity Press International; Borg, M. (Ed.) (1997). *Jesus at 2000.* New York: Westview Press; Borg, M. and Wright, N. (1999). *The meaning of Jesus: Two visions.* New York: HarperSanFrancisco; Charlesworth, J. and Weaver, W. (Eds). (1994). *Images of Jesus today.* Valley Forge, PA: Trinity Press International; Charlesworth, J. and Weaver, W. (Eds.) (2000). *Jesus two thousand years later.* Harrisburg, PA: Trinity Press International; Chilton, B. and Evans, C. (Eds.) (1994). *Studying the historical Jesus: Evaluations of the state of current research.* Leiden: E. J. Brill; Crossan, J. D. (1991). *The historical Jesus: The life of a Mediterranean Jewish peasant.* New York: HarperCollins; Evans, C. (1989). *Life of Jesus research: An annotated bibliography.* Kinderhook, NY: Brill; Meier, J. (1991/1994). *A marginal Jew: Rethinking the historical Jesus* (2 volumes). New York: Doubleday; Reumann, J. (1989). Jesus and Christology. In E. Epp and G. MacRae (Eds.). *The new testament and its modern interpretation.* Atlanta, GA: Scholars Press, pp. 501-564; Sanders, E. P. (1993). *The historical figure of Jesus.* New York: Penguin Books; Vermes, G. (1993). *The religion of Jesus the Jew.* Minneapolis, MN: Fortress Press; Witherington, B. (1995). *The Jesus quest: The third search for the Jew of Nazareth.* Downers Grove, IL: InterVarsity Press; Wright, N. T. (1992). *The New Testament and the people of God,* vol. 1 of *Christian origins and the question of God.* Minneapolis, MN: Fortress Press; Wright, N. T. (1996). *Jesus and the victory of God,* vol. 2 of *Christian origins and the question of God.* Minneapolis, MN: Fortress Press.

8. There has been a consensus for several years among New Testament theologians that the "kingdom of God" was the central theme of Jesus' teachings: Bultmann, R. (1951). *Theology of the new testament* (Vol. 1). New York: Charles Scribner's Sons, p. 4; Bornkamm, G. (1960). *Jesus of Nazareth.* New York: Harper and Row, p. 64; Perrin, N. (1967). *Rediscovering the teaching of Jesus.* London: SCM Press, p. 54; Jeremias, J. (1971). *New testament theology: The proclamation of Jesus.* New York: Charles Scribner's Sons, p. 96; Sanders, E. P. (1993). *The historical figure of Jesus.* New York: Penguin Books, pp. 70, 169; Vermes, G. (1993). *The religion of Jesus the Jew.* Minneapolis, MN: Fortress Press, p. 119; Wright, N. T. (1996). *Jesus and the victory of God.* Minneapolis, MN: Fortress Press, pp. 198-368, 663-670.

The Greek word *basileia* in the New Testament has been translated as kingdom, empire, sovereignty, rule, reign, realm, dominion, or domain of God. All translations affirm a real sphere of influence under God, and in which God acts to liberate and reconcile humankind. See for example, Patterson, S. (1996). Shall we teach what Jesus taught? *Prism, 11*(1), 40-57; and Throckmorton, B. H. (1987). Evangelism and mission in the new testament. *Prism, 2*(1), 30-41.

9. As a worldview, humanism emerged in the fourteenth and fifteenth centuries in the period known as the Renaissance. Unlike naturalistic humanists who are atheistic, most humanists of the Renaissance were religious, and especially in Italy, they were Catholic. Their aim was not to undermine or oppose Christianity, but to "humanize" and renew it via a return to the Patristic writings (100-451 C.E.) and to the Greek classics. For discussion, see McGrath, A. (1997). *Christian theology: An introduction.* Oxford, England: Blackwell Publishers, pp. 37-42.

10. For a Christian psychologist, the dominant biopsychosocial model of behavior expresses only half the picture, and not the most important half. A second tripartite model is needed to understand the nature and destiny of humans in terms of spiritual, moral, and historical dimensions.

11. All four sources have been included in the Wesleyan Quadrilateral. See Gunter, W., Jones, S., Campbell, T., Miles, R., and Maddox, R. (1997). *Wesley and the quadrilateral: Renewing the conversation.* Nashville, TN: Abingdon Press, pp. 9-142.

12. By definition a "liberal" Christian manifests "a willingness to use historical-critical tools in the interpretations of scripture, an appreciation of the contributions of the post-Enlightenment natural and social sciences in our anthropological and sociological analyses, a willingness to work ecumenically with the denominations and sympathetically with the world religions, and an inner tendency to be active for peace, human rights, and social justice." See Stackhouse, M. (1986). Obedience to Christ and engaged in the world. *Prism, 1*(2), p. 9.

13. Funk, R., Hoover, R., and The Jesus Seminar (1993). *The five Gospels: The search for the authentic words of Jesus.* New York: Macmillan, p. 128. The first surviving copies of "Bibles" have been dated between 300 and 350 C.E.

14. Genuine letters of Paul and their estimated dates include 1 Thessalonians (50-51 C.E.), Philippians (54-55), Philemon (54-55), Galatians (50-56), 1 Corinthians (54), 2 Corinthians (55-56), and Romans (56-57), according to Bultman, R. (1951). *Theology of the New Testament,* Vol. I. New York: Charles Scribner's Sons,

p. 190; Division of Christian Education of the National Council of Churches of Christ in America (1989). *The HarperCollins study Bible: New revised standard version.* New York: HarperCollins, pp. 2113 and 2210. Others have accepted Ephesians and Colossians based on their use of the concept of the body *(soma),* which is consistent with Paul's other letters. See, for example, Robinson, J.A.T. (1952). *The body: A study in Pauline theology.* London: SCM Press, p. 10. Most exegetes do not accept 1 and 2 Timothy, Hebrews 1, and 2 Titus, Ephesians, Colossians, or 2 Thessalonians as genuine letters of Paul, and I have not counted them in the citations in Section Two.

15. Harnack, A. (1900/1989). *What is Christianity?* Philadelphia: Fortress Press, p. 30. The Protestant theologian, Paul Tillich rejected the reliance on the three Synoptics as sources of the message given *by* Jesus in contrast to the fourth Gospel and Epistles as the message *about* Jesus. See Taylor, M. K. (1991). *Paul Tillich: Theologian of the boundaries.* Minneapolis, MN: Fortress Press, pp. 134, 220-221, 231-232. Nevertheless, Tillich agreed that a difference between the Synoptic portraits and John's Gospel is the kingdom-centered sayings of Jesus in the Synoptics versus the Christ-centered sayings in John. See Tillich, P. (1957). *Systematic theology* (Vol. 2). Chicago: University of Chicago Press, pp. 136-138. A contemporary New Testament scholar, Marcus Borg, noted that the Christ of faith and Jesus of history are by and large very different, "if by the Christ of faith one means the Son of God who came and died for our sins on the cross and rose again from the dead." Cited by Witherington, B. (1995). *The Jesus quest: The third search for the Jew of Nazareth.* Downers Grove, IL: InterVarsity Press, p. 102.

16. For references concerning the dates of the gospels, see Olson, R. P. (1997). *The reconciled life: A critical theory of counseling.* Westport, CT: Praeger, p. 88, n. 54. A recent panel of independent biblical scholars has confirmed these approximate dates for the four Gospels: Mark (70 C.E.), Matthew (85 C.E.), Luke (90 C.E.), and John (90 C.E.). The earliest version of the fifth Gospel of Thomas has been estimated between 50 to 60 C.E., prior to the earliest versions of the other four Gospels. See Funk, R. W., Hoover, R. W., and The Jesus Seminar (1993). *The five Gospels: The search for the authentic words of Jesus.* New York: Macmillan, pp. 18, 128, 474. This group of New Testament scholars has suggested that about 80 percent of the 1,500 versions of about 500 sayings ascribed to Jesus in twenty-two different Gospels written before 325 C.E. were probably not actually spoken by him (Ibid., pp. ix, 5; cf. Funk, R. and the Jesus Seminar (1999). *The Gospel of Jesus according to the Jesus Seminar.* Santa Rosa, CA: Polebridge Press, pp. 107-110. The database accepted by the Jesus Seminar includes thirty parables and sixty-one sayings for a total of ninety-one authentic citations of Jesus. This listing includes about 50 percent of the sayings attributed to Jesus by the four Gospels in the New Testament. For a listing see Cain, M. (1999). *Jesus the man: An introduction for people at home in the modern world.* Santa Rosa, CA: Polebridge Press, pp. 150, 159-162.

17. Funk, R., Hoover, R., and The Jesus Seminar (1993). *The five Gospels: The search for the authentic sayings of Jesus.* New York: Macmillan, pp. 15-16, 470, 474.

18. Meeks, W., Bassler, J., Lemke, W., Niditch, S., and Schuller, E. (Eds.). (1993). *The HarperCollins study bible: New revised standard version.* London: HarperCollins; Kohlenberger, J.R. (1991). The *NRSV concordance unabridged.*

Grand Rapids, MI: Zondervan Publishing House; Crim, K., Bailey, L., Furnish, V., and Bucke, E. (Eds.). (1976). *The interpreter's dictionary of the bible: An illustrated encyclopedia.* Nashville, TN: Abingdon Press. See also Beasley-Murray, G. R. (1986). *Jesus and the kingdom of God.* Grand Rapids, MI: Eerdmans; Saucy, M. (1997). *The kingdom of God in the teachings of Jesus in 20th-century theology.* Dallas: Word Publishing. The three books by Marcus J. Borg are *Jesus—A new vision: Spirit, culture, and the life of discipleship.* New York: HarperSanFrancisco, 1987; *Jesus in contemporary scholarship.* Valley Forge, PA: Trinity Press International, 1994; and *Meeting Jesus again for the first time: The historical Jesus and the heart of contemporary faith.* New York: HarperSanFrancisco, 1994. A classic existential interpretation of Jesus' teachings is Bornkamm, G. (1959). *Jesus of Nazareth.* New York: Harper and Row. A conservative Christian critique of historical-critical research on Jesus and his message is Johnson, T. (1996). *The real Jesus: The misguided quest for the historical Jesus and the truth of the traditional gospels.* New York: HarperSanFrancisco.

19. Tillich, P. (1963). *Systematic theology* (Vol. 3). Chicago: University of Chicago Press, pp. 13-17.

20. The principle of functional autonomy was ascribed by Gordon Allport to human motives and dispositions, which both emerge from biological drives and transcend them. For discussion, see Allport, G. (1968). *The person in psychology: Selected essays.* Boston: Beacon Press, pp. 78, 167-169, 394.

21. A "realm" is a metaphor to indicate an aspect of life in which a particular dimension is predominant. Tillich, *Systematic theology* (Vol. 3), p. 16.

22. As illustrated by the personalistic theory of William Stern, including several motivational concepts provides a comprehensive theory of personality dynamics. Stern employed such terms as instinct, impulse, motive, need, disposition, goal-striving, urge, interest, inclination, wish, will, drive, volition, entelechy, and personal energy. Cited by Allport, *The person in psychology,* p. 283. A more parsimonious list includes needs, values, and goals, will, choose, and decide. Including more than one motivational concept avoids succumbing to the model of the individual as merely a set of reactive responses to environmental stimuli. Human persons are characterized by free, creative, intentional, conscious, spontaneous action.

23. Olson, *The reconciled life,* p. 176.

24. Rychlak, J. (1981). *Introduction to personality and psychotherapy.* Boston: Houghton Mifflin Company, p. 294. This is an important insight which should help us avoid a judgmental moralism.

25. Viktor Frankl advocated "freedom of will" and "the will to meaning" as central postulates of Logotherapy. See Frankl, V. (1969/1988). *The will to meaning: Foundations and applications of logotherapy.* NewYork: Meridian Books, pp. 15-49.

26. Bultmann, *Theology of the New Testament,* Vol. 1, p. 14.

27. Olson, *The reconciled life,* p. 179.

28. Bultmann, *Theology of the New Testament,* Vol. l, p. 11.

29. Olson, *The reconciled life,* p. 179. The relative frequencies of cognates of motivational terms appearing in the New Testament as a whole are approximately as follows: want, 121, will, 81, need, 71, choose, 61, desire, 53, wish, 45, purpose, 29, decide, 25, intend, 17, drive, 15, strive, 14, value, 13, goal, 2, and motive, 2. All

of these terms presuppose human freedom, though not absolute freedom. Human freedom is conditional and finite.

30. Allport, *The person in psychology,* p. 73.

31. Rychlak, *Introduction to personality and psychotherapy* (Second edition), pp. 788-798.

32. Cited by Hall, C. and Lindzey, G. (1970). *Theories of personality.* New York: John Wiley and Sons, p. 276.

33. Emmons, R. (1999). *The psychology of ultimate concerns: Motivation and spirituality in personality.* New York: The Guilford Press, p. 4.

34. Two recommended books about the therapeutic role of hope include Capps, D. (1995). *Agents of hope: A pastoral psychology.* Minneapolis: Fortress Press, esp. pp. 52-78; Lester, A. (1995). *Hope in pastoral care and counseling.* Louisville, KY: Westminster John Knox Press, esp. pp. 125-152.

35. Self-actualization has been a primary goal of humanistic therapy espoused by Carl Rogers and Abraham Maslow. An example is Patterson, C. H. and Hidore, S. (1997). *Successful psychotherapy: A caring, loving relationship.* Northvale, NJ: Jason Aronson, pp. 23-40. As a counterpoint, the Catholic theologian, Daniel Helminiak advocated that any theory of human motivation must include "the inherent human need for authenticity," which he describes as a need of the human spirit. Helminiak, D. (1996). *The human core of spirituality: Mind as psyche and spirit.* Albany, NY: State University of New York Press, p. 267.

36. Helminiak, D. (1996). *The human core of spirituality: Mind as psyche and spirit.* Albany, NY: State University of New York Press, p. 142.

37. For a concise summary of emergent strengths or virtues of each stage of faith development, see Fowler, J. (1981). *Stages of faith: The psychology of human development and the quest for meaning.* New York: HarperSanFrancisco, Figure 5.3, p. 290.

38. Ibid., p. 300.

39. An interface of Kohlberg's theory of moral development with religion and clinical practice is L. Kuhmerker (Ed.) (1991). *Kolberg legacy for the helping professions.* Birmingham, AL: Religious Education Press, esp. pp. 157-210.

40. I concur with Marcus Borg's view that a significant element of Jesus' unique vision of life was his emphasis upon personal transformation. This occurs through the religious experience of God within a compassionate community of Jesus' disciples. Borg, *Jesus in contemporary scholarship,* pp. 151-155. I have chosen to describe this transformation as a movement toward a more reconciling life. This is not merely a quantitative change occurring across time (as stimulus-response theories and mediational theories of learning view change). Rather, consistent with Gestalt-phenomenological theories, to become more reconciling is a qualitative change as a direct result of patterns occurring within time. It is an emphasis upon formal causation rather than efficient causation. For discussion of these distinctions, see Rychlak, *Introduction to personality and psychotherapy,* pp. 768-773.

41. United States Catholic Conference (1994). *Catechism of the Catholic Church.* Mahwah, NJ: Paulist Press, p. 450.

42. Ibid., p. 450.

43. Ibid., pp. 446-451. Tillich subsumes hope under faith, and emphasizes faith and love as the manifestations of the Spirit. Tillich, *Systematic theology* (Vol. 3), pp. 130f.

44. Galatians 5:22-23. Goodness, modesty, and chastity are added in the *Catechism of the Catholic Church*, p. 451.

45. Tillich, *Systematic theology* (Vol. 2), pp. 176-180, and (Vol. 3), pp. 129-138, 362-423. Chicago: University of Chicago Press. Tillich wrote that the question arising out of the human condition of estrangement is "the question of a reality in which the self estrangement of our existence is overcome, a reality of reconciliation and reunion, of creativity, meaning, and hope. We shall call such a reality the 'New Being'. . . . It is based on what Paul calls the 'new creation'. . . ." (*Systematic theology*, Vol. 1. Chicago: University of Chicago Press, p. 49). Since Tillich describes the Christian message as the message of "New Being," and because he equates this with "a power and reality of reconciliation," his theological system can be characterized as an existential theology of reconciliation.

46. Tillich, *Systematic theology* (Vol. 3), p. 221f. The notion of transformation and growth is grounded philosophically. The ontic polarity of "dynamics" is effective in the function of life called "self-creativity" through the principle of "growth" (p. 50).

47. As an important concept in his theoretical formulation of client centered therapy, Carl Rogers defined the self-ideal as the self-concept of the individual that depicts who one would like to become, and upon which one places highest value for oneself. See Rogers, C. (1959). A theory of therapy, personality, and interpersonal relationships, as developed in the client-centered framework. In S. Koch (Ed.). *Psychology: A study of science. Volume 3: Formulations of the person in the social context.* New York: McGraw-Hill, p. 200.

48. Kress, R. (1986). The Catholic understanding of human nature. In F. Greenspahn (Ed.). *The human condition in Jewish and Christian traditions.* Hoboken, NJ: KTAV Publishing House, pp. 45-49, 54, 58. The consequences of sin do not include abandonment by God, but divine forgiveness (p. 61).

49. Tillich, *Systematic theology.* (Vol. 3), p. 276.

50. American Psychiatric Association (1994). *Desk reference to the diagnostic criteria from DSM-IV.* Washington, DC: Author, pp. 37, 300.

51. Lazarus, A. (1989). *The practice of multimodal therapy.* Baltimore: The Johns Hopkins University Press, pp. 13-18.

52. For a popular expression of this theme, see Kushner, H. (1981). *When bad things happen to good people.* New York: Basic Books.

53. According to yoga psychology, the fundamental cause of human suffering is the incorrect identification with the ego as if it were one's true nature and personal center. One must become disidentified with this illusion of the ego and reidentified with the Self (Atman), which is God (Brahman) incarnate as the One in the many. See Swami Ajaya (1983). *Psychotherapy East and West: A unifying paradigm.* Honesdale, PA: The Himalyan International Institute of Yoga Science and Philosophy of the USA, pp. 127-182. The application of the disidentification process in psychotherapy is found also in Assagioli, R. (1973). *The act of will.* New York: Viking Press, pp. 214-217.

54. Kress, "The Catholic understanding of human nature," p. 50.

55. Olson, *The reconciled life,* pp. 97-166.

56. Burton, A. (1972). *Interpersonal psychotherapy.* Englewood Cliffs, NJ: Prentice-Hall, pp. 10-11. For discussion of goals from a variety of theoretical orientations, see Mahrer, A. (Ed.) (1967). *The goals of psychotherapy.* New York: Appleton-Century-Crofts. Each of these stated purposes of psychotherapy functions as a nonmoral value, that is, as a good (end) one seeks to bring into being through the means of psychotherapy. Where the social sciences once defensively insisted they were "value-neutral," they now tend to present themselves as unavoidably "value-loaded." Robinson, D. N. (1985). *Philosophy of psychology.* New York: Columbia University Press, p. 142.

57. An improved quality of life is another stated purpose. For measures see Lawton, M. (1997). Operational definitions of quality of life and subjective well-being. *Generations, 21,* 45-47; and Frisch, M., Cornell, J., Villanueva, M., and Retzlaff, P. (1992). Clinical validation of the Quality of Life Inventory: A measure of life satisfaction for use in treatment planning and outcome assessment. *Psychological Assessment, 4,* 92-101.

58. Lazarus, A. (1989). *The practice of multimodal therapy.* Baltimore: The Johns Hopkins University Press, p. 13.

59. Tillich, *Systematic theology* (Vol. 3), pp. 321-324. Joseph Rychlak discusses Aristotle's four meanings of change as first, teleological change, and three types of accidental change (quantitative, local, and qualitative). Rychlak, *Introduction to personality and psychotherapy,* pp. 268-270.

60. Tillich, *Systematic theology* (Vol. 3), p. 277.

61. In Tillich's existential anthropology, the ontic polarity of *individualization* is expressed in the function of life called "self-integration" through the principle (or quality) of centeredness. The ontic polarity of *dynamics* is expressed in the function of life known as "self-creativity" through the principle of growth. The ontic polarity of *freedom* is effective in the function of life called "self-transcendence" through the principle of finitude. Tillich, *Systematic theology* (Vol. 3), pp. 33, 50, 86.

62. Clinebell, H. (1984). *Basic types of pastoral care and counseling.* Nashville, TN: Abingdon Press, pp. 25-46. A further development of this model is Malony, H. N. (Ed.). (1983). *Wholeness and holiness: Readings in the psychology/theology of mental health.* Grand Rapids, MI: Baker Book House; and Malony, H. N., Papen-Daniels, M., and Clinebell, H. (Eds.) (1988). *Spirit centered wholeness: Beyond the psychology of self.* Lewiston, New York: Edwin Mellen Press.

63. Olson, *The reconciled life,* p. 99. Several implications of this definition are outlined in pages 99-100 and are discussed throughout chapters four through six of that book.

64. For discussion of these characteristics of a reconciling life and their foundations in Jesus' teachings, see Olson, *The reconciled life,* pp. 119-202.

65. Cowdell, S. (1996). *Is Jesus unique? A study of recent Christology.* New York: Paulist Press, p. 160.

66. In psychological language, a moral ideal functions as an "ego-ideal" or "ideal-self," not merely as an incorporation of parental values as in Freud's concept of the "superego." A moral ideal forms one's conscience and provides it content.

The Catholic Church utilizes the inspiring power of moral ideals in its veneration of saints as human examples of faith-filled virtue. The therapeutic value of a moral ideal was recognized and applied in the approach developed by Assagioli, R. (1965). *Psychosynthesis: A collection of basic writings.* New York: Arkana, pp. 166-177. It is a strategy employed in Christian humanistic therapy.

67. Paul Tillich's term is "New Being," a reality of reconciliation and reunion. Tillich wrote that the question arising out of the human condition of estrangement is "the question of a reality in which the self estrangement of our existence is overcome, a reality of reconciliation and reunion, of creativity, meaning, and hope. We shall call such a reality the 'New Being'. . . It is based on what Paul calls the 'new creation.' " Tillich, Systematic theology (Vol. 1), p. 49. Perhaps Rogers' concepts of "organismic valuing" and "organismic actualization" could serve as psychological indicators of the imago dei. Items from the Personal Orientation Inventory (POI) might be used as a partial measure.

68. The reconciling personality is more open to experience, hence more of experience is available to awareness; one's flexible self-structure assimilates new experience, and the self-concept becomes congruent with one's experience. The individual becomes a locus of evaluation, and relatively free of influence from conditions of worth set by others. For the Christian, this new freedom occurs due largely to the acceptance of God's acceptance of oneself. Finally, one lives with others in greater harmony because of the mutually rewarding character of reciprocal positive regard. Rogers, *A theory of therapy, personality and interpersonal relationships,* pp. 234-235.

69. Tillich, *Systematic theology* (Vol. 3), p. 281.

70. Ibid., p. 282.

71. Ibid., p. 281. Three types of existential anxiety and three correlated types of courage were discussed by Tillich, P. (1952). *The courage to be.* New Haven, CN: Yale University Press, pp. 40-56. In the latter work he used "courage" as a translation for "faith."

72. Tillich, *Systematic theology* (Vol. 3), p. 281.

73. Olson, *The reconciled life,* p. 77.

74. Ibid., p. 78.

75. In contrast to the traditional focus of psychotherapy upon an individual's self-interest and self-fulfillment, William Doherty suggests therapists must serve as moral consultants to deal with client issues of moral responsibility. Doherty, W. (1995). *Soul searching: Why psychotherapy must promote moral responsibility.* New York: Basic Books, pp. 3-20.

76. Tillich, *Systematic theology* (Vol. 3), p. 49.

77. Ibid., p. 240. This emphasis on the healing of character points to the voluntaristic and teleological emphasis in Christian humanism. This approach highlights the roles of both "will" and decision in the therapeutic process. A phenomenological study of the experience of willing, its aspects, qualities, and stages, was provided by Assagioli, *The act of will,* pp. 19-84, 135-198. Practical suggestions for therapeutic development of the will were provided in this book and Assagioli, *Psychosynthesis,* pp. 125-142.

78. A developmental model of the psychotherapy change process based on stages of assimilation was illustrated in an analysis of the same case study included in the present chapter. See Field, S., Barkham, M., Shapiro, D., and Stiles, W. (1994). Assessment of assimilation in psychotherapy A quantitative case study of problematic experiences with a significant other. *Journal of Counseling Psychology, 41,* 397-406.

79. The author has written an extensive monograph which critiques managed mental health care in Minnesota's Health Maintenance Organizations.

80. Tillich, *Systematic theology* (Vol. 3), p. 282.

81. Contemporary psychological studies of conversion include Paloutzian, R., Richardson, J., and Rambo, L. (1999). Religious conversion and personality change. *Journal of Personality, 67*(6), 1047-1079; Stromberg, P. (1993). *Language and self-transformation: A study of the Christian conversion narrative.* New York: Cambridge University Press; Zinnbauer, B., and Pargament, K. (1998). Spiritual conversion: A study of religious change among college students. *Journal for the Scientific Study of Religion, 37,* 161-180; H. Malony and S. Southard (Eds.) (1992). *Handbook of religious conversion.* Birmingham, AL: Religious Education Press; Gillespie, V. (1991). *The dynamics of religious conversion.* Birmingham, AL: Religious Education Press.

82. A contemporary discussion of compassion and forgiveness in counseling is Sapp, G. (1993). *Compassionate ministry.* Birmingham, AL: Religious Education Press. The old adage has some truth to it: "Confession is good for the soul." O. H. Mowrer emphasized the counselor's own confession as central to a therapeutic outcome in Integrity Therapy. See Mowrer, O. H. (1960). Sin, the lesser of two evils. *American Psychologist, 15,* 303; and Mowrer, O. H. (Ed.). (1972). Integrity groups: Basic principles and objectives. *The Counseling Psychologist, 3,* 7-32. Another saying of Andean Indians is equally germane: "Unconfessed sins cause epidemics." Cited by Gilke, L. (1986). The Protestant view of sin. In G. Greenspahn (Ed.). *The human condition in the Jewish and Christian traditions.* Hoboken, NJ: KTAV Publishing House, p. 153.

83. For discussion of various approaches to therapy integration, see Norcross, J. and Goldfried, M. (Eds.) (1992). *Handbook of psychotherapy integration.* New York: Basic Books. Common therapeutic factors have been identified. See for example, Grencavage, L. and Norcross, J. (1990). Where are the commonalities among the therapeutic common factors? *Professional Psychotherapy: Research and Practice, 21,* 372-378.

84. An example from experiential psychotherapy is Greenberg, L., Rice, L., and Elliott, R. (1993). *Facilitating emotional change: The moment-by-moment process.* New York: The Guilford Press, pp. 12-34, 101-117.

85. For discussion of research on the therapeutic alliance, see Henry, W., Strupp, H., Schacht, T., and Gaston, L. (1994). Psychodynamic approaches. In A. Bergin and S. Garfield (Eds.). *Handbook of psychotherapy and behavior change.* New York: John Wiley and Sons, pp. 480-489; Horvath, A. and Greenberg, L. (1994). *The working alliance: Theory, research, and practice.* New York: John Wiley and Sons, pp. 13-130, 259-286.

86. Helminiak, *The human core of spirituality,* p. 188.

87. For discussion of the Spirit-consciousness of Jesus, see Borg, *Meeting Jesus again for the first time,* p. 42, n.26, and p. 43, n.28. Borg characterizes Jesus' central teaching as a Spirit-centered compassion (Ibid., p. 46). He interprets the admonition to be perfect like God as "Be compassionate as God is compassionate" (Luke 6:36).

88. See Taylor, M. K. (1991). *Paul Tillich: Theologian of the boundaries.* Minneapolis, MN: Fortress Press, p. 121. What qualifies the theory of psychotherapy presented in this chapter as a theonomous psychology is the ultimate concern and transcending meaning of reconciliation. To describe psychotherapy as theonomous does not mean the acceptance of theology as the higher authority imposed upon psychology; rather, it refers to an autonomous psychology united with its own transcendent dimension of being and meaning. The form of theonomous psychotherapy presented here attempts to disclose the spiritual dimension of therapy as the liberating experience of reconciliation. In this manner, therapeutic insight is complemented by spiritual insight, but not replaced by it. See Tillich, *Systematic theology* (Vol. 1), pp. 72-73, 85, 95-96, 110, 121-123, 147.

89. Tillich, *Systematic theology* (Vol. 3), pp. 249-250.

90. Cited by Cowdell, *Is Jesus unique?,* p. 196.

91. Gestalt-phenomenological theories emphasize qualitative change as the direct result of patterns occurring within time as a formal cause. See Rychlak, *Introduction to personality and psychotherapy,* pp. 768-773. The concept of creative change is discussed by Tillich, *Systematic theology* (Vol. 3), p. 324.

92. Schleiermacher, F. (1830/1989). *The Christian faith* (trans. by H. R. Mackintosh and J. S. Stewart). Edinburgh: T. and T. Clark, pp. 77, 262-264, 425.

93. Barbour, I. (1966). *Issues in science and religion.* New York: Harper Torchbooks, p. 212.

94. Ibid., p. 213.

95. See the section on personality dynamics for discussion of the "telosponse."

96. Janus, I. and Mann, L. (1977). *Decision making: A psychological analysis of conflict, choice, and commitment.* New York: The Free Press, p. 333. Two somewhat related models of the psychotherapy process are Curtis, J. and Silberschatz, G. (1997). The plan formulation method; and Nezu, A., Nezu, C., Friedman, S., and Haynes, S. (1997). Case formulation in behavior therapy: Problem-solving and functional analytic strategies. Both appear as chapters in T. Eells (Ed.). *Handbook of psychotherapy case formulation.* New York: The Guilford Press, pp. 116-136, 368-401.

97. Greenberg, L., Rice, L., and Elliott, R., *Facilitating emotional change,* pp. 115; cf. 72, 75.

98. Compare Rogers, C. (1942). *Counseling and psychotherapy.* Boston: Houghton Mifflin, with Rogers, C. (1961a). *On becoming a person.* Boston: Houghton-Mifflin, pp. 132-159, and with Rogers, C. (1961b). The process equation of psychotherapy. *American Journal of Psychotherapy, 15,* 27-45.

99. Mathieu-Coughlan, P. and Klein, M. (1990). Experiential psychotherapy: Key events in client-therapist interaction. In L. Rice and L. Greenberg (Eds.). *Patterns of change.* New York: Guilford Press, p. 214.

100. The term "felt meanings" suggests that the emotional (felt) dimension and cognitive (meaning) dimension are inseparable in actual human experience. Feelings are meaningful, and meanings are felt, not merely thought. For a theoretical and empirical perspective on the therapeutic relationship, see Patterson, C. H. (1985). *The therapeutic relationship: Foundations for an eclectic psychotherapy.* Monterey, CA: Brooks/Cole. For practical skills see Brammer, L. and MacDonald, G. (1996). *The helping relationship: Process and skills.* Boston: Allyn and Bacon; and Egan, G. (1990). *The skilled helper: A systematic approach to effective helping.* Pacific Grove, CA: Brooks/Cole.

101. Fowler, J. (1987). *Faith development and pastoral care.* Philadelphia: Fortress Press.

102. A practical workbook is Foster, R. and Yanni, K. (1989). *Celebrating the disciplines: A journal workbook to accompany Celebration of Discipline.* New York: HarperSanFrancisco. An excellent recent review of approaches and instruments for assessing spirituality is Gorsuch, R. and Miller, Wm. (1999). Assessing spirituality. In Wm. Miller (Ed.). *Integrating spirituality into treatment.: Resources for practitioners.* Washington, DC: American Psychological Association, pp. 19-46.

103. Various approaches to assessing spiritual needs and levels of spiritual maturity within the Christian tradition are found in Fitchett, G. (1993). *Assessing spiritual needs: A guide for caregivers.* Minneapolis, MN: Augsburg Press; Tan, Siang-Yang (1991). *Lay counseling: Equipping Christians for a helping ministry.* Grand Rapids, MI: Zondervan Publishing House, pp. 102-106, 169-171. One example is the Spiritual Well-Being Scale by Bufford, R., Paloutzian, R., and Ellison, C. (1991). Norms for the spiritual well-being scale. *Journal of Psychology and Theology, 19*(1), 56-70. Two forgiveness scales were developed by Hebl, J. and Enright, R. (1993). Forgiveness as a psychotherapeutic goals with elderly females. *Psychotherapy, 30*(4), 658-667, and by Mauger, P., Perry, J., Freeman, C., and Grove, D. (1992). The measurement of forgiveness: Preliminary research. Special Issue: Grace and forgiveness. *Journal of Psychology and Christianity, 11*(2), 170-180. A comprehensive review of about 100 validated measures of various dimensions of religiosity is P. Hill and R. Hood (Eds.) (1999). *Measures of religiosity.* Birmingham, AL: Religious Education Press. A concise review of ways of assessing spirituality in psychotherapy is Gorsuch, R. and Miller, W. (1999). Assessing spirituality. In Wm. Miller (Ed.). *Integrating spirituality into treatment.* Washington, DC: American Psychological Association, pp. 47-64.

104. Three resources for treatment planning based on the biopsychosocial model are Berman, P. (1997). *Case conceptualization and treatment planning: Exercises for integrating theory with clinical practice.* Thousand Oaks, CA: Sage Publications; Jongsma, A. and Peterson, M. (1995). *The complete psychotherapy treatment planner.* New York: John Wiley and Sons; and Wiger, D. (1999). *The psychotherapy documentation primer.* New York: John Wiley and Sons. A therapy-by-objectives (TBO) approach is an application of the principles of management-by-objectives (MBO) for the purposes of therapeutic case management. These are goal-

directed, teleological approaches. Examples are Odiorne, G. (1965). *Management by objectives: A system of managerial leadership.* New York: Pitman, see pp. 54-79; and Humble, J. (1973). *How to manage by objectives.* New York: AMACOM, a Division of American Management Associations, see pp. 31-77.

105. As a mechanism of therapeutic change, a corrective emotional experience was emphasized originally by Alexander and French as a balance to Freud's intellectual, insight-oriented theory. Alexander, F. and French, T. (1946). *Psychoanalytic therapy: Principles and applications.* New York: Ronald Press. It has been incorporated into a form of integrative psychotherapy by Wachtel, P. and McKinney, M. (1992). Cyclical psychodynamics and integrative psychodynamic therapy. In J. Norcross and M. Goldfried (Eds.). *Handbook of psychotherapy integration.* New York: Basic Books, pp. 335-370, especially pp. 338 and 343. See also Godlman, R. and Greenberg,L. (1997). Case formulation in process-experiential therapy. In T. Eells (Ed.), *Handbook of psychotherapy case formulation.* New York: Guilford Press, pp. 402-430.

106. For practical discussion of decisional counseling, see Ivey, A., Ivey, M., and Simek-Downing, L. (1987). *Counseling and psychotherapy: Integrating skills, theory, and practice.* Englewood Cliffs, NJ: Prentice-Hall, pp. 25-48. See also Levenson, H. and Strupp, H. (1997). Cyclical maladaptive patterns: Case formulation in time-limited dynamic psychotherapy. In T. Eells, (Ed.). *Handbook of psychotherapy case formulation.* New York: The Guilford Press, pp. 84 -115.

107. Both the concept of "spiritual intelligence" and its competencies have been articulated by Emmons, R. (1999). *The psychology of ultimate concerns: Motivation and spirituality in personality.* New York: The Guilford Press, p. 164.

108. Kiresuk, T., Smith, A. and Cardillo, J. (Eds.) (1994). *Goal attainment scaling: Applications, theory, and measurement.* Hillsdale, NJ: Lawrence Erlbaum.

109. See the section on evaluation in this chapter for further discussion of the criteria for an effective decision-making process.

110. For definitions and distinctions of terms such as spiritual discernment, spiritual formation, and spiritual guidance and direction, see May, G. (1992). *Care of mind—care of spirit: A psychiatrist explores spiritual direction.* New York: HarperSanFrancisco, pp. 7-14.

111. These spiritual disciplines are "classic" not because they are ancient, but because they are central to experiential Christianity. Foster, R. (1981). *Freedom of simplicity.* New York: HarperSanFrancisco, p. 186, n.5. See also Foster, R. (1998). *Streams of living water: Celebrating the great traditions of Christian faith.* New York: HarperSanFrancisco, pp. 3-272.

112. See Mark 12:28-31, Matthew 22:34-40, and Luke 10:25-28. Another prayer central to later Rabbinic Judaism is the Amidah. See Rabbi L.A. Hoffman (Ed.). (1998). *My people's prayer book: Traditional prayers, modern commentaries, Vol. 2—The Amidah.* Woodstock, Vermont: Jewish Lights Publishing, pp. 38-42.

113. Merton, T. (1960). *Spiritual direction and meditation.* Collegeville, MN: The Liturgical Press, see pp. 3-48; Higgins, J. (1975). *Thomas Merton on prayer.*

Garden City, NY: Image Books, see pp. 19-26, 79-88; Pennington, M. (1980). *Centering prayer: Renewing an ancient Christian prayer form.* Garden City, NY: Image Books, see pp. 61-84; Oliver, F. (1976). *Christian growth through meditation.* Valley Forge, PA: Judson Press, see pp. 13-96.

114. The Greek term *pneuma* means both breath and spirit. Pneumogenic phrases are Spirit-directed rather than self-directed, and their focus is on one's relationship with God rather than a physiologically directed focus that characterize autogenic phrases. Their application is an example of a structured meditation of the inner way, which focuses on one's inner-life and experience (particularly one's spiritual experience), and which defines what the inner activity is that one strives for in the practice of meditation. See LeShan, L. (1974). *How to meditate.* New York: Bantam Books, pp. 41, 45, 69-72. Pneumogenic phrases are prayers of affirmation that complement prayers of petition and intercession, thanksgiving, and praise.

115. The method is described fully in Schultz, J. and Luthe, W. (1969). *Autogenic Therapy (Vol. 1): Autogenic methods.* New York: Grune and Stratton. Applications in psychotherapy with neurotics, psychotics, and personality disorders are discussed in Luthe, W. and Schultz, J. (1969). *Autogenic Therapy (Vol. 3): Applications in psychotherapy.* New York: Grune and Stratton. The technique includes passive concentration and standard exercises involving physiologically directed phrases (e.g., "my right arm is heavy and warm"), but also methods of autogenic meditation and visualization.

116. For discussion of this topic, see Wimberly, E. (1994). *Using scripture in pastoral counseling.* Nashville, TN: Abingdon Press.

117. Capps, D. (1981). *Biblical approaches to pastoral counseling.* Philadelphia: The Westminster Press, see pp. 147-205; Capps, D. (1990). *Reframing: A new method in pastoral care.* Minneapolis, MN: Fortress Press, see pp. 9-54.

118. Themes include initiative and freedom, fear and faith, conformity and rebellion, death and rebirth, and risk and redemption. Oglesby, W. (1980). *Biblical themes for pastoral care.* Nashville, TN: Abingdon, see pp. 45-220.

119. Assagioli, *The act of will,* pp. 19-84, 135-198.

120. Lester, A. (1995). *Hope in pastoral care and counseling.* Louisville, KY: Westminster John Knox Press, see pp. 125-152. Another practical book on this topic is Capps, D. (1995). *Agents of hope: A pastoral psychology.* Minneapolis, MN: Fortress Press, see pp. 52-78.

121. Olson, *The reconciled life,* pp. 99-101.

122. Wells, D. (1986). The Protestant perspective on human nature. In F. Greenspahn (Ed.). *The human condition in the Jewish and Christian traditions.* Hoboken, NJ: KTAV Publishing House, p. 94.

123. Janus, I. and Mann, L., *Decision making,* p. 11.

124. One example of this type of research is Propst, R., Ostrom, R., Watkins, P., Dean, T., and Mashburn, D. (1992). Comparative efficacy of religious and non-religious cognitive-behavioral therapy for the treatment of clinical depression in religious individuals. *Journal of Consulting and Clinical Psychology, 60,* 94-103.

Another illustration is Johnson, W., Devries, R., Ridley, C., Pettorini, D., and Peterson, D. (1994). The comparative efficacy of Christian and secular rational-emotive therapy with Christian clients. *Journal of Psychology and Theology, 22*(2), 130-140. Note that both studies used cognitive-behavioral approaches, not an experiential approach to counseling with religious clients.

125. For reviews of outcomes from pastoral counseling, see Johnson, W. (1993). Outcome research and religious psychotherapies: Where are we and where are we going? *Journal of Psychology and Theology, 3*(2), 297-308; Gartner, J., Larson, D., and Vaclar-Mayberry, C. (1990). A systematic review of the quantity and quality of empirical research published in four pastoral counseling journals, 1978-1984. *Journal of Pastoral Care, 44,* 115-123; Strunk, O. (1988). Research in the pastoral arts and sciences: A reassessment. *Journal of Pastoral Psychotherapy, 2,* 3-12. For a review of psychological literature, see Worthington, E., Kurusu, T., McCullough, M., and Sandage, S. (1996). Empirical research on religion and psychotherapeutic processes and outcomes: A 10-year review and research prospectus. *Psychological Bulletin, 119,* 448-487.

126. See Lambert, M. and Bergin, A. (1994). The effectiveness of psychotherapy. In A. Bergin and S. Garfield (Eds.). *Handbook of psychotherapy and behavior change.* New York: John Wiley and Sons, pp. 143-228.

127. One application of reconciliation is conflict resolution with victims of clergy malpractice. See Hunter, M. (1996). Ritual of reconciliation—another way. *The ISTI Sun, 2*(2), 3. Published by the Interfaith Sexual Trauma Institute at Saint John's University and Abbey in Collegeville, MN, 56321-2000.

128. See Norcross, J. and Goldfired, M. (1992). *Handbook of psychotherapy integration.* New York: Basic Books, see pp. 3-45, 94-129.

129. Illustrations of empirical research on the therapeutic efficacy of forgiveness are provided by Enright, R. (1995). *The psychology of forgiveness.* Paper presented at the National Conference on Forgiveness, Madison, WI, March 1995; McCullough, M. and Worthington, E. (1994). Models of interpersonal forgiveness and their applications to counseling: Review and critique. *Counseling and Values, 39*(1), 2-14; McCullough, M. and Worthington, E. (1994). Encouraging clients to forgive people who have hurt them: Review, critique, and research prospectus. *Journal of Psychology and Theology, 22*(1), 3-20; Pingleton, J. (1989). The role and function of forgiveness in the psychotherapeutic process. *Journal of Psychology and Theology, 17*(1), 27-35; Phillips, L. and Osborne, J. (1989). Cancer patients' experiences of forgiveness therapy. *Canadian Journal of Counseling, 23*(3), 236-251; Fitzgibbons, R. (1986). The cognitive and emotive uses of forgiveness in the treatment of anger. *Psychotherapy, 23*(4), 629-633. A number of relevant articles appeared in the Special Issue: Grace and Forgiveness (1992). *Journal of Psychology and Christianity, 11*(2), 125-216. See also Halling, S. and Rowe, J. (1996). *The implications of a phenomenological understanding of forgiveness for psychotherapy.* Paper presented at the Second National Conference on Forgiveness in Clinical Practice. Baltimore, MD, April 26, 1996; Enright, R. and Fitzgibbons, R. (2000). *Helping clients*

forgive: An empirical guide for resolving anger and restoring hope. Washington, DC: American Psychological Association. Finally, two helpful books written for clients are Affinito, M. (1999). *When to forgive: A healing guide to help you.* Oakland, CA: New Harbinger Publications; Smedes, L. (1996). *The art of forgiving: When you need to forgive and don't know how.* Nashville, TN: Moorings, A Division of the Ballantine Publishing Group.

130. Bergin, A. and Garfield, S. (1994). *Handbook of psychotherapy and behavior change.* New York: John Wiley and Sons, see pp. 3-18, 143-376.

131. Garfield, S. (1992). Eclectic psychotherapy: A common factors approach. In J. Norcross and M. Goldfried (Eds.). *Handbook of psychotherapy integration.* New York: Basic Books, pp. 169-201.

132. Olson, *The reconciled life,* pp. 204-226. Measurement of the construct of reconciliation will benefit from comparable efforts to measure the construct of forgiveness. Current examples are: Brown, S., Gorsuch, R., Rosik, C., and Ridley, C. (2001). The development of a scale to measure forgiveness. *Journal of Psychology and Christianity, 20*(1), 40-52; McCullough, M., Pargament, K., and Thoresen, C. (Eds.) (2000). *Forgiveness: Theory, research, and practice.* New York: The Guilford Press.

133. Kiresuk, T., Smith, A., and Cardillo, J. (Eds.) (1994). *Goal attainment scaling: Applications, theory, and measurement.* Hillsdale, NJ: Lawrence Erlbaum Associates.

134. Current books on clinical and religious measures include Fischer, J. and Corcoran, K. (1987/1994). *Measures for clinical practice: A sourcebook. Vols. 1 and 2.* New York: The Free Press; Hill, P., and Hood, R. (1999). *Measures of religiosity.* Birmingham, AL: Religious Education Press; Maruish, M. (1999). *The use of psychological testing for treatment planning and outcomes assessment.* Mahwah, NJ: Lawrence Erlbaum Associates; Ogles, B., Lambert, M., and Masters, K. (1996). *Assessing outcome in clinical practice.* Boston: Allyn and Bacon.

135. Rice, L. and Greenberg, L. (1990). Fundamental dimensions in experiential therapy: New directions in research. In G. Lietaer, J. Rombauts, and R. Van Balen (Eds.). *Client-centered and experiential psychotherapy in the nineties.* Louvain, Belgium: Leuven University Press, pp. 397-444.

136. Rice and Greenberg discussed a variety of research approaches to the study of the essential mechanisms of change occurring in psychotherapy, which are based on discovery-oriented, intensive analyses of recurring patterns of client performance within its in-session context. Rice, L. and Greenberg, L. (1984). *Patterns of change.* New York: Guilford Press, pp. vi, 2, and 8.

137. See Stackhouse, M. (Ed.) (1976). *James Luther Adams: On being human religiously.* Boston: Beacon Press, p. xxiii.

138. Cowdell, S. (1996). *Is Jesus unique? A study of recent Christology.* New York: Paulist Press, pp. 195, 203. To affirm that truth, wisdom, and saving grace is present in other religions does not necessitate the view that all the religious traditions of humanity are equally valid paths to an identical religious reality, or that they

are all particular, concrete instances of a common encounter with God. There are for example, nontheistic religious traditions such as Advaitin Hinduism and Theravada Buddhism. In this respect, Christian humanism presented here is closer to Christian "inclusivism" illustrated by the Catholic theologian, Karl Rahner, than the "pluralism" defined by McGrath, A. (1997). *Christian theology: An introduction.* Malden, MA: Blackwell Publishers, pp. 534-537.

139. Ibid., p. 290.

140. Cited by Livingston, J. (1971). *Modern Christian thought: From the enlightenment to Vatican II.* New York: Macmillan, p. 496. The view that salvation is mediated exclusively through the Roman Catholic Church is a more narrow version of "Christian particularism," which holds that only those who hear and respond to the Christian gospel may be saved. See McGrath, *Christian theology: An introduction,* pp. 532-534. By contrast, McGrath notes that in *Nostra Aetate, 28,* (Oct., 1965), the Second Vatican Council acknowledged revelation in other religions, yet limited salvation to the Christian way, for reconciliation between God and humans was achieved in Christ (Ibid., p. 536).

141. A more inclusive position has been developed by several other Catholic theologians. See Dupuis, J. (1997). *Toward a Christian theology of religious pluralism.* Maryknoll, NY: Orbis Books, pp. 185-202, 330-357.

142. Christian humanism is compatible with the inclusive pluralism expressed in the Unitarian-Universalist vision. See Frost, E. (Ed.). (1998). *With purpose and principle: Essays about the seven principles of Unitarian Universalism.* Boston: Skinner House Books. Christian pluralism is not, however, the same as religious relativism, and remains Christian, not Unitarian.

143. Wright, N. T. (1996). *Jesus and the victory of God.* Minneapolis, MN: Fortress Press, p. 91.

144. The fundamental structures of the Jewish worldview were the concepts of monotheism and covenant. Witherington, B. (1995). *The Jesus quest.* Downers Grove, IL: InterVarsity Press, pp. 222-223. These continue as central ideas in contemporary Judaism: God is one, not two, not three or more. See Steinberg, M. (1975). *Basic Judaism.* New York: Harcourt Brace, pp. 42-45. In the liberal Protestant tradition, covenantal theology affirms reconciliation as its aim, expressed as unity of heart and spirit, a just peace church, and a church united and uniting. See Fackre, G. (1990). Christian doctrine in the United Church of Christ. In D. Johnson and C. Hambrick-Stowe (Eds.). *Theology and identity: Traditions, movements, and polity in the United Church of Christ.* Cleveland, OH: United Church Press, p. 142; Shinn, R. (1990). *Confessing our faith: An interpretation of the statement of faith of the United Church of Christ.* Cleveland, OH: United Church Press, pp. xi, 3, 82, 85.

145. For a Christian Quaker's discussion of these Jewish concepts, see Foster, R. (1981). *Freedom of simplicity.* New York: HarperSanFrancisco, pp. 24-32. Another contemporary dialogue is Zannoni, A. (1994). *Jews and Christians speak of Jesus.* Minneapolis, MN: Fortress Press.

146. Both Abraham Heschel's philosophical anthropology and Viktor Frankl's Logotherapy are rooted in their shared Jewish faith. See Macquarrie, J. (1988). *20th century religious thought.* Philadelphia: Trinity Press International, p. 394. Another Torah scholar with psychological insights is Rabbi Abraham Twerski (1993). *I am I: A Jewish perspective—from the case files of an eminent psychiatrist.* Brooklyn, NY: Shaar Press.

147. Chilton *Pure kingdom: Jesus' vision of God,* pp. 56-101. Jesus' vision was more personal, relational, inclusive, non-violent, earthly, and urgent (Ibid., pp. 29-30.)

148. The persistent preaching of Christian exclusivism in mainline Protestant churches may be one of the causes for their declining membership among educated Americans. In this respect, the corollary rise in membership among more conservative, evangelical, and fundamentalist churches is a cause of concern for interfaith relations.

149. McGrath, A. E. (1994/1997). *Christian theology: An introduction.* Molden, MA: Blackwell, pp. 242-248.

150. Troeltsch, E. (1925/1991). *The Christian Faith.* Minneapolis, MN: Fortress Press, p. 122. The name that Hindus give to the supreme reality is *Brahman,* which has a dual etymology derived from both *br,* "to breathe," and *brih,* "to be great." The chief attributes to be linked with the one divine name and reality are *sat, chit,* and *ananda:* God is being, awareness, and bliss. Smith, H. (1991). *The world's religions.* New York: HarperSanFrancisco, p. 60.

151. See Wells, D. (1986). Protestant views of sin. In F. Greenspahn (Ed.). *The human condition in the Jewish and Christian traditions.* Hoboken, NY: KTAV Publishing House, pp. 83-86. The distinctions drawn by Wells seem to lose the more dialectical nature of the theologies he classifies as "monistic," hence his categories lead to misunderstandings.

152. Troeltsch, E. (1925/1991). *The Christian faith.* Minneapolis, MN: Fortress Press, p. 122. A contemporary apology for a nontheistic Christianity has been offered by an American, Episcopal Bishop. See Spong, J. (1998). *Why Christianity must change or die: A bishop speaks to believers in exile.* New York: HarperSanFrancisco.

153. A Buddhist perspective on wisdom and the will warrants further exploration. A Western translation is Humphreys, C. (1971). *A Western approach to zen.* Wheaton, IL: The Theosophical Publishing House. A contemporary comparison with Christianity is Borg, M. (1997). *Jesus and Buddha: The parallel sayings.* Berkeley, CA: Ulysses Press. A therapeutic application is Brazier, D. (1995). *Zen therapy: Transcending the sorrows of the human mind.* New York: John Wiley and Sons.

154. Smith, *The world's religions,* p. 60.

155. A concise discussion of these four pathways to liberation from finite being, limited knowledge, and human sorrow is provided by Smith, *The world's religions,* pp. 26-50. The ultimate goal is *samadhi,* the state in which the human mind is completely absorbed in God (p. 49).

156. For discussion, see Macquarrie, *20th century religious thought,* pp. 416-418.

157. Cited by Cowdell, *Is Jesus unique?*, pp. 267-268.

158. Advocates of a Christian, personal realism include Henry Nelson Wieman, Douglas C. Macintosh, H. Richard Niebuhr, and the neothomist theologian Jacques Maritain. See Livingston, J. C. (1971). *Modern Christian thought from the enlightenment to Vatican II.* New York: Macmillan, pp. 385-456. Several others have been included in this approach: Harry Emerson Fosdick, Nicolas Berdejaev, John Macmurray, Charles Hartshorne, James Ward, Bordon Bowne, and Edgar Brightman. See Macquarrie, *20th century religious thought*, pp. 63-68, 186-209, 258-277, 438.

159. Borg, *Jesus—a new vision*, pp. 137; 143, n.5 and n.8; 148, n.63 and n.66.

160. Macquarrie, *20th century religious thought*, p. 418. For discussion of the Christian image of a suffering God, see also McGrath, *Christian theology: An introduction*, pp. 248-254.

161. Borg, *Jesus—a new vision*, pp. 104; 117, n.1; 118, n.21; 125, n.75.

162. Cited by Livingston, *Modern Christian thought*, pp. 480-482. A similar emphasis upon service as an expression of the Christian gospel's "reverence for life" was given by Albert Schweitzer. See Chilton, B. (1996). *Pure kingdom: Jesus' vision of God.* Grand Rapids, MI: William B. Eerdman, pp. 1-6.

163. Ibid., p. 471.

164. Rand, A. (1964). *The virtue of selfishness.* New York: NAL-Dutton.

165. This definition was provided by the personalistic psychologist, William Stern, quoted by Allport, G. (1968). *The person in psychology: Selected essays.* Boston: Beacon Press, p. 280. Allport contrasted Stern's definition with Titchener's: "Psychology is the study of experience considered as dependent on some person." The latter seemed a rhetorical expression of deference to the person, whereas Stern considered the person the most significant fact in all of science. Ibid., p. 297, n.4. Redefining psychology as "the systematic study of personal experience" opens its horizons to the insights from other scientific disciplines, the humanities, arts, and religion.

166. Allport, *The person in psychology*, p. 280.

167. The need for a holistic, idiographic, and ethical model of the individual in medical science and practice was recommended recently by Bolletino, R. C. (1998). The need for a new ethical model in medicine: A challenge for conventional, alternative, and complementary practitioners. *Advances in Mind-Body Medicine, 14,* 6-28. The author added the spiritual and historical dimension, but contrary to the title of the article, he minimized the moral dimension.

168. Emmons, *The psychology of ultimate concerns*, pp. 89-156.

169. See Paul Tillich, "Theology is not anthropology and when studied as if it were it surrenders itself into the hands of Feuerbach and his psychological and sociological followers. But theology is the solution of the anthropological question, which is the problem of the finiteness of man." Quoted in Taylor, M. K. (1991). *Paul Tillich: Theologian of the boundaries.* Minneapolis, MN: Fortress Press, p. 112.

170. Cited by Livingston, *Modern Christian thought*, pp. 402-403.

171. Madill, A. and Barkham, M. (1997). Discourse analysis of a theme in one successful case of brief psychodynamic-interpersonal psychotherapy. *Journal of Counseling Psychology,* extract 12, session 5, line 6.

172. Ibid., p. 233.

173. Task analysis research with Gestalt therapy clients indicates that a shifting in attitude from self-criticism to self-acceptance takes place in resolving conflicts. See Greenberg, L. (1984). A task analysis of intrapersonal conflict resolution. In L. Rice, and L. Greenberg (Eds.). *Patterns of change.* New York: Guilford Press, p. 120.

174. Freud, S. (1917/1957). Mourning and melancholia. In J. Strachey (Ed.). *Standard edition* (Vol. 14). London: Hogarth Press.

175. Selye, H. (1976). *The stress of life.* New York: McGraw Hill.

176. Rogers, *A theory of therapy, personality and interpersonal relations,* p. 213.

177. Madill and Barkham, Disclosure analysis of a theme . . . , extract 2, session 3, lines 8-12; extract 3, session 7, lines 5-11; extract 14, session 7.

178. Bibring, E. (1968). The mechanism of depression. In W. Gaylin (Ed.). *The meaning of despair.* New York: Aronson, pp. 163-164.

179. Tillich, P. (1952). *The courage to be.* New Haven, CN: Yale University Press.

180. Luborsky, L., Singer, B., Hartke, J., Crits-Christophy, P., and Cohen, M. (1984). Shifts in depressive state during psychotherapy: Which concepts of depression fit the context of Mr. Q's shifts? In L. Rice and L. Greenberg (Eds). *Patterns of change.* New York: The Guilford Press, pp. 157-193.

181. Beck, A. (1972). *Depression: Causes and treatment.* Philadelphia: University of Pennsylvania Press.

182. This definition is an expansion of the discussion by May, G. (1992). *Care of mind—care of spirit: A psychiatrist explores spiritual direction.* New York: HarperSanFrancisco, pp. 7- 14. A practical guide to spiritual disciplines written by a Christian Quaker is Foster, R. (1988). *Celebration of discipline: The path to spiritual growth.* New York: HarperSanFrancisco.

183. The presence of the spirit in Jesus' life was a particular emphasis of the Gospel of Luke. For commentary and various portraits of Jesus, see Borg, *Jesus—A new vision,* pp. 51, 54 n.30.

184. Smith, H. (1976). *Forgotten truth: The primordial tradition.* New York: Harper and Row. See also Smith, H. (1982). *Beyond the post-modern mind.* New York: Crossroad.

185. John Macquarrie characterized the founders of the world's religions as spiritual geniuses who had an inspiring vision of holy being, and whose visions of God have been and still are among the most powerful factors shaping human existence. Macquarrie, J. (1996). *Mediators between human and divine: From Moses to Muhammad.* New York: Continuum.

186. Eells, T. (1997). Psychotherapy case formulation: History and current status. In T. Eells (Ed.). *Handbook of psychotherapy case formulation.* New York: The Guilford Press, pp. 1-25.

Chapter 6

Islamic Psychology

Zehra Ansari

INTRODUCTION

"Today have I perfected your religious law for you, and have bestowed upon you the full measure of My blessings, and willed that self-surrender unto Me shall be your religion" (Quran 5:3).[1]

Islam is one of the three monotheistic religions of the world. The word "Islam" is derived from two Arabic words: *taslim* (submission) and *salam* (peace).[2] Followers of Islam (Muslims)[3] profess to gain peace in their lives in this world and in the hereafter through a complete submission to the will of God.[4]

A monotheistic belief in the oneness of God is the essence of Islam, summarized in Chapter 112 of the Quran: "Say: He is the One God; God is Eternal, the Uncaused Cause of All That Exists; He begets not, and neither is He begotten; and there is nothing that could be compared with Him" (Quran 112:1-4). Muslims believe that God, and God alone, created the universe; he has no partner and no offspring; and it is his divine will that governs all occurrences.

Muslims also believe that God transmitted his divine will to humanity by way of prophets, including Adam, Noah, Abraham, David, Moses, and Jesus. The last of these prophets, and the one to whom the sacred Quran was revealed, was Muhammad.

The Islamic creed is: "There is no god except Allah, and Muhammad is His Messenger."[5] In addition to emphasizing the oneness of God, this statement makes clear Muhammad's status as a human being, not a divine being. As the seal of the prophets, Muhammad's role was to transmit God's message to humanity. Because of his role in revealing divine truth and the will of God, Muhammad holds a sacred place in the hearts of Muslims as the one whose sayings and practices are to be emulated in order to please God.

Islam is a complete system of beliefs—indeed, a complete way of life. It governs the relationship between a human being and the Creator as well as the relationships among human beings themselves. There are approximately one billion Muslims in the world today, and they are found among the members of every nationality, race, and culture worldwide. Approximately six million Muslims live in the United States where Islam is currently the fastest growing religion.[6]

A Brief History of Islam

The history of Islam centers on the life and teachings of Muhammad. Muhammad was born in Mecca, in what is today Saudi Arabia, in the year 570 A.D. Muhammad's father, Abdullah, died before his birth and his mother, Amina, died shortly afterward. Muhammad was raised by his paternal uncle, Abu Talib, who was the leader of the respected Quraish tribe in Mecca. Early in his life, Muhammad earned the title of "Al-Amin" because of his truthfulness, generosity, and sincerity. He was described by his contemporaries as calm and meditative, and he was sought after as an arbitrator of disputes. He was known to meditate frequently in the Cave of Hira, near the summit of Jabl-e-Nur (the Mountain of Light) just outside Mecca. "At the age of forty," while meditating there, "Muhammad received his first revelation from God through the Angel Jibrael (Gabriel)."[7] "Read in the name of thy Sustainer who created men out of a germ-cell" (Quran 96:1-2). Muhammad continued to receive such revelations for the next twenty-three years until his death. These revelations make up the Islamic scripture known as the Quran.

Muhammad was very distressed and perturbed by the decadence of his society. Muhammad began sharing his revelations with his close relatives and friends, and preaching the prophetic message of Islam. He and his followers were bitterly persecuted by the people of Mecca. The persecution became so unbearable that God commanded Muhammad and his followers (called Muslims) to Medina, a city 260 miles north of Mecca. This migration, known as the Hijra, was more than just a geographical relocation. Once in Medina, Muhammad established the first Islamic society that has served as a model for all Islamic societies since. As a result of the Hijra, Muslims were transformed from a persecuted minority fleeing their Meccan homes to a major political power with control and influence reaching far beyond the borders of Medina. The Hijra is such an important event in Islamic history that it marks the beginning of the Islamic calendar.[8]

After several years in Medina, Muhammad was able to return to Mecca peacefully and establish Islam there. The greater part of Arabia was Muslim before Muhammad's death at the age of sixty-three (632 A.D.) Within a century of his death, Islam had spread to Spain in the West and to China in the Far East.

Basic Islamic Beliefs and Practices

The practice of Islam consists of five basic acts of worship, known as the Five Pillars of Islam. These are based on the teachings of the Quran, and on the sayings and actions of Muhammad. These Five Pillars are: (1) a two-fold affirmation of faith *(shahadah)* in which a Muslim states the Islamic creed, "There is no god except Allah, and Muhammad is His Messenger"; (2) the five daily prayers *(salat);* (3) fasting *(sawm)* from dawn to sunset throughout the Islamic month of Ramadan; (4) the pilgrimage to Mecca *(hajj),* which Muslims are required to perform once in a lifetime if health and finances permit; and (5) paying a 2.5 percent tax *(zakat)* on one's savings and possessions in excess of one's needs for the benefit of the community and the poor. These five acts of worship are obligatory for all Muslims unless performance of them incurs physical or financial harm.

The basic articles of faith in Islam include believing in God, his angels, his prophets, his scriptures, and the Day of Judgment. Muslims believe that every human being will be judged based on his or her deeds and will correspondingly earn his or her way to heaven or hell. As God's unseen servants, angels are each charged by God with a specific duty to perform. The angel Gabriel was charged with the duty of transmitting God's revelations to the prophets.

Muslims also believe that throughout history, since the creation of Adam, God has sent numerous prophets and messengers to implant in the human mind awareness of his existence. Some of these prophets are mentioned in the Quran (Quran 42:13). All are believed to be human beings who preached a common religion of submission and accountability to one God. The last three major prophets were Moses, Jesus, and Muhammad, who founded respectively: Judaism, Christianity, and Islam. All three were descendants of the patriarch Abraham and his two sons, Ishmael and Isaac. Hassan Hathout writes: "Islam is the final expression of the Abrahamic tradition. One should in fact properly speak of Judeo-Christian-Islamic tradition, for Islam shares with the other Abrahamic religions their sacred history, the basic ethical teachings contained in the Ten Commandments, and above all, belief in One God."[9]

Muslims believe that God gave some prophets scriptures to share the revealed message of divine guidance with their fellow human beings, and some were given the power to perform miracles. Muslims believe in several revealed scriptures, namely the Psalms of David, the Torah, the Bible, and the Quran.[10] It is often surprising for people of other religions to hear that Muslims not only believe in the existence of prophets such as Moses and Jesus, but that Muslims also hold these prophets in very high esteem and even believe in the original messages of their scriptures. Because of their common ancestry and shared theology and ethics, Muslims have a great reverence for Judaism and Christianity.

Although Muhammad was not given the power of specific miracles as Moses and Jesus were, the revelation of the Quran itself is considered to be a miracle performed through Muhammad. He did not know how to read or write, and yet the Quran was written in the most literary and poetic form of the Arabic language. As the Quran itself challenged (Quran 17:88, 11:13-14), its literary excellence could not be duplicated even by the best poets of the time or later. These facts attest to the divine source of the Quranic text and refute assertions by some historians that the Quran was written by Muhammad.

The Quranic verses revealed by God were memorized by Muhammad and dictated to his companions as they were revealed. To this day, Muslims believe the Quran is preserved in its original words as the divine revelation to Muhammad 1,400 years ago. It is this one text that is followed by all Muslims regardless of sect or school of thought. The practice and traditions *(Sunnah)* of Muhammad, which include his sayings *(Hadith),* are additional guides for Muslims in understanding the Quran, and they are the primary sources of Islamic principles and law *(Shariah).*[11]

The performance of good deeds and abstinence from evil actions are basic expectations of Islamic teachings. Some examples of Muhammad's *Hadith* are:

- "God has no mercy on one who has no mercy for others"
- "None of you truly believes until he wishes for his brother what he wishes for himself"
- "He who eats his full while his neighbor goes without food is not a believer"
- "Powerful is not he who knocks the other down, indeed powerful is he who controls himself in a fit of anger"
- "God does not judge according to your bodies and appearances, but scans your hearts and looks at your deeds"
- " There is a reward for kindness to every living thing."[12]

Through its insistence on the importance of knowledge, thinking, and striving for perfection, the Quran instilled among its early followers the intellectual curiosity, independent inquiry, and aesthetic sensitivity that is behind the legacy that Islam gave to world civilization. Islam incorporated the science and culture of the old civilizations "into its own world view, as long as they were consistent with the principles of Islam." Each ethnic or racial group that embraced Islam contributed toward the single Islamic civilization to which all Muslims belonged. Universal solidarity took precedence over attachments to a particular tribe, race, culture, or language. People of all ethnic origins worked together to cultivate various arts and sciences.[13]

As Islam grew, universities and libraries flourished, probably in part because of Muhammad's hadith. Seeking knowledge is considered an obligation of every Muslim man and woman. Great advances in medicine, physics, astronomy, architecture, and literature were made in Córdoba and Baghdad. Many important systems such as algebra, the Arabic numerals, and the concept of zero were transmitted to medieval Europe from the Islamic world. Early Muslims developed sophisticated navigational instruments that made several European explorations possible. Greek philosophy was transmitted to Europe through Arabic translations.[14]

There are several other unique features of Islam that need to be mentioned in order to understand it. These include expressions of God consciousness, dualism, innocence at birth, the place of worship, holidays and the Islamic calendar, the relation of religion and the state, the absence of a priesthood, women's rights in Islam, polygamy, prohibitions, Islamic sects, and schools of thought.

Expression of God Consciousness

God consciousness *(Taqwa)* is a very fundamental concept in Islam. Consequently, Muslims remember God in everything they do. Certain common expressions are *Bismillah* (In the Name of Allah) before beginning any task; *Alhamdulillah* (Praise be to Allah) when one is pleased with something; *Inshaallah* (If Allah Wills) when one intends to do something in the future; and *Allahu Akbar* (God is Great) when witnessing or experiencing anything that is awesome.

Dualism

An important concept that recurs in the Quran is that of dualism in creation. "And in everything have We created opposites" (Quran, 51:49). Every entity has two coexisting forms that may be different in characteristics and function, but are congruent parts of the same whole.[15] Examples of such duality in the universe are human sexuality (male and female), animals and plants, light and darkness, hot and cold, good and evil, positive and negative magnetism, happiness and sadness, and so forth. God alone is one. All other realities are dual.

Innocence at Birth

Though imbued with the potentials for both God-consciousness and moral failings (Quran 91:7-8), and the freedom to choose between good and evil, humans are born innocent and free of sin (Quran 95:4). Accountability for one's actions begins after puberty. Thereafter, each individual is considered to be responsible for his or her own behavior, good and bad, saintly and sinful. God is by nature most forgiving so he will forgive those who sincerely repent for their sins.

Place of Worship

A Muslim's place of worship is called a *masjid* or mosque. Muslims believe that worship is not limited to a mosque, however. In other words, the whole world is a mosque. Three particularly holy places for Muslims are the Kaaba, in Mecca, Saudi Arabia; Masjid-al-Nabi (the Prophet's Mosque) in Medina, Saudi Arabia; and Masjid Aqsa in Jerusalem.

Holidays

Muslims have two major holidays: Eid-ul-Fitr, the day following the fasting month of Ramadan; and Eid-al-Adha, the Holiday of Sacrifice, following Hajj, the pilgrimage to Mecca. Hajj is in part a commemoration of the trials that Abraham and his wife, Haggar, experienced in the Arabian desert with their baby Ishmael.

Islamic Calendar

Muslims follow the Lunar calendar in which each month starts with the new moon. The lunar year is ten days shorter than the Gregorian calendar.

State and Religion

Islam is a total way of life. It encourages a holistic approach to living. Muslims believe that the entire universe is governed by God's will; therefore, religion and politics should not be separated. Islam encourages an economic, social, and political way of life that leads toward the one unifying goal—acceptance of the will of God.

No Priesthood

There is no priesthood in Islam. Every individual is required to establish a direct link with God through worship and piety. A person who leads congregational prayer is called the imam. Any male who is respected for his piety and knows how to pray may be chosen by the congregation to be the imam.

Women's Rights in Islam

Islam emphasizes the common origin and equal value of men and women in many verses (e.g., Quran 30:21; 7:189; 9:71-72; 4:1; 33:35). The identity of a woman is fully protected in Islam. When she marries, a woman keeps her maiden name and has the right to keep her religion, provided she believes in one of the revealed religions. She also receives inheritance, and she may own and manage property. Similar rights were granted to married women in Europe as late as the fourteenth century.

Furthermore, a man and a woman are equally obligated to seek knowledge, and a woman may pursue any occupation or profession. She may spend her earnings in any way she wishes, and she has no financial obligation to support her family.

Polygamy

Polygamy is permitted for men in Islam as a "conditional permission."[16] Polygamy is more an exception than the rule. A relevant verse is Quran 4:129: "You are never able to be just and fair as between women." Many Islamic scholars interpret this verse to mean that monogamy is the preferred form of marriage in Islam.[17] Polygamy, when practiced under prescribed conditions, such as a high number of widows due to war, is a means of giving legitimate status to women and children who could become victims of extramarital affairs.

Prohibitions

Islam prohibits all intoxicating substances (wine, liquor, and drugs), meat and products from swine (pork, bacon, ham, lard), and meat from carrion. Islam also forbids all forms of gambling and any sexual relationships outside of marriage.

Islamic Sects

Islam has two major sects, Sunni and Shiite. Sunnis are the majority. There are no fundamental differences in their basic theological beliefs; however, they disagree over the rightful successor of Muhammad. Shiite Muslims believe that Ali, Muhammad's cousin, was the rightful successor of Muhammad, hence the leader of the Muslim state after Muhammad, whereas Sunni Muslims believe that Abu Bakr, Muhammad's closest friend, was the rightful successor.

Schools of Thought

Different schools of thought *(madhahib)* follow variations in details of Islamic practice based on the various interpretations of Islamic law by different scholars of Islam. Currently, there are four existing Sunni schools of thought (Hanafi, Hanbali, Maliki, and Shafi'i) and one Shiite school of thought (Jafari), each one named after the Islamic scholar upon whose interpretations the school is based.

PERSONALITY THEORY

Personality Structure: A Dialectical Unity of Body, Mind, and Spirit

All human beings have a common origin, the *nafs* (self or "living entity"). The *nafs* is an integrated whole of biological, psychological, and spiritual domains of life granted by the Creator.[18] Its usage in the Quran refers to "the common origin of all humankind."[19] The Quran addresses the origin and the process of creation in general, including the creation of human beings in particular (Quran, 4:1; 38:71-72; 15:29; 51:49; 36:36). For instance, in one verse the Quran states: "O Mankind! Be conscious of your Sustainer, who has created you out of one living entity *[nafs]* and out of it created its mate *[zawj]*, and out of the two spread abroad a multitude of men and women. . . ." (Quran, 4:1). Sometimes in Islamic literature, *naf* refers to the basic pleasurable instincts in human beings. It is more commonly translated as the "self."

Personality is viewed as a complex and multifaceted unity. Its three major components of body, mind, and spirit interact with one another to form a whole.[20]

The Islamic view of human nature is dialectical. The body with its biological instincts and needs is one pole, and the spirit with its abstract and subliminal (spiritual) goals is the other. The psychological component of human personality, referred interchangeably in Islamic philosophy as soul, self *(nafs)*, overlaps the body and spirit, and acts as a mediator between the two. Consisting of body, mind, and spirit, the total human being as God intended is called *nafs wama sawwaha* (Quran, 91:7-8). For consistency and clarity, the psychological component of personality is referenced as the mind in the following discussion.

Islamic personality theory follows the four types of causes identified by Aristotle: material, efficient, formal, and final.[21] There are many references in the Quran about the biological components (material causes) that constitute a human being. Some of the recurring elements are clay (Quran, 6:2), soil (22:5), molded mud (15:26), sticky clay (37:11), water (25:54), germ-cell (96:1) or clot of blood (2:14).[22] Heredity (genetics) also contributes toward the biological aspects of human personality. All of these may be considered as material causes symbolized structurally as the body.

Human beings are biological creatures with basic needs for survival and pleasure (sex) as suggested by Maslow's concept of basic (deficiency) needs. Fulfillment of these needs is necessary for life to be sustained. These human needs are fulfilled through learning and experience (an efficient cause). When the fulfillment of the needs arising from the biological domain becomes one's primary objective and reaches the level of passion, the individual's soul is referred to in Islamic literature as *nafs Ammarah,* that is, a "soul addicted to passion."[23] Such a personality type may be considered an example of a formal cause. Exclusive indulgence in this biological domain of life inhibits the growth of the psychological and the spiritual domains of personality. Islam prescribes as the ultimate purpose of life acceptance of the will of Allah. This ultimate purpose is a final cause which, when chosen as one's life purpose, leads toward a balance between the bodily needs and spiritual aspirations.

The psychological domain of personality, the mind, consists of three primary attributes or functions with which humans are endowed by God: intelligence, will or volition, and emotions (affective/intuitive). These three functions (subdomains) represent the human mind and constitute the psychological domain. These personality characteristics may be considered as formal causes of behavior; that is, personality is formed by intelligence, will, and emotion. Besides these unique psychological attributes, the mind subsumes the attributes of the body as well as the spirit, and acts as an intermediary between them.[24]

Spirit is the third domain of personality. Spirit is that human domain which connects humans to their Creator.[25] In describing the process of human creation, the Quran states: "[For] Lo, thy Sustainer said unto the angels, 'Behold, I am about to create a human being out of clay, and when I have formed him fully and breathed into him of My spirit, fall you down before him in prostration!'" (Quran 38:71-72). In another verse the Quran states: "Consider the human self *[nafs]* and how it is formed in accordance with what it is meant to be *[wama sawwaha]*, and how it is imbued with moral failings as well as with consciousness of God!" Muhammad Asad interprets this verse as referring to the extremely complex human personality consisting of bodily urges, emotions and intellect so "closely intertwined as to be indissoluble." He also points out the polarity in human nature that allows human beings either to behave like the lowest animal or to achieve the highest form of spirituality and closeness to God.[26] Striving for this close relationship with God in obedience to God's will is a final cause and the ultimate purpose of all human life and action.

The step of breathing the Spirit of Allah *(nafkhat-al-ruh)* into human beings elevates them above the rest of creation and creates the spirit *(ruh),* the eternal component of personality.[27] While God has endowed humans with many of his own attributes, such as knowledge, will, and compassion, Islam clearly differentiates between the creator and the created.[28] Affirmation of the oneness of God *(Tawhid),* is the essence of Islam.[29] As the ultimate goal of human life, *Tawhid* would be considered a final cause (purpose) of human creation.[30] It is for *Tawhid* that man exists. Faruqi and Faruqi express this concept well. They write that *Tawhid* is the teleology of life from the Islamic perspective: ". . . the act of affirming Allah to be the One, absolute, transcendent Creator, Lord and Master of all that exists. *Tawhid* gives Islamic civilization its identity. It binds all its different constituents together into a harmonious and meaningful whole." This view is expressed in the phrase: *La ilaha illa Allah,* which means, "There is no god but God." Though this phrase may be considered a "negative statement, brief to the utmost limits of brevity . . . ," nevertheless, ". . . all the diversity, wealth and history, culture and learning, wisdom and civilization of Islam is compressed in this shortest of sentences."[31]

The body, mind, and spirit together form the total human being *(nafs wama sawwaha)* as God intended. In Islam, the body is finite and will end with death. The finite mind is the executive, or agent of action and thought, and functions as the mediator between the body and the spirit. The distinct functions of the mind are manifested in various forms of actions and thoughts *(aamaal),* and move humans in the direction of the final cause, which is bearing witness to the oneness of God and actualization of his will.

The spirit *(ruh)* is the entity that gives life to the organic body. It is the eternal component of human personality. Upon physical death, the spirit leaves the body and transcends into the next world (hereafter). There it will face the consequences of the choices that the individual made during his or her earthly life. During this earthly life, if the mind chooses thoughts and actions that are in harmony with both the spirit and the body, the individual will experience harmony and balance in this world as well as the next.[32]

Because this section of the chapter focuses on personality structure, the three psychological components of the mind will be stressed: intelligence *(Aql/Ilm)* will *(Qadar)* and feeling-intuition *(Qalb).* All three have been analyzed in great detail by two renowned Muslim philosophers, Ibn Sina (980-1037 A.D.) and Imam Al Ghazali (1072-1135 A.D.).[33] Ibn Sina is known as Avicenna in the West, and the one who systematized Aristotelian philosophy, filling "the void between God and man" that was left out by Aristotle.[34] These authors suggest that personality structure consists of intellect, will, and heart.

Aql/Ilm *(Intellect/Knowledge)*

The first verse that was revealed to Muhammad was: "Read in the name of thy Sustainer, who has created man out of a germ-cell! Read—for thy Sustainer is the Most Bountiful One who has taught [man] the use of the pen—taught man what he did not know" (Quran 96:1). Al Ghazzali points out that knowledge is the content of intellect, and God created knowledge first. Knowledge *(Ilm)* and intellect *(Aql)* are sometimes used interchangeably in Islamic philosophy.

Hassan Hathout points out, "Our brain is equipped to observe, imagine, rationalize, analyze, experiment, and conclude."[35] These human abilities are emphasized in the Quran many times in the form of reminders to observe, to listen, to think, to ponder, to reason, and to strive to understand the truth. Implicit in these admonitions is a phenomenological approach to learning, based upon what one actually experiences and perceives.

According to Al Ghazzali, there are two kinds of knowledge: one pertaining to the affairs of this world and the other pertaining to knowledge about God. He says that worldly knowledge is useful, praiseworthy and desirable; however, knowledge about God brings true guidance and success both in this world and the hereafter.[36]

Besides knowledge, humans have an inherent moral capacity to differentiate between good and evil.[37] However, the choice between the two is not always simple. As Satan's primary occupation is to present evil as more appealing and the good as less attractive from a worldly perspective, an individual has to exercise higher reasoning and self-discipline to make the right choice that brings him or her closer to truth.[38] In order to do the good, good must be known. As the good is ultimately of a spiritual nature, both knowledge and moral judgment are viewed as spiritual capacities.

Qadar *(Will)*

The capacity to choose is the one human attribute that differentiates them from other animals. Faruqi and Faruqi state, "Man is the only creation in which the will of God is actualized not necessarily, but with man's own personal consent."[39] Thus the concept of the will is a reference to the human capacity to make choices and decisions. These authors note that the biological aspects of human life, and certain psychological factors, are governed by the laws of nature established by God. However, as the spiritual functions of human life and personality, understanding and moral judgment are not solely determined by natural causes or laws; rather, they are directed by human will. Therefore, a human is capable of changing oneself, one's fellow beings, and one's environment so as to "actualize the divine pattern."[40] This explanation sounds similar to an existential approach with the exception that the final cause is God's will and striving to be accountable to God, not merely actualization of one's self as contemporary existential theorists would suggest.

Qalb *(Heart)*

The heart *(Qalb)* is referenced in the Quran 132 times. The "heart" symbolizes intuitive wisdom, which according to Jalal-al-Din Rumi, another medieval Muslim philosopher, brings an individual into contact with aspects of reality other than those open to observation through the senses.[41] The Quran states that if properly understood, what the heart perceives and conveys can never be untrue.[42] A contemporary social scientist, Zafar Afaq Ansari, states that from an Islamic point of view the heart is a "source of illumination, as it provides understanding of the substances that our sensual organs fail to comprehend."[43] This seems to refer to the intuitive function of the heart, and to knowledge acquired through intuition. Intuitive wisdom serves as a sixth sense.

Moreover, medieval Muslim philosophers as well as the twentieth century philosopher and poet, Mohammed Iqbal, state that the heart is the source of mystical and spiritual knowledge. Iqbal suggests that spiritual knowledge cannot be measured empirically, yet neither can it be rejected as a mere fiction or myth. In order to understand reality, one needs to utilize both intuitive and phenomenological experiences along with reason and observation. Salvatore Maddi describes a similar process in discussing the kinds of knowledge that lead to truth through scientific research.[44] The Quran states in one of the verses addressing humans' creation: ". . . and He endows you with hearing and sight and feelings as well as mind: [yet] how seldom are you grateful!" (Quran 32:7-9). It exhorts humans again and again to use both their senses and their heart (intuition) as guides to understanding truth (Quran 22:46).

Sachiko Murata writes in her book, *The Tao of Islam*, that the Quran pictures the heart as "the center of human personality, the place where they [humans] meet God. The meeting has both a cognitive and a moral dimension." Murata explains that "God pays special attention to it [one's heart] and less attention to the actual deeds that people do."[45] In the Quran this idea is expressed in several places. "If God finds any good in your hearts, He will give you something better than all that has been taken from you, and will forgive your sins; for God is much forgiving, a dispenser of grace" (Quran 8:70, 33:5, 2:118 and 2:225). While the heart is a place of vision, understanding, and remembrance of God *(dhikr),* it is also the place of doubt, denial, and unbelief. Consequently, the heart is the most vulnerable part of a human psyche that can succumb to the evil influences of Satan's misguidance.[46]

The heart's intuitive and affective functions seem to operate within both the psychological and spiritual domains of human personality. Human knowledge about the spiritual domain is limited. However, God may bestow the secrets of this domain to individuals of His choice. The more one is conscious of God *(Taqwa),* the greater the chance that one will be chosen for spiritual endowments and illumination.

Personality Dynamics

According to Islam, the Oneness of God *(Tawhid)* is not only the essence of Islam; it is the primary motivating force, the innate drive behind human behavior, and the ultimate purpose of life. It is for *Tawhid* that humans exist. Thus, the cosmos is viewed teleologically, and *Tawhid* is: ". . . the first principle governing the universe. To witness that there is no god but God is to hold that He alone is the Creator Who gave to everything its being. He is the First and the Last."[47]

God instilled in humans an innate thirst for knowledge. This inborn drive has made them become explorers, scientists, inventors, philosophers, historians, and futurists. It motivates humans to reach the highest limits of any knowledge base and to attain their highest potential. *Tawhid* affirms that God created humans for the purpose of knowing and worshiping him (Quran 51:56). This purpose is fulfilled when, as viceroys on earth, humans actualize the divine pattern in themselves, in others, and in the universe (Quran 2:30; 6:165; 10:14).

It is logical to believe that with the ability to choose, humans would be held accountable for the choices they make. This is true in the religious as well as secular realms. Hassan Hathout notes that in a religious context, the concept of accountability implies that one should not face consequences on the Day of Judgment unless one has the ability to make choices. Nor should one be held responsible for events that are outside the sphere of human choice. Animals are exempt from the continuous battle of the will within the self, because animals simply follow the laws of nature. Angels are created by God to do only good and are not capable of evil.[48] Humans have the choice to do either good or evil.

The ability to choose is what makes humans *ashraf ul-maqhlooq* (the noblest of creatures). God has given humans power over all his creation and the freedom to use its resources for human benefit, to satisfy their rightful needs and wishes. Everything on earth is subservient to humans. Human beings are responsible not only for satisfying their own personal needs, but similar needs of other humans as well. Human beings are also responsible for making the world a better place in every respect for all creation, and they must not abuse or exploit natural resources for their own private advantage without consideration for others.

Humans have been innately equipped with the ability to choose and the ability to discern good from evil. When choices are not very clear, or wrong choices have been made, God sends guidance through messengers and revealed scriptures. However, humans are constantly struggling between their primal and pleasure instincts (including associated feelings of anger, jealousy, hubris, and greed) and their more subtle spiritual urges, which are transcendent and endurable, though with delayed gratifications. This constant striving for self-improvement or actualization is called *jihad* in Islamic terminology. *Jihad* is an obligation for all humans because it is the duty to "enjoin good and forbid evil" (Quran 3:104). *Jihad* denotes human striving toward the good. Unfortunately, it is often translated into English as "Holy War," hence it has been misunderstood and misrepresented by some non-Muslims.

Jihad is a struggle against oppression and injustice. When it is within oneself to overcome ones weaknesses (e.g. control of anger) it is called *Jihad bil Nafs*. The outer striving to bring justice to the community is called

Jihad fi Sabeel Allah (for Allah's sake). Such *jihad* may be carried out through speaking or writing. If oppression continues toward oneself or others, one may resort to physical force, but inflicting harm on others for selfish reasons is against the essence of Islam, against *Tawhid,* and contrary to actualizing the will of God.

The prophet of Islam is quoted as having said after returning from a battle with unbelievers that he had returned from a lesser *jihad* to a greater *jihad,* referring to the inner struggle against temptation which every individual experiences personally. Muslims believe that there is always a negative force, personified as Satan *(Iblis),* tempting humans away from the right path. This negative force of evil finds root in human shortsightedness and the failure to see the signs of God.[49] The Quran and Hadith have many supplications asking God to protect one from Satan's evil (Quran 113:1-5, 114:1-6).

Personality Development

Islam is a religion that encourages discovery and understanding of natural phenomena through observation, reason, and scientific research. In Islam, science and religion are not opposed. To the contrary, Islam supports scientific inquiry and experimentation. Islam encourages humans to optimize their own natural tendencies and the natural resources around them. In this respect, Muslims characterize Islam as a natural religion.

There are several references in the Quran and Hadith on the importance of both nature and nurture (heredity and environment) in human development. Neither one is emphasized over the other. In this respect, Islam is compatible with contemporary biosocial and developmental theorists of maturation, such as Bandura and Piaget, which take into account both innate and environmental factors. In fact, several verses of the Quran describe the developmental stages of a human being from conception to death in physiological, cognitive, and moral dimensions (Quran 40:67; 32:7-9; 22:5).

In addition to the factors of heredity and environment (nature and nurture), an important third factor that cannot be ignored in Islam is divine intervention. Ultimately, what determines the interacting effects of nature and nurture in forming an individual's personality is God's will. The Quran states that for something to come into existence, God has to merely say, "Be" and it will happen, *"Kun faye koon"* (Quran 36:82).

All phenomena in the universe follow certain divine principles that are referred to in Islamic literature as "the *Sunnan* of Allah." These principles or laws are universal and nondiscriminatory, and may be specific to certain situations. Examples include: (a) everything happens in stages, (b) there is a stage of gestation and maturity in every process, and (c) with every hardship there is ease.[50]

Moral Development

In this section and the next, moral and spiritual development of personality are addressed from an Islamic perspective because these are the most important facets of personality in Islam. The whole purpose of human existence in Islam is to achieve submission to God. It is through total submission to his will that one attains peace in this world and the next. "Morality is a primary factor in the development of a sound, well-balanced personality and is a major determinant of a just society . . . with equal opportunity to all."[51]

God has created humans in the "best of molds" (*ahsan-i-taqwin,* Quran 95:4). However, a human can choose from a range of options available to him or her, from the least favorable (evil) to the most favorable (good). Evil is the most harmful and degrading. Alternatively, choosing the good earns self-respect and God's pleasure (Quran, 58:11, 49:13).

The concept of morality in Islam centers around seven basic beliefs:

1. God is the Creator and source of all goodness.
2. Humans are respectable and responsible agents of God.
3. All of God's creation in heaven and on earth are in the service of humans.
4. God does not expect the impossible from humans, does not forbid them to enjoy the good things in life, and God does not hold them responsible for things beyond their control.
5. God has forbidden certain things that in his wisdom are harmful to humans, hence they will serve themselves better by avoiding these things.
6. God has also made some actions obligatory, the observation of which will benefit humans.
7. Humans' ultimate return is to God and their highest goal is to please Him.[52]

When an individual holds these beliefs, his or her relationship with God is characterized by trust, obedience, and love. Consequently, human acts are performed with God consciousness. Needless to say, achieving the highest level of piety or morality involves not only faith *(Iman),* but also practice *(Ibadat).* Doctrine without deeds, or beliefs without behavior, do not bring the fulfillment human potential or peace with God and with one another.

There is no concept of original sin in Islam. Islam professes that every human is born innocent and is solely responsible for developing his or her relationship with God based on the choices he or she makes.

The Five Pillars of Islamic faith and practice, while on the surface may seem ritualistic, render a very balanced way of life when they are observed.

They are a sound prescription for a healthy body, mind, and spirit because they take into account a human's relationship (rights and obligations) with God, other humans, society at large, and the rest of creation. In so doing, these Five Pillars permit and encourage the fulfillment of both worldly and spiritual needs. Islam emphasizes balance and moderation. It is essential to be in touch with the real world and to live a natural life with its share of pleasurable and painful experiences. This is true piety in Islam. Neither extreme of a worldly or other-worldly lifestyle is good. Neither hedonism nor hermitage is encouraged in Islam; neither a libertine life nor a cloistered life of a nun or a monk is considered ultimate piety.

As mentioned earlier, the belief in One God *(Tawhid)* is the essence of Islam. The first pillar, which includes belief in God's Unity (oneness) and in Muhammad as God's prophet, implies that a Muslim believes the Quran is a sacred book of divine guidance, and accepts Muhammad as the human role model concerning how to put the Quran's injunctions into practice. Hammudah Abdulati, in his book *Islam in Focus,* writes: "The range of morality in Islam is so inclusive and integrative that it combines at once faith in God, religious rites, spiritual observances, social conduct, decision making, intellectual pursuits, habits of consumption, manners of speech and all other aspects of human life."[53]

It is impossible to address the complete code of moral conduct enjoined of a Muslim in this chapter. However, to illustrate what the Quran enjoins, a translation of one of the verses is included here.

> And worship God (alone), and do not ascribe divinity, in any way, to ought beside Him. And do good unto your parents, and near of kin, and unto orphans, and the needy, and the neighbor from among your own people, and the neighbor who is a stranger, and the friend by your side, and the wayfarer, and those whom you rightfully possess. Verily, God does not love any of those who, full of self-conceit, act in a boastful manner; [nor] those who are niggardly, and conceal whatever God has bestowed upon them out of His bounty; and so We have readied shameful suffering for all who thus deny the truth. (Quran 4:36-37)

By way of interpretation, piety in Islam is God-consciousness *(taqwa)* expressed in righteous conduct. Both belief and behavior counts. This is the only dimension of human endeavor that brings honor to the individual in the hereafter. In order to attain piety, one has to strive continuously to overcome one's *nafs Ammarah* (pleasure instincts and hubris). This striving is the *jihad bil nafs* explained previously. Muhammad had many suggestions about how to be triumphant in this inner struggle. Knowledge is essential to success: "knowledge is protection against lust and vain desires."[54]

Spiritual Development

On the basis of various Quranic references, Al Ghazzali postulated a three-stage theory of spiritual development of the human personality. The first stage is referred to as *nafs Ammarah*—the passionate soul (Quran 12:53). This soul inclines one toward sensual pleasure, passion, self-gratification, anger, greed, and envy. If this *nafs* is not checked it would lead to distress. The second stage is called *nafs Lawwamah*—the reproaching soul (Quran 75:1; 9:102) which has a similar role as that of Freud's superego.[55] This soul is conscious of evil and resists it, and asks for God's grace and pardon, and guides an individual toward righteousness. The third stage of spiritual development is called *nafs Mutmainnah*—the satisfied soul. "This is the highest stage of spiritual development. A satisfied soul is in a state of bliss, contentment and peace. The soul is at peace because it knows that in spite of its failures in this world it will return to God."[56]

As a Muslim, this author believes that observing God consciousness, daily prayers, fasting, *zakat* and *Hajj* (the Five Pillars of Islam), makes the struggles of life easier and more successful. Regular adherence to these forms of worship imparts a balance in one's life and protects one from over indulgence of material needs and desires. Simultaneously, one develops patience, honesty, humility, compassion, and other moral traits encouraged universally by the world's major religions.

Yasser Haddad[57] described spiritual development in five stages. The first stage is *Islam,* the state of striving, when you do things required of you by God, but you have not internalized the faith. The second stage is *Iman,* when faith truly enters your heart. The third stage is *Ahsaan,* which means excellence. In this stage you worship God as though you see Him, knowing that even though you do not see Him physically, He is always seeing you. The fourth stage is *Taqwa,* when the interaction of the first three stages has matured to the point that you are aware of Allah and obey Him all the time. *Taqwa* means living a life without sin. The final stage of spiritual growth is attainment of gratitude *(Shukr).* Gratitude is the pinnacle of faith attained when you dedicate your entire life in thanksgiving to God, and see only the good in whatever he wills for you.

When individuals put forth effort to gain God's pleasure, he rewards them by increasing their honor: "God will exalt by [many] degrees *[darajat]* those of you who have attained to faith . . ." (Quran, 58:11). Many other verses express a similar theme (Quran, 4:95; 9:20; 20:75; 6:132; 46:19). However, besides this blessing, which is contingent on human effort and belief, there is another level of blessing from God. This blessing *(faddala)* is unconditional and "cannot be earned by performing certain deeds. It can only be given by Allah, who has it and grants it to whom He wishes and in the form He wishes."[58] A God-conscious person prays unceasingly that God will grant his gracious gift of *fadl.*

Different people attain different levels of spirituality. Some may follow the sacred commands more ritualistically and others may practice them to the highest level of actualization. Whatever the level of an individual's belief and practice may be, God is the only one who can judge if that individual has worked up to one's potential or not.

Individual Differences

Although all human beings were created from a common living entity and they have a common biological origin, God's plan for the universe includes diversity among human beings: "And among His wonders is the creation of the heavens and the earth and the diversity of your tongues and colors: for in this behold, there are messages indeed for all who are possessed of [innate] knowledge!" (Quran 30:22). A related Quranic verse states: "O men! Behold, We created you all out of a male and a female and have made you into nations and tribes, so that you might come to know one another. Verily, the noblest of you in the sight of God is the one who is deeply conscious of Him. Behold, God is all-knowing, all aware" (Quran 49:13).

Besides cultural and national diversity, the Quran affirms that God bestows individual differences among human beings in capabilities, wealth, social status, power, family and knowledge (Quran, 43:32). Simultaneously, it emphasizes that none of these differences matter. What counts is one's attainment of righteousness expressed in an ethical life and religious devotions grounded in one's consciousness of God.

As discussed in the preceding section, the Quran addresses the two ways in which God bestows his blessings on human beings in order to establish differences among them. One is by giving them different ranks *(darajat)* in different domains, and the other is by bestowing God's preference *(faddala)* on whomever God wills. "We do raise to [high] degrees *[darajat]* [of knowledge] whomever We will—but above everyone who is endowed with knowledge there is One who knows all" (Quran 12:76). This verse refers to the spectrum of individual differences in cognitive abilities, which God has ordained and designed.

The Quran allows for individual differences in the understanding and expression of faith by emphasizing that each individual should use his or her own abilities of observation and reason to reach the truth. While basic tenets of Islamic belief and practice are derived from the Quran and *Sunnah,* many matters of life are open to individual interpretations of the religious scriptures. This flexibility is all the more possible since there is no authoritative clergy in Islam who set dogmatic rules.

Individual capabilities and expectations are also recognized in Islam from a developmental perspective. Consequently, the rights and responsibilities of children, adults, and elderly, are compatible with their corresponding capabilities and developmental levels.

Islam recognizes clear differences among individuals and groups of people. It not only encourages tolerance, but respectful understanding of differences. The most important point to make here, though, is that God will hold people accountable for their deeds based on only what they are capable of doing: "We do not burden any human being with more than he is well able to bear" (Quran 6:152).

THEORY OF DISTRESS

Health and illness, comfort and distress, ecstasy and suffering are the essential polarities of the dialectical nature of human life. If one did not experience sadness, one could not recognize happiness, and without knowing distress and suffering one could not appreciate comfort and ecstasy. The primary reason for the creation of humans is that God wanted to be known, and only human beings can know God in his fullness.[59] The polarities of human experience move human beings toward the ultimate purpose *(Tawhid),* the realization of the supremacy and oneness of God. This is the teleology of Islam, which renders harmony and balance in human lives and in the universe. Every entity exists for a purpose. According to Rumi, even sinfulness had to exist in order for God's quality of forgiveness to be revealed.[60]

In his infinite wisdom, which transcends time and space, God did not just permit negative human states, such as pain and suffering. God also equipped humans with the ability to deal with these conditions. As the Quran states: "Verily God does not change men's condition unless they change their inner selves" (Quran 13:11). God has given humans certain power over their destiny through the use of their will. The choices an individual makes in life either aggravate the negative states or restore positive states of being.

Another belief about suffering and affliction is that they are atonement for one's sins *(Kaffara).* Accepting pain and suffering with the belief that it is part of God's plan brings a person closer to salvation. "No calamity can ever befall [man] unless it be by God's leave . . ." (Quran 64:11). For a Muslim enduring difficulty, another statement restores faith and sustains hope: "And, behold, with every hardship there is ease: verily with every hardship there is ease!" (Quran 94:5-6).

THEORY OF THERAPY

Purpose of Therapy

Islamic perspective on psychotherapy is grounded in its view of health as a gift from God, ". . . and when I fall ill, is the One [God] who restores me to health" (Quran 26:80). A Muslim therapist must believe that the art and science of healing are not merely the result of the therapist's knowledge, experience and skill, "but rather a divinely revealed science whose results are ultimately and essentially the outcome of the mercy and the decree of God."[61] This quote is from Jalalú Din As-Suyuti who practiced medicine based on his knowledge of the Quran and Hadith 500 years ago.[62] This belief is based on the verse: "If God should touch thee with misfortune, there is none who could remove it but He; and if He would touch thee with good fortune—it is He who has the power to will anything" (Quran 6:17).

Islam encourages humans to find cures and remedies for illnesses. Muhammad is reported to have instructed people to take medicine, as Allah has not created a disease without creating a cure.

Since the body, mind, and spirit interact to form the human personality, the Islamic approach to treatment of any type of ailment—physical, psychological, or spiritual—is holistic. A therapist attends to the whole person, and not merely to parts of a person. A contemporary model of an Islamic approach to treatment is the Institute of Islamic Medicine in Panama City, Florida.[63] One of its founders, Ahmed Elkadi, states six basic criteria for Islamic Medicine, two of which are: (1) "It must submit to Islamic teachings and ethics, and (2) it must be comprehensive in its concerns, giving equal attention to body, mind and spirit and to the individual and society."[64]

As an intermediary between body and spirit, the mind exercises executive powers. In this respect it is somewhat comparable to the Western, psychoanalytic concept of "ego," except the latter mediates between instinctual drives (sex and aggression) and societal injunctions internalized as the superego. In Islam, the ego (mind) mediates between the physical and spiritual dimensions of the personality, not between biological and social morality.

By virtue of its mediating role, the mind is crucial in the maintenance of a healthy balance between body and spirit. When this balance is reached one attains *nafs mutmainnah* (the satisfied soul), characterized by an inner sense of peace and emotional strength, which in turn, enables one to cope with the hardest of life's tribulations with a manageable degree of distress. Helping a Muslim client achieve this state would be the optimum goal for a Muslim therapist.

Psychological distress and/or mental illness can be caused by a deficiency or dysfunction of one or more of the aspects of the human mind: cognition *(Aql),* volition *(Qadr),* and intuition/affective (*Qalb,* heart). These aspects of human problems in living become the major focus of treatment for a psychotherapist. However, this cannot be done effectively without considering the effects of psychological distress upon body and spirit as well.

One can reclassify all the mental disorders identified in the *Diagnostic and Statistical Manual of Mental Disorders,* Fourth Edition (DSM-IV) under the three psychological subdomains of the mind previously listed. For instance, mental retardation and the pervasive developmental disorders would be considered cognitive deficits; an oppositional defiant disorder or disruptive disorder would be volitional (conative) disorders; and mood disorders (anxiety, anger, depression) would be examples of disorders related to the heart (the affective domain). However, it would not be consistent with Islamic psychology for any mental disorder to be categorized primarily under one aspect or subdomain of mind, since all three are interdependent and must interact for the mind to function as a whole. Consequently, from an Islamic perspective, not just the somatoform disorders, but every mental disorder listed in the DSM-IV has physical, psychological, and spiritual dimensions and implications for treatment.

A healthy mind is essential for an individual to be triumphant over temptations of one's own *nafs,* and over those temptations from Satan that lead one's spirit away from God's pleasure. A therapist using Islamic principles in treating mental disorders or emotional distress would draw upon the client's strengths and resources in all three facets of personality—body, mind, and spirit. In addition, since Islam emphasizes the individual's responsibility to bring out the best in self and others, a Muslim therapist would encourage self-enhancement in a client, and include family and community support whenever possible.

Specific techniques that lend themselves well to the Islamic viewpoint because of their holistic nature are biofeedback, progressive relaxation, positive thinking, imagery, visualization, and sound therapy, such as the relatively new Heart Math technique. The Institute of Heart Math in Boulder Creek, California, has developed special music called Heart Zones, which, research shows, reduces stress and enhances positive energy in an individual when listened to while focusing attention around the area of one's heart. To assist the client in self-understanding, culture free, standardized measures of personality, intelligence and learning styles can be used without compromising Islamic values. Ideally, therapy or healing in Islam would be conducted in the context of the family or community through emotional, social, economic, and moral support and religious guidance. The concept of therapy provided by a paid therapist in an outpatient clinical setting is foreign to most Muslim cultures from the Eastern hemisphere. However, with the change in family dynamics and the challenges faced by Muslims living in the West, some Muslims are finding the outpatient model of therapy as their only option and are adapting to it.

Providing psychotherapy in a truly Islamic style would entail knowledge, understanding, and belief in the central creed of Islam: "There is no god but Allah and Muhammad is His Messenger," and belief in the unique themes derived from it. This belief entails placing all one's trust in God and God alone, and involves commitment to follow Quranic wisdom. The extent to which a therapist brings religious practices into the healing process ought to be decided only after assessing a client's level of religious conviction. It would be unethical for a therapist to impose one's own beliefs on clients since the Quran says that there is no compulsion in religion (Quran 109:1-6).

PRACTICE OF THERAPY

Because Islam is a comprehensive way of living, it is difficult to draw all the implications of the Islamic creed for the practice of therapy. Important themes include trust in God, the power of prayer and meditation, fasting, pilgrimage, charity, recitation of the Quran, moderation and balance, various behavioral prohibitions, the importance of knowledge, including self-knowledge, the central role of the "heart," and the functioning of family and community.

Trust in God

Constant reminders in good times and bad of God's omnipresence and omnipotence, and his attributes such as compassion, love, wisdom, power, justice, and mercy, all instill hope, courage tolerance, forgiveness, thankfulness, and many other reconciling traits in individuals. In times of suffering or affliction, a Muslim would recite verses or supplications from the Quran and Hadith that would remind him or her of God's power over all things. This belief frees a person from blaming self or others for things going wrong, and sets the stage for conflict resolution both within one's self and with others.

Power of Prayer

Muslims believe that, ultimately, only prayer can change human destinies. The Quran and Hadith are rich with prayers for all situations, including specific prayers to overcome psychological symptoms such as anxiety, panic, and anger. The prayer that is considered most acceptable to God is one in which humans ask for God's blessings for their well-being in this world and in the next.

The five daily, obligatory prayers *(salat)* are a very distinctive feature of Islamic practice. Through different physical postures, verbal recitation of the Quran, and total physical, mental, and spiritual attention toward God, these prayers involve the whole person. *Salat* is believed to be a shield from all evil, and relaxes the body, mind, and spirit of a Muslim with conviction.

Dhikr *(Meditation)*

Reciting any of God's names repeatedly, *dhikr,* is a form of meditation with powerful psychological effects. The Quran says, "Verily in the remembrance of God [men's] hearts do find their rest" (Quran). *Dhikr* brings one spiritually close to God and is practiced commonly by Muslims.

Saum *(Fasting)*

Fasting is an exercise in self-restraint. It consists of a person refraining from eating, drinking, and sexual acts from dawn to sunset. Recent research has shown that Islamic fasting has beneficial effects on metabolism.[65] The psychological and spiritual effects of fasting include inner peace and tranquillity. Besides the obligatory fasting in the month of Ramadan, fasting is also recommended at other times as atonement for one's sins, and to suppress one's pleasure instincts if a person feels that they may interfere with one's spiritual aspirations.

Hajj *(Pilgrimage)*

If affordable, the pilgrimage to Kaaba in Mecca is prescribed once in a person's lifetime as another form of atonement for sins. Following *hajj,* a Muslim believes that all past sins are forgiven and one becomes as innocent as a newborn baby. *Hajj* could be an effective healing process for clients ridden with extreme and persistent guilt. A pilgrimage to Kaaba, Mecca, at times other than the designated month for *hajj* is known as *Umrah,* and it is another form of worship, which is practiced by Muslims as a means of atonement of their sins.

Sadaqa *(Charity)*

Sharing your blessings with those in need, whether it is in the form of money, food or clothing or through pleasant manners, is considered in Islam as a gesture of gratitude to God, which will be rewarded by God's pleasure. It is a common therapeutic practice among Muslims to give charity or to sacrifice a lamb on behalf of a sick person, along with supplications to God for the person's recovery.

Quran

In addition to the many direct and indirect injunctions that the Quran contains relevant to coping with life's various circumstances, the acts of listening to or reciting the Quran in Arabic have been proven to have therapeutic effects. Ahmed Elkadi of the Institute of Islamic Medicine in Panama City, Florida, studied the heart rate, muscle tension, and blood pressure of subjects while they listened to Quranic recitations. A significant number showed a decline, whether the individual was a practicing Muslim or not; however, the stress-reducing effect of Quranic recitation increased when the listener understood the recited text.[66]

Moderation and Balance

Moderation and balance in all aspects of life is an essential rule in Islam. As mentioned earlier, there are limits set on piety as well, hence one cannot abandon his or her worldly duties and physiological needs in pursuit of the hereafter. Islam does not encourage celibacy; rather, strong approval is given for a legitimate conjugal relationship between a man and a woman.

When performed with the intention of pleasing God, even secular acts become worship, thereby bridging the gap between spiritual and secular domains. Promoting balance in daily human activities is illustrated by the following: "Partake of the good things We have provided for you as sustenance, but do not transgress therein the bounds of equity . . ." (Quran 20:81); ". . . eat and drink [freely] but do not waste; verily He does not love the wasteful!"(Quran 7:31). In another Quranic verse God directs human beings to be balanced in their spending so that they are neither miserly nor so careless that they end up being destitute. (Quran 17:29). Islam suggests repeatedly that personal and community wellness are attained through balance and moderation, in a manner somewhat similar to Aristotle's golden mean, which counsels moderation in all matters. This notion is very relevant to psychotherapy with clients suffering from low self-esteem and depression. The concept of moderation and balance encourage clients to enjoy the pleasures of a good life, which they may not believe they deserve or allow themselves to enjoy.

Behavioral Prohibitions

Islam prohibits the use of intoxicating drugs, alcohol, and gambling. The wisdom in these prohibitions is apparent, knowing both the addictive nature of these habits and the far reaching, negative effects they have on individuals, families, and communities across generations.

Importance of Knowledge

The Quran exhorts its readers to use all their senses, as well as their cognitive and intuitive abilities in the pursuit of truth and wisdom. Moreover, Muhammad said that ignorance is an enemy of the soul (mind). Therefore, a Muslim therapist must encourage clients to be adequately informed and knowledgeable before making choices. Accurate religious knowledge eliminates irrational thoughts, superstition, and fears.

Self-Knowledge

Muhammad said, "He who knows his own soul knows his Lord." Al-Ghazzali wrote that you cannot know another if you do not know yourself. These thoughts suggest that insight and self-knowledge are prerequisites to spiritual growth and good interpersonal relationships, hence they are considered critical mechanisms of change in psychotherapy.

The Heart

The feelings and intuitions arising from the heart are emphasized numerous times in the Quran as pivotal to spiritual growth. For instance, ". . . God knows what is in your hearts" (Quran 33:51); "It is He who from on high has bestowed inner peace upon the hearts of the believers so that . . . they might grow yet more firm in their faith" (Quran 48:4). Affirming feelings and recognizing intuitions in clients is crucial to the therapeutic process. The heart is the focal point of techniques such as meditation, relaxation, *dhikr,* and imagery (interventions for stress, anxiety, fear, and anger). Muslims of the Sufi order give a great deal of importance to the heart, since they say that it is the place where humans meet God.[67]

Family and Community

The Quran and Hadith enumerate in detail the rights and responsibilities of individuals, specific family members, particularly parents, and the community at large. Social etiquette and boundaries among different members of the family and community *(ummah)* are clearly established. There is a corpus of Islamic law governing various situations such as marriage, divorce, inheritance, and other matters of importance. Following these rules allows for mutual respect, fairness, care, and predictable interdependence among people. Family involvement in therapy is a common practice. Encouraging clients to perform community service is another useful strategy for increasing their self-worth.

As mentioned earlier, the extent to which a psychotherapist incorporates Islamic principles in treating individuals should be determined only after a sound assessment of the client's own faith. While the therapist may serve as a spiritual guide, psychotherapy needs to be client-centered, allowing the client to make appropriate choices that bring healing. The Islamic practice of therapy would follow the usual stages of rapport building, assessment, enlisting commitment to a treatment plan, implementing the plan, and evaluating progress, but with a few additional features. Assessment would include checking not only the physical health and psychological status of the client, but also his or her spiritual condition and religious inclinations and affections. Depending upon the client's religious affections, the therapist and client could begin and end each session with a brief supplication to God for his mercy and guidance toward complete trust in him to enhance hope and healing from suffering.

Every therapist working with Muslim clients in the West needs to be keenly aware of the unique dynamics that are created as a consequence of the minority status of Muslims in this culture. Many Muslim clients in the United States are not in therapy due to their religious faith or lack of it, but rather because of the stress they experience in adjusting to a mainstream culture that does not understand them. The scope of this chapter does not allow for elaboration on this important aspect of practice. An interested therapist can learn more from a recent model of psychotherapy known as "Multicultural Person-Environment Fit World View" developed by Manuel Ramirez III. This model helps the victims of mismatch by empowering them to create a better world, a world in which individual, cultural and religious differences are respected and viewed positively as a "resource for the development of mutual understanding, cooperation, and self-actualization."[68]

EVALUATION

Human endeavors to present divine knowledge and wisdom are always imperfect, and never do justice commensurate with one's intent, however noble. An attempt has been made to portray the Islamic theory as precise, comprehensive, integrative, operational, and heuristic. If this has not happened, it is a reflection of the author's limitations and not of Islam.

No empirical research has been done to establish the theory of personality and psychotherapy described in this chapter, although there is ongoing study and research being done on various aspects or constructs of the theory.[69] Though empirical research remains to be done, the practicality of the Islamic theory of life has been endorsed by millions of people across the world who follow Islam in its true spirit and experience the self-actualization it brings them. The chapter was written with the hope that future students of psychology will conduct further research on the Islamic perspective of personality and psychotherapy.

According to standard criteria for evaluating a theory, Islamic psychology is certainly important because it is relevant to life. The theory is also understandable and internally consistent. Basic assumptions are identified, and both an inductive and deductive approach help to make this theory clear and experiential.

An Islamic theory of personality and psychotherapy is also comprehensive and integrative. It addresses a range of human concerns, it is consistent with much known data in the field, and it is sensitive to cross-cultural diversity. It strives for a multidimensional perspective, and ideally, an interdisciplinary point of view, which integrates psychology and religion.

An Islamic theory of personality and psychotherapy is empirically verifiable in principle, though causal and teleological hypotheses derived from the theory are supported presently by limited scientific research. As the theory develops more operational definitions, further study can be conducted on independent, intervening, and dependent variables, which are measurable and publicly verifiable.

Islamic theory may be considered heuristic and practical. It stimulates thinking and the development of holistic concepts (body, mind, spirit), and it can generate new knowledge. Practitioners may find that this theory helps them to organize their thinking, and that it serves as a guide to their clinical work, particularly with Muslim clients. Techniques can be derived logically from Islamic beliefs and principles rather than approaching therapy by trial and error. The theory encourages the psychotherapist to function as a professional, not merely as a technician.

POINTS OF DIALOGUE

With Other Religions

As with Judaism and Christianity, Islam affirms a monotheistic theory. God is the Creator of the universe, and is other than the universe. In this respect, Islam is a more Western religion than an Eastern monistic worldview. God is conceptualized as a personal agent of action, not as a static, impersonal being identical with the universe. Moreover, the Islamic emphasis upon the sovereign will of God is akin to the Jewish and Christian images of God as King and the Kingdom of God. The prophet Muhammad is known for his transforming consciousness of God, similar to Judeo-Christian portrayals of prophetic figures such as Abraham, Moses, and Jesus.

Islamic anthropology views the human personality in multidimensional terms, similar to other religious theories. The tripartite personality structure (body, mind, spirit) is similar to Christian anthropology particularly, yet also compatible with a holistic perspective on the person as a unified whole. Contrary to Eastern perspectives, the individual is viewed as a separate entity apart from both other people and from God, not as a part of one single reality, such as the Atman/Brahman concepts in Hindu psychology. A real, human self is affirmed, contrary to the Buddhist notion of no self *(anatta).*

As with other world religions, Islam provides a cosmology; a definition of the good life; an ultimate purpose for living (obedience to the will of God); and guidelines for living a healthy, moral, and spiritual life. The dialectical concepts of polarities, and the emphasis upon living a balanced life of moderation have affinities with Taoism.

Dialogue with Other Theories of Personality/Psychotherapy

Contemporary theories that include constructs recognized in the Islamic worldview and have approaches that can be adapted to Islamic beliefs and practices would be recognized as valid and appropriate in Islamic practice of therapy. Islamic psychology emphasizes the intellect, emotion, and will.

Muslim psychotherapists employ these concepts in cognitive behavior therapy, rational-emotive therapy, reality therapy, along with client-centered therapy and other existential therapies informed by the ultimate purpose of *Tawhid* (oneness of God). An Islamic perspective adds the moral and spiritual dimensions of both personal functioning and therapeutic healing to the dominant biopsychosocial model that undergirds Western clinical psychology. Consequently, spiritual disciplines may be incorporated with Muslim clients, including such "techniques" as prayer and meditation, fasting, charity, recitation of the Quran, and certain behavioral prohibitions consistent with a balanced life of moderation. Self-knowledge and the affective and volitional dimensions of experience are particular emphases in an Islamic theory of the process of therapeutic change.

CASE STUDY*

As with other chapters in this book, the identical case study is being used to illustrate the application of personality theory and psychotherapy in this instance, derived from this author's interpretation of Islamic principles. The client is married and has taken care of her eighty-four-year-old mother in her home for seventeen years, while being employed full time outside the home. The client is experiencing guilt over a decision to move her mother to a nursing home on a permanent basis. The client is a dutiful daughter despite her mother's critical and unkind treatment of her. There is even a suggestion that the client was an unwanted child who the mother attempted to abort before birth. An additional dimension is that the client was molested during her childhood by someone, and she may be carrying feelings of shame, guilt and low self-worth associated with this experience. In this chapter, an assumption is made that the client is a Muslim.

In the intake process, a therapist using the holistic, Islamic approach would assess the client's strengths and needs in the three domains of personality: biological, psychological, and spiritual. In addition, the therapist would also explore the resources available to the client in the personal as well as the family and community spheres.

From the inception of the therapeutic process, empathetic listening and unconditional positive regard for the client would be essential to develop rapport and a trusting relationship between the therapist and the client. The next step would be to formulate goals of therapy with the client and enlist her commitment to work toward them with the help of the therapist. Ideally

---

*The case selected is the analysis of a forty-two-year-old, married, employed, Caucasian woman suffering from a major depressive episode. Madill and Barkham (1997). From "Discourse analysis of a theme in one successful case of brief psychodynamic-interpersonal psychotherapy," *Journal of Counseling Psychology, 44* (2), 232-244.

these goals would be to reduce the client's depressed mood; eliminate her feelings of anxiety, guilt, and shame; restore her sense of self-worth; and promote an overall sense of well-being. In Islamic terms, the ultimate goal would be to attain the final stage of *nafs mutmainnah* (satisfied soul). It would be critical to set realistic intermediate goals, and pace the treatment process in a manner that the client is encouraged and not overwhelmed.

The concepts and techniques recommended in this case are not categorized as biological, psychological, or spiritual, since all three overlap. If the client's depression is at a clinical level, pharmacological treatment would be recommended, in the form of prescribed, antidepressant medications to supplement psychotherapy. If, when, and how this recommendation is made is critical because a Muslim therapist needs to be sensitive to the implications of this recommendation to the client. The goal would be to empower the client to problem solve and facilitate healing and not to convey a sense of despair or helplessness.

Physical aspects of maintaining health such as proper diet, exercise, and rest would be encouraged and reviewed in every session. Reframing the concept of self-care as a religious duty, since it means proper use of God-given resources, would hopefully motivate the client toward self-enhancing behaviors. Also, since the client appears to be a selfless, conscientious, and "dutiful" person, it would appeal to her to point out that keeping herself healthy would allow her to be a better companion to her husband while being able to take better care of her ailing mother.

The client would be trained in deep breathing, progressive relaxation techniques, and imagery. Meditation on the attributes of God *(dhikr)* would be introduced. These practices would not only raise the client's awareness about herself and her relationship with God, but also give her holistic coping skills to overcome stress, anxiety, and depression.

The client would be encouraged in self-examination using a combination of cognitive and rational-emotive methods, and relevant Islamic knowledge. She would be made aware of possible irrational thoughts and beliefs that if harbored, would contribute to her guilt and low self-worth. She would be guided to explore and to use her cognitive, intuitive, and conative abilities to find ways of resolving the conflicts and problems she was facing at the time, and to cope with the stress of her decision in particular. In an Islamic context, she would need to learn to trust her heart *(Qalb)* or intuition, since, "the heart never lies," use her intelligence *(Aql)* and knowledge *(Ilm),* and her ability to make choices *(Qadar)* so they all lead toward a satisfying resolution.

The client would be guided toward putting all her trust in God, remembering that nothing happens without his will. The therapist would gently remind her that God knows best and his love for her is more than the love of seventy mothers as the prophet had said. She would overcome her difficulties with God's help and guidance. Continued patience and perseverance would be encouraged in dealing with her mother's temperament by suggesting that she exercise inner *jihad,* for which she will be rewarded. The Islamic belief that God's justice will not hold her responsible for happenings out of her control, would hopefully lead toward restoring her self-worth, which may have been negatively impacted by the childhood molestation.

Certain Islamic practices such as regular prayers and specific Quranic supplications to overcome anxiety and sadness would be suggested to instill hope in the client. The extent to which the spiritual aspect of therapy would be developed would depend on the level of sophistication of the client's spirituality.

Finally, including the client's husband in therapy at an appropriate point would be critical to help resolve the possible tension in their relationship due to the stressful circumstances they were experiencing, and also to recruit his support for the client. The therapist would guide the couple toward exploring more community resources to check out the possibility of less-restrictive alternatives than a nursing home for the mother. Some possibilities that may arise from such exploration are home health care, or friends and relatives providing respite to the client and her husband by visiting the mother according to a planned schedule, or a long-term elderly foster care in a home that is sensitive to the family's cultural and religious needs and sentiments. Through these interventions, the client can begin to experience God's gracious blessing of peace.

NOTES

1. Asad M. (1984) *The message of the Quran.* Lahore, Pakistan: Maktaba Jawahar ul uloom, p. 141. All Quranic translations in this chapter are from Muhammad Asad's translation of the Quran. The first number refers to the sura (chapter); the second number refers to the verses.

2. Yamani, S. (1995) Foreword to H. Hathout, *Reading the Muslims mind.* Plainfield, IN: American Trust Publications, pp. xi-xii.

3. People who follow Islamic teachings are called Muslims, not Muhammadans, as the latter name suggests incorrectly that they worship Muhammad or that they believe that Muhammad wrote the Quran.

4. Most of the historical background in this chapter was summarized from Embassy of Saudi Arabia publications, *Islam a global civilization* and *Understanding Islam and Muslims.*

5. "Allah" is the Arabic word for God.

6. Yamani, Foreword to *Reading the Muslim mind,* pp. xi-xii.

7. Embassy of Saudi Arabia. Washington, DC. (1989). *Understanding Islam and Muslims.* Cambridge, UK: Islamic Texts Society.

8. In the Islamic world, dates are often described with the suffix "A.H." for "After Hijra."

9. Hathout, H. (1995) *Reading the Muslim mind.* Plainfield, IN: American Trust Publications, pp. 9-10.

10. It is important to note that Muslims believe in messages of the *Psalms* revealed to David, the *Torah* revealed to Moses, and the Bible revealed to Jesus in their original forms. Muslims consider those texts as they exist today to be tainted by man-made alterations. Only the Quran remains in its pure and original form.

11. *Shariah* is Islamic law derived primarily from the primary sources (the Quran and *Sunnah).* Juristic reasoning *(ijtihad)* is applied where an issue is not clearly stated in either of the primary sources.

12. The Hadith quoted here were printed in the booklet, *Understanding Islam and Muslims.*

13. Embassy of Saudi Arabia. Washington, DC. *Islam a global civilization,* p. 10.

14. Faruqi, I. and Faruqi, L. (1986). *The cultural atlas of Islam.* New York: Macmillan, p. 305. Check this reference for further details on Islamic contributions to world civilization.

15. Wudud-Muhsin, A. (1994). *Quran and woman.* Kuala-Lumpur, Malaysia: Penerbit Fajar Bakti Sdn. Bhd., p. 21.

16. Abdulati, H. (1990). *Islam in focus.* Salimah, Kuwait. International Islamic Federation of Student Organizations, p. 166.

17. Wudud-Muhsin, *Quran and woman,* p. 83.

18. Asad, *The message of the Quran.* Lahore, Pakistan: Maktaba Jawaharul uloom, p. 100.

19. Wudud-Muhsin, *Quran and woman,* p. 19.

20. Haneef, S. (1996). *What everyone should know about Islam and Muslims.* Chicago: Kazi Publications, p. 104.

21. Rychlak, J. (1981). *Introduction to personality and psychotherapy,* Second Edition. Boston: Houghton-Miffin, p. 7.

22. Bucaille, M. (1986). *What is the origin of man?* Paris, France: Seghers Publisher, pp. 1-220. In this book Bucaille examines the frequent references in the Quran to the origin of man from clay, water, etc. He explains that this is a reference to the chemical composition of the human body and also a symbolic reference to man's return to the earth before being raised on the Day of Judgment for accountability of his deeds.

23. Ghazzali, Imam. (1996). *Ihyaulum-id-din-the book of religious learnings, Book III.* (trans. by Al-Haj Maulana Fazlul-Karim). New Delhi, India: Islamic Book Services, p. 5.

24. Murata, S. (1992). *The Tao of Islam.* New York: State University of New York Press, p. 237.

25. In critiquing this chapter, Professor Ibrahim Al Dharrab of King Abdul Aziz University, Saudi Arabia, drew a distinction between spirit and spiritual. As the entity that gives life, spirit in this sense cannot be a dynamic component of personality. The present author is using the term "spirit" in this chapter to represent the spiritual aspect of personality.

26. Asad, *The message of the Quran,* p. 954.

27. Wudud-Muhsin, *Quran and woman,* p. 17.

28. Faruqi and Faruqi, *The cultural atlas of Islam,* p. 73.

29. Ibid., pp. 89-90.Faruqi and Faruqi point out that *"Tawhid* distinguishes itself from Sufism and some sects of Hinduism, where reality of the world is dissolved into God and God becomes the only reality, the only existent.

30. Rahman, A. (1988). *Muhammad encyclopedia of Seerah,* Vol. VI. London, UK: Seerah Foundation, p. 583.

31. Faruqi and Faruqi, *The cultural atlas of Islam,* pp. 73-74.

32. Murata, *The Tao of Islam,* p. 238.

33. Abu Ali al Husayn ibn Sina (980-1037 A.D.), known in the Western world as Avicenna, was born in Afshana, near Bukhara. He produced the first systematic statements of philosophy titled *Ahwal al Nafs.*

34. Rahman, *Muhammad encyclopedia of Seerah,* Vol. VI, p. 582.

35. Hathout, *Reading the Muslim mind,* p. 6.

36. Rahman, *Muhammad encyclopedia of Seerah,* Vol. III. London: Seerah Foundation, p. 7.

37. Hathout, *Reading the Muslim mind,* p. 7.

38. Satan, according to Muslim belief, is a Jinn, a species similar to humans but created by God from fire. Jinns are invisible to the human eye and have a universe of their own parallel to the human universe. There are both good Jinns and evil Jinns. Satan (also known as Iblis) is the leader of the evil Jinns.

39. Faruqi and Faruqi, *The cultural atlas of Islam,* p. 75.

40. Ibid.

41. Jala al-Din Rumi (d. 1273 A.D.) was one of the most famous Persian Sufi poets, translated and studied in the West by several scholars.

42. Rahman, *Muhammad encyclopedia of Seerah,* Vol. VI, p. 540.

43. Ansari, Zafar (1992). *Quranic concepts of human psyche.* Paper No. 118. Islamabad, Pakistan: International Institute of Islamic Thought, p. 61.

44. Maddi, S. (1996). *Personality theories of comparative analysis,* Sixth edition. Pacific Grove, CA: Brooks/Cole Publishing Company, p. 9.

45. Murata, *The Tao of Islam,* p. 289.

46. Ibid., p. 290.

47. Faruqi and Faruqi, *The cultural atlas of Islam,* pp. 80-81.

48. Hathout, *Reading the Muslim mind,* pp. 7-8.

49. Murata, *The Tao of Islam,* p. 323.

50. Information of the *Sunnans* of Allah comes from a lecture at the Muslim Youth Camp in San Jose, California, in August 1999, by Professor Fouad M.A. Dehlawi, King Abdul Aziz University, Saudi Arabia.

51. Khouj, A. (1990). *Essentials of human understanding.* ISBN 0-9628292-0-X. p. 33.

52. Abdulati, *Islam in focus,* p. 40.

53. Ibid., p. 43.

54. Rahman, A. (1988). *Muhammad encyclopedia of Seerah,* Vol. II. London: Seerah Foundation, p. 4.

55. Al-Ghazzali's (1072-1135 A.D.) description of the three kinds of *nafs: nafs Ammarah, nafs Lawwamah, and nafs Mutmainnah,* are very similar to Sigmund Freud's (1856-1939) id, superego, and ego, respectively. One wonders how much influence Al-Ghazzali's work had on Freud's thinking since Al-Ghazzali's philosophy had reached Europe during his lifetime.

56. Athar, S. (1993). *Islamic perspectives in medicine.* Indianapolis, IN: American Trust Publications, p. 138.

57. Haddad, Y. (1999). *The Stages of Iman.* Lecture delivered at the Muslim Youth Camp, San Jose, California, August 19, 1999.

58. Wudud-Muhsin, *Quran and woman,* p. 69

59. Murata, *The Tao of Islam,* p.34

60. "Allah" is the all-comprehensive name of God. God's qualities are reflected in the ninety-nine names of God referred to in the Quran as the *Asma-al-Husna* (the Beautiful Names). Some of these are Ar-Rahman (the Beneficent), Ar-Rahim (the Merciful), Al-Jabbar (the One who Compels), Ar-Razzaq (the Provider), Al-Wahhab (the One who Bestows), and Al-Qawi (the Strongest).

61. As-Suyuti, J. (1997). *Medicine of the prophet.* London: Ta-Ha Publishers Ltd., p. v.

62. Jalalu'Din Abd'ur-Rahman As-Suyuti (1445-1505 A.D.) was a scholar of Islamic sciences and wrote on a variety of subjects, of which *Tibb an-Nabbi* (medicine of the prophet) was one of the most popular. He was of Persian and Turkish descent and had memorized the Quran at age eight. He was very familiar with the works of the early Muslim philosophers, including Ibn Sina.

63. The Institute of Islamic Medicine, Panama City, Florida, offers a Multi-modality Immunotherapy Program (MIP), which uses natural remedies such as herbs and minerals, nutritional programs, rational emotive therapy such as guided imagery and visualizations, biofeedback, and Quranic recitations to enhance the immune system.

64. Elkadi, A. (1995). *Contemporary definition of Islamic medicine.* Institute for Islamic Medicine for Education and Research, Panama City, Florida. Paper presented at the Fifth International Conference on Islamic Medicine, Orlando, Florida, April 1995, p. 2.

65. Athar, *Islamic perspectives in medicine,* pp. 146-147.

66. Ibid., p. 139.

67. Murata, *The Tao of Islam,* p. 289.

68. Ramirez III, M. (1991). *Psychotherapy and counseling with minorities.* New York: Pergamon Press, p. 14.

69. The Association of Muslim Social Scientists based in Herndon, Virginia, and the International Institute of Islamic Thought (IIIT) based in Malaysia, together publish a quarterly journal, *The American Journal of Islamic Social Sciences.* This journal publishes original research on topics of social and psychological nature related to the Islamic perspective and experience.

Chapter 7

Convergence and Divergence

R. Paul Olson
Bruce McBeath

This chapter highlights both the similarities and differences among the religious theories of personality and psychotherapy presented throughout this book. It follows the format of the previous chapters, but with some variance. The very striking similarities among these theories warrants prominent attention to their shared themes. These general commonalities structure the initial sections, within which differences are also acknowledged. More specific comparisons are addressed in the subsequent sections on personality structure, dynamics and development, individual differences, psychopathology, and psychotherapy.

We acknowledge limitations to the approach taken here. The various religious constructs selected for comparison are derived from the religious psychologies presented. Since the latter are based on the interpretations of individual adherents in each tradition, the convergences and divergences drawn here are subject to their selections and interpretations, in addition to our own biased viewpoints as American, male psychologists who are more familiar with a Western worldview. Variability in the amount of our discussion about the views of different religious psychologies is partially a function of the different emphases found within particular chapters in this volume.

PERSONALITY THEORY

General Commonalities

Points of convergence among these religious psychologies include the following:

1. Ethical, spiritual, and historical dimensions of personal experience are emphasized.
2. A behavioristic reductionism is rejected.
3. A critical realism is implicit, if not explicit.

4. A phenomenological perspective is common.
5. Religious psychologies are optimistic.
6. Human freedom is a shared premise.

Moreover, these religious psychologies are normative, teleological, and dialectical; they affirm paradox and appreciate the mystery of life; they are existential and holistic; they affirm the priority of the spiritual dimension of life; and finally, religious psychologies sanctify personhood.

Ethical, Spiritual, and Historical Dimensions Are Emphasized

None of these religious psychologists rejects the dominant biopsychosocial model of human behavior that characterizes contemporary clinical psychology. This commonality is predictable in light of the contributors' secular graduate training in the corpus of scientific psychology, and in light of their chosen clinical professions. All of them acknowledge the biological, psychological, and social dimensions of human experience. These dimensions are taken seriously both in their theories and practice.

Equally striking is that the anthropological insights about the human condition derived from each religious tradition are also taken seriously, and to a much greater degree than is evident in secular, scientific theories of personality. This characteristic distinguishes these theories as *religious* or *spiritual* psychologies. Consequently, although their commitment to the biopsychosocial model prevents the contributors from lapsing into a speculative idealism, none of them considers a biopsychosocial model of personality as sufficient to comprehend human being, human experience, and human behavior. All of them add ethical and spiritual dimensions as essential perspectives for the description and understanding of who a person is, what one thinks, feels, wants, or does, and how one grows, relates, or becomes maladjusted and healed. Western religious theories seem to have a greater emphasis upon the historical dimension than Eastern psychologies, but this distinction can be drawn only on a continuum, not as a categorical contrast.

A Behavioristic Reductionism Is Rejected

None of these theories could be faulted for advocating a reductionistic behaviorism. Internal constructs such as self, mind, or spirit symbolize realities related to behavior, but distinct from behavior. The contributors recognize that there is more to a person than his or her overt behavior. Personality cannot be reduced to performance, though it is manifested partially through one's actions. Nor are the antecedents or consequences of behavior limited to measurable, environmental contingencies. Rather, internal perceptions and interpretations, intentions and intuitions, spiritual experiences and spiritual strivings, desires and decisions, values and virtues are all accepted as legitimate constructs in personality theory, even though they may not be directly observable from an external frame of reference. The contributors share the conviction that there is a legitimate role for hypothetical constructs which are theoretically heuristic, though presently they may lack precise operational definitions. The main point here is that the contributors agree that human beings cannot be reduced to human behavior. Consciousness is not subsumed by conduct. Stated another way, the Lockean-Skinnerian conceptualizations of the personality as a "blank slate" or as an "empty black box" are rejected. The internal contents postulated by these religious anthropologies qualifies them as genuine personality theories.

A Critical Realism Is Implicit, if Not Explicit

Consistent with their rejection of a behavioristic reductionism, none of these theories advocate a philosophical position of either radical empiricism or logical positivism. While they all affirm the crucial importance of experience, including experiential learning, they do not limit the scope of their theories to constructs and phenomena that can be analyzed solely in quantitative measurements.

This is not to say these theories reject realism as a philosophical position. Rather, they reject a naïve realism that views a concept as a sign with a one-to-one correspondence to the reality it references. Instead, most of these religious psychologies seem to favor a critical realism that appreciates the symbolic nature of language, yet affirms simultaneously that an objective reality is being symbolized. Critical realism "recognizes that no theory is an exact description of the world, and that the world is such as to bear interpretation in some ways and not in others."[1] As Ian Barbour observed, "Against the positivist, the realist asserts that the real is not the observable. Against the instrumentalist, he affirms that valid concepts are true as well as useful. Against the idealist, he maintains that concepts represent the structure of events in the world. The patterns in the data are not imposed by us, but originate at least in part in objective relationships in nature" (p. 168).

There are some differences in this respect. That is, some religious psychologies seem more "realistic" than others. The Hindu-Buddhist notions of maya suggest an illusory quality to the "real" world, including the illusion of a stable, phenomenal self. Nevertheless, these traditions are as realistic as Western religious psychologies in affirming the reality of natural laws, human existence, and human suffering. Indeed, all of these religious psychologies can be construed as strategies for coping with real problems experienced by real people.

A Phenomenological Perspective Is Common

One may postulate an objective reality and simultaneously affirm that the reality which counts for the individual is the reality which that person perceives. Most of these religious psychologies acknowledge this principle. In this regard they may be construed as perceptual or phenomenological theories.

They are phenomenological in another respect. The common aim of these religious psychologies is to describe and understand the human condition. Prediction and control are goals associated with causal-scientific explanations, but these aims are not paramount in religious psychologies. Moreover, consistent with a phenomenological approach, these religious theories emphasize subjective experience and internal states. Meaning matters more than measurement, just as being precedes knowing.

Religious Psychologies Are Optimistic

All of the theories presented in this book affirm the possibility of change. People are not viewed as captives of their circumstances nor as pawns of fate, even if spiritual laws such as karma, or innate predispositions, place limits on their ultimate destinies. The individual is viewed as an agent of action, with the capacity to transcend his or her life circumstances despite the limitations due to heredity, environment, or constitutional predispositions toward self-defeating attitudes and maladaptive behavior. These religious psychologies affirm the possibility of human happiness, liberation, or peace in such concepts as nirvana, moksha, shalom, or the kingdom of God. Moreover, these positive states can be known at least partially in real, spiritual experiences, here and now, whether these are associated with meditative states of unitive consciousness, or described as liberating experiences of reconciliation. Promises of an improved quality of life characterize every religious psychology. Although abuse, injustice, and violence are acknowledged as part of the human condition, along with tragic, natural disasters, people who experience such conditions need not view themselves as helpless, hopeless victims. So long as they survive, they have the capacity to effect some change, if only in the meaning they give or discover in the midst of their tragic circumstances. Meaning matters; spiritual meanings are life-enhancing and life-sustaining. These religious psychologists help their clients look toward the future with hope.

Human Freedom Is a Shared Premise

The possibility and hope for change is affirmed as a logical consequence of another shared belief about personality. All of these religious psychologies affirm human freedom. This is not an absolute freedom, but a finite freedom. There is a shared recognition that human freedom is limited by the exigencies and vicissitudes of life. As an embodied existence, human life is natural, hence subject to both natural laws and natural forces. Spiritual and moral laws, such as the predictable negative effects of misidentifications, dualistic thinking, or human selfishness are also affirmed along with the limitations imposed by historical contingencies of time, place, and events. Human freedom is a conditional freedom.

Despite the limitations of a contingent existence, these theories affirm that humans have both the freedom and responsibility to make choices and decisions that lead to action and change. An individual's intentions and decisions are considered important antecedents of behavior. Though an individual might be unable to alter circumstances, one can always choose how to perceive and interpret circumstances, and thereby change one's response, and perhaps the outcome. More than that is affirmed, however. One may initiate change proactively, rather than merely react reflexively. As a creature with conditional freedom, a person has the capacity to choose, to decide, to set goals, and to function as an agent of self-directed action. This empowering insight is common to all of the religious psychologies presented here and fundamental to their therapeutic applications.

The affirmation of human freedom, and the view that decisions are "causes" to be considered in any explanation of human behavior, makes these religious theories *voluntaristic*. Voluntarism is the view that human behavior involves freedom to choose between alternative forms of conduct. Voluntaristic action is (a) goal-directed (teleological), (b) takes means into consideration, (c) is normatively regulated with respect to the choice of ends and means, and (d) depends upon reason and choice. In a voluntaristic theory, human intentions, desires, or acts of will are viewed as salient causes and explanations of social behavior, though not the sole causes of conduct. Voluntaristic theories are advocated by classical sociologists more than by academic psychologists.[2] The psychologists who have contributed to this book are exceptions, based on both their religious convictions and clinical experience.

Religious Psychologies Are Normative

According to these religious psychologies, the causes of human distress are diverse and multiple. Included among them are ignorance, insatiable desires, inordinate attachments, misidentifications, predispositions to do both good and evil, bad choices, sin and estrangement from God, others and self, and disobedience to the will of Allah.

These differences may be viewed as variations of a common theme: A self-centered life is a major cause of human misery. The attendant greed, pride, and lust for pleasure, power, or privilege condemns the narcissistic individual and those with whom he or she relates to an unhappy life of frustration and conflict, disillusionment and despair. A lifestyle characterized by egoistic hedonism is renounced by all of these religious psychologies. This seems to be a fundamental consensus.

This common characteristic can be expressed by describing religious psychologies as normative or explicitly ethical. The moral dimension of human experience is acknowledged by all of them. Human beings are described as moral beings, whose choices, decisions, and actions are influenced by their commitments to values, and by the goals that express their values. Construing human behavior ethically makes these religious theories of personality explicitly value-laden. None would pretend to be value-free or value-neutral. The claim of value-neutrality is a pretense that has been dropped by many secular psychologists as well, particularly in the areas of personality and psychotherapy.[3]

The ethical nature of religious psychologies is evident in another respect. These psychologies are normative theories, not merely descriptive theories. They advocate in common an approach to life grounded in two fundamental values—wisdom and compassion. Consequently, as normative theories, religious psychologies focus on the development of moral character, not merely on personality development. Duties are defined as guiding principles, along with the virtues (moral traits) that one must acquire to fulfill one's moral obligations or divine commandments. As with most ethical theories, these religious psychologies also envision the good life and how it should be lived. In this respect, they are "critical theories" of personality,[4] which not only describe, but also prescribe dispositions and behaviors conducive to growth, healing, and harmony.

Religious Theories Are Teleological

Values may be construed as formal causes, and when they are embedded in goals they function as final causes,[5] for the sake of which behavior is intended. While religious theories of personality do not deny material and efficient causes such as heredity and learning, a defining and common characteristic is their addition of formal and final causes, which are characteristic of teleological theories.

Examples of *formal causes* are the tripartite layers within the personality in Hindu psychology related to various types of motivations; the five personality types or styles postulated in Tantric Buddhism (logical, expansive, passionate, active, and meditative); the Taoist concepts of temperament (*jing*) and the Sage personality type with its associated traits such as humbleness, flexibility, adaptability, persistence, and acceptance; the form of relationship called "I-Thou" in Jewish psychology; the formation of faith and character in Christian humanism, and the three cardinal virtues of faith, hope, and love, which characterize a reconciled life; the Muslim notion that people manifest different levels of spirituality, and the form of personality called the *nafs wama sawwaha,* which represents the authentic human being as God intended.

Final causes function as purposes, for the sake of which behavior is intended. These purposes are evident particularly in the ultimate goals which are advocated in these religious psychologies: nirvana, moksha, oneness with Tao, an accurate perception of reality, wisdom and compassion, bringing holiness into the world, a liberating reconciliation, and obedience to the will of Allah.

Incorporating final causes in explanations of behavior is what distinguishes teleological theories. A teleological perspective is evident in the view shared by the contributors of this book that human behavior is goal-directed, hence oriented to changing the present by making choices based on an anticipated future. For example, the more immediate goal of establishing a therapeutic relationship, and intermediate goals such as reduction of psychological distress function as purposes (final causes), for the sake of which therapists and clients engage in problem-solving conversations and therapeutic interventions.

Religious Theories Are Dialectical

A linear logic that maps human experience onto Cartesian coordinates is generally rejected by these religious psychologies. An unidirectional line of causation from past to present, or from a stimulus to a response, is considered simplistic and contrary to lived experience. Reciprocity, mutuality, and the complexity of personal life are more characteristic affirmations.

Dichotomous thinking in black-and-white categories is considered problematic and a cause of human distress in most of these religious psychologies. Dualism is denied explicitly by the monistic theories of Hinduism, Buddhism, and Taoism, but they share with Judaism, Christianity, and Islam an appreciation for dialectical reasoning and polar constructs. There are several illustrations of dialectical reasoning in these religious psychologies. An example from Eastern spiritual traditions is the Buddhist who affirms the determining influences of both the laws of karma and the three primary drives of greed, hatred, and delusion, yet who also affirms human freedom, illustrating the dialectical assertion of a "both/and." The Taoist notion of *yin* and *yang* polarities synthesized in the Tao is another example of dialectic thought.

Western religious psychologies are grounded in a theological view that God is the ultimate reality, separate from, yet dwelling within the world and within human souls, as the One Spirit dwelling within many spirits, but not identical with any of them. To assert that God is both immanent in human life and a transcendent Other is a form of dialectical reasoning. To affirm that God is Being Itself with personal attributes (the One who acts in freedom to love) reflects the dialectics of personal theism. Trinitaritarian concepts of the one divine reality in both Hindu theology (Brahma, Vishnu, and

Shiva) and in Christian theology (Creator, Christ, Spirit) are additional examples of dialectical distinctions within unity.

The three layers (gross, subtle, and causal) within one unified personality described in Hindu psychology, and the tripartite conceptions of personality in Taoist psychology (*chi, jing,* and *shen*), and in Christian and Muslim psychologies (body, mind, spirit) are additional examples of dialectical concepts. The idea that the psychological dimension/layer mediates and synthesizes the biological and spiritual dimensions is a dialectical concept explicit in Hindu and Muslim psychologies, and implicit within Christian anthropology. The Jewish notion of dual predispositions to do both good and evil, and the view that while the human and divine are distinct and separate, they are intimately connected in an "I-Thou" relation is another example. Religious psychologies are dialectical and synthesizing.

Religious Theories Affirm Paradox and Appreciate the Mystery of Life

The dialectical nature of the religious theories of personality presented here is related to another characteristic of these religious psychologies—their affirmations of paradox and mystery. A comparison with Western logic will help to clarify this distinguishing feature.

Aristotelean logic is categorical and discrete: "If A is A, then A is not-B." Discursive reasoning is considered the pathway to truth, guided by the rules of a linear logic which employs unipolar concepts. By contrast, the religious psychologies of both the West and East claim that reality cannot be boxed into discrete, mutually exclusive categories. One can affirm that "A is both A *and* B" without lapsing into nonsense, if one can appreciate the multidimensional nature of reality and human life. Thus life is both physical *and* spiritual, humans are both saintly *and* sinful. The Jewish concepts of *yetzar hator* and *yetzar harvar* reflect this paradoxical quality of human dispositions toward both good and evil. "Either/or" constructs are replaced by "both/and" constructs; unipolar concepts which function as signs in a one-to-one correspondence with reality are replaced by bipolar concepts or multidimensional symbols.

The role of paradox seems most apparent in Eastern religious psychologies. The Buddhist practice of meditation on koans, such as "what is the sound of one hand clapping?" appears to be not only paradoxical, but nonsensical, if not irrational. Everyone knows it takes two hands to make a clapping sound! Or do we? Buddhist psychology invites us to perceive our experience differently, from a more comprehensive perspective. As a strategy designed to show the limits of both our perceptions and rational thinking, the practice of koans becomes more understandable. Implicit in the practice is the premise that there is more to reality and life than what we perceive through our senses or comprehend through discursive reasoning. There is more to life than our dichotomous categories could ever capture; there is mystery. In the presence of mystery, religiously committed individuals experience reverence, awe, and a sense of the holy.[6]

By implication, these religious psychologies affirm alternative ways of knowing reality besides reason alone. Although highlighted in the chapter on Taoism, intuition is affirmed by most religious psychologies as a non-rational way to understand the felt-meanings associated with human experience. The implication is that feelings are meaningful sources of insight and knowledge, including religious affections experienced in meditative states, acts of worship, and loving relationships. Simultaneously, our meanings have affective dimensions; they are meanings we feel.

The truths disclosed in human feelings and revealed in spiritual intuitions challenge the dogmatic claims made in the name of either reason or tradition, and they help us to avoid identifying our concepts with the realities they reference or name. Ultimate reality remains a mystery, though we give it a name to relate with it—Brahman, Tao, Yahweh, God, or Allah. Intuition can help one appreciate the mystic's experience of "a cloud of unknowing" as an antidote to the kind of intellectual pride that would dismiss a unitive experience as a defacto symptom of a pathological dissociative state.

Religious Theories Are Existential

Insofar as these religious psychologies address concerns about human existence and its boundary situations such as suffering and death, or peak spiritual experiences such as unitive consciousness, forgiveness and reconciliation, they may be construed as existential theories. To call them existential is not to say that they affirm no human essence; neither is Sartre's dictum that "existence precedes essence" endorsed by all religious psychologies. Rather, all of these theories assume an essential human nature, and they take seriously the challenges and struggles of human existence. All of them address concrete experiences of unique individuals as they struggle to create and fulfill their personal destinies. Additional existential themes evident in these theories are their shared affirmations about human freedom, the necessity of making decisions, the fundamental challenge of finding meaning in life, the appreciation for personal selfhood, the principle that one knows authentic human existence only by being personally involved as concrete individuals making free decisions, and the accent upon human agency and responsibility. An existential premise common to these religious psychologies is that the most significant aspects of human life are understood only through decisions, commitment, and involvement in life, not through a detached, logical attitude of impersonal objectivity.

Religious Theories Are Holistic

The title of Gordon Allport's book, *The Person in Psychology,*[7] symbolizes his call for psychology to regain a sense of the uniqueness of the individual and to focus on the person as a whole. The religious theories of personality within this volume have made significant contributions on both counts.

Their resistance to various forms of reductionism noted previously, and their addition of the moral, spiritual, and historical dimensions of human experience take into account both the wholeness and the uniqueness of human personality. With the exceptions of the Taoist and Buddhist theories of no separate self *(anatta),* these religious psychologies are all explicit theories of personality. Most of these theories affirm the real existence of a unique, separate individual, who is considered holistically as a multidimensional or multilayered unity. Cognitive, affective, conative, behavioral, and interpersonal dimensions are recognized in constructs such as intellect, mind, heart, emotion, desire, will, action, and relationships. The individual is portrayed as a unitary being who makes decisions, who strives toward goals, and who is the locus of action and change. Concepts such as the ego, "I," self, person, soul, or spirit all reflect holistic and ideographic conceptions of personality and human being. For example, the individual soul *(jiva)* affirmed in Hindu psychology provides an ideographic perspective that complements the more nomothetic principle of the divine reality (Brahman) incarnate in all human beings as their essential self *(Atman).*

Religious Theories Affirm the Priority of the Spiritual Dimension of Life

When he sailed across the seas to America, Columbus proved that the world was not flat, and that one would not fall off the edge where the sea meets the horizon. With his discovery and many others preceding and following him, the Western view of the world changed. Western culture was said to have experienced such a radical transformation from Newtonian, Darwinian, and Freudian insights, that the modern epoch has been described by historians as the post-Enlightenment period. Despite descriptions of our current epoch as "post-modern," many individuals continue to perceive the world as flat in a metaphorical sense, and even in an ontological sense. There is only one reality—the world we see, hear, touch, taste, and smell, and above all, the one we can measure. What we cannot measure does not exist! There is no other world, not even in the expanse of outer space nor in the depths of inner space explored by those who meditate. Reality is one-dimensional; it is material, not material *and* spiritual.

In contrast, religious psychologies share in common the belief in another reality—a spiritual reality. This does not commit one to a kind of spiritualism, or even to the notion of spirit-beings such as angels or demons. To avoid confusion, perhaps a better way of saying it is that these religious psychologies affirm a spiritual dimension of reality, including the human personality. They share the conviction that spiritual experiences are real, relevant, powerful, transforming, and potentially therapeutic. Humans are described as spiritual beings, not merely in biological or psychological categories. These religious psychologists suggest that the varieties of religious experience are more nuanced than William James' contrast between once-born and twice-born believers.[8]

Despite some important differences in their spiritual and theological perspectives, all of these religious psychologies address the human spirit in a manner that secular psychologies do not. Several of them incorporate the concept of spirit or soul as one of the constituents of personality structure, or as a symbol for the person as a whole, and in some instances, as the essential being of human persons.

This contrast between religious and secular psychologies is not a dichotomous (either/or) distinction. The reality of this material, phenomenal world can be affirmed, and is affirmed in most religious psychologies. Simultaneously they affirm the reality and relevance of a broader vision that acknowledges spiritual dimensions of reality, and spiritual experiences as real, informing, and transforming. Spiritual disciplines such as meditation and prayer, the study of sacred texts, worship and service, and struggles for liberation and justice are affirmed in these religious psychologies as transforming media or vehicles for the development of an authentic humanity, both individually and collectively. One becomes who one truly is by conforming to spiritual principles and laws, by responding to a Spiritual Presence of compassionate wisdom, and by actualizing one's essential spiritual identity. Nurturing a spiritual life is considered vital to becoming fully human. Not only psychological insight, but spiritual insight is required and viewed as paramount. Not merely consciousness, but a *spiritual* consciousness is advocated by all religious psychologies, albeit with unique meanings of the term "spiritual." Matters of ultimate loyalty and trust, ultimate meaning and concern are addressed by religious psychologies to a greater degree than by the secular theories of scientific psychology. Each of these religious psychologies qualifies as a psychology of ultimate concerns. They affirm the reality and priority of spiritual dimensions of human personality including spiritual experience and spiritual strivings.

Religious Psychologies Sanctify Personhood

Albert Schwietzer translated Jesus' vision of the kingdom of God into an ethical "reverence for life." Schweitzer's work as a medical missionary in Africa was religiously motivated by his own reverence for all of life. Each of the religious psychologies in this book resonates with a reverence for life. They claim with one voice that life is sacrosanct.

By construing life as sacred and holy, each of these religious psychologies sanctify life more explicitly than secular psychologies grounded in naturalistic theories. This is not to deny that secular psychologies affirm human worth and dignity; however, we wish to assert that these religious psychologies have the potential to lead clinicians to view their clients with both reverence and compassion, and to view themselves as vessels of healing grace. Therapeutic encounters affirm and express the sanctity of life.

Moreover, human development itself can be construed religiously as a process of sanctification. Whether the aim is unitive consciousness, enlightenment, harmony, holiness, reconciliation, or obedience to God's will, the journey depicted is toward a greater good, toward a more meaningful life of greater value, and toward social relations characterized by love, justice, and peace. All of these religious psychologies affirm a virtuous life of wisdom and compassion, which is much more than merely an adjusted life. Each theory provides an answer to the question of what it means to be a good person, to be a real human being, and to live a meaningful life. Each aims to help its followers to thrive and grow, not merely to survive or cope. The ultimate aims are life-affirming, promoting the dignity and worth of individuals, and placing human existence in a scared shroud. They are to be commended on these grounds alone as sources of inspiration based on their visions of not only who and what we are, but who we might become.

More Specific Comparisons

The general commonalities previously described are paramount in these religious psychologies. They have been highlighted to encourage dialogue based upon their multiple shared convictions. There are other similarities (and differences) related to personality structure, dynamics, and development, individual differences, human distress, and psychotherapy. To these more specific comparisons we now turn.

Personality Structure

At the time of this writing, a considerable amount of construction of various commercial buildings was occurring in our city. After huge steel girders are driven into the ground to provide a secure foundation, they are connected with more cross beams to which joists for floors are attached and constructed with reinforced concrete. Gradually more floors are added, and eventually the ceiling and outside walls enclose the building. Internal spaces are divided and framed, while wiring, plumbing, heating and air-conditioning are all connected. Finally, the building becomes a whole, unified, distinct structure.

The image of a building can serve as a metaphor for understanding the structure of personality. Theories of personality structure describe what elements, constituents, dimensions, or aspects provide the foundation for stability and integration into one whole unit called the person. What accounts for the continuity of persons across time and situations? Habits or traits? Self-concept or object-relations? Memory or perceptions? Thoughts, intentions, or feelings?

Concepts such as personality, self, person, "I," spirit, or soul express the structure of individual human life in several of the religious theories presented in this collection. However, the meaning of these terms, and particularly the "self" varies considerably, and in some instances the existence of a self as a separate entity or identity is denied.

For example, the goal of Self-realization in Hindu psychology is not the same as self-actualization in Western humanistic psychologies. Their differences are grounded in various meanings of the self. In Hindu psychology, one Supreme Soul (Brahman) is manifest as *Atman* in the individual soul *(Jiva)*. In this sense, one's real self is not the conscious "I" or ego, but is essentially the one, infinite, eternal self. Human consciousness is a manifestation of Absolute Consciousness, a part of it, and identical with it. This notion expresses the principle of the One in the many, and the many who are the One. Self-realization is the awareness of this connection or unity. This Hindu view of personality structure is a consistent application of its fundamental monism: All reality is one Infinite Consciousness and "That Thou Art." The spiritual center of the personality is the divine life. Hence the individual is essentially united with the eternal and infinite Brahman.

Just as there are multiple floors in a building, the structure of personality in Hindu psychology consists of "layers" within which there are various "sheaths." The three major layers represent the biological aspects (gross layer), psychological aspects (subtle layer), and spiritual aspects (causal layer) of personality. This suggests a tripartite model of personality structure. Insofar as the subtle layer mediates a balance between the other two, the psychological functions of mind and intellect are decisive for human functioning.

In Taoist psychology, the Tao symbolizes a unitary, absolute reality. It is an all-encompassing energy, nature itself, or the universe as a whole. All that exists is a part of the integral force of Tao. Insofar as all that exists is a part of the Tao, this religious theory of personality structure is more similar to Hindu psychology than any of the others presented here.

Since human personality is part of the Tao, the fundamental principles of the Tao apply also to understanding both personality structure and personality dynamics. These basic tenets of Taoist psychology are natural simplicity, spontaneity, harmonious action, personal power (virtue), and the *yin-yang* polarity.

Analogous to the tripartite model of personality structure in Hindu psychology, three additional Taoist concepts appear to provide structure to personality. *Chi* is the energy of life derived from the food we eat and the air we breathe; *jing* provides our basic temperament and personality characteristics; and *shen* (spirit) is the essence of what makes us human. *Shen* is consciousness, and includes thinking, reasoning, and memory.

Although these three aspects of personality are present in Taoist psychology, a holistic perspective on personality is also affirmed in Taoist psychology. This is expressed in an appreciation for the individual as a whole, and in a comprehensive, biopsychosocial and spiritual model of personality structure.

Similar to Taoism, Buddhism affirms no personal God. Unlike Hindu psychology, Buddhism also denies a Supreme Self. Even more striking is the Buddhist's denial of any enduring, separate self as either a real phenomenon or the structure of human personality. One's sense of a separate self (ego) is considered an illusion. Zen Buddhism appears to be even less of a personality theory than the Tibetan Buddhism presented in this book. Nevertheless, both affirm that a continuous identity or stable structure of personality is an illusion, a misperception, a false belief. There is no such thing as a real self, which is separate from other selves; only an illusory ego.

What then contributes to the continuity and stability of personality over time and across situations? The answer is past actions (karma). Past actions create predispositions, tendencies, and attitudes, which influence the present and future. Insofar as past actions provide the structure of personality, Buddhist psychology may be construed as a behavioral psychology, which appreciates influences of the past. Perceptual, cognitive, and affective dimensions are also acknowledged in the development of the fictitious self. Nevertheless, behavior is fundamental, and evident in the view of the ego as consisting of habitual patterns and delusions. The concept of "habit" is a key term in behavioral psychology, which is derived from learning theory and experimental psychology.

Since the ego is no substantial reality, neither is it an inherent structure of the individual personality. One is not born with a separate self, a distinct ego, or an individual soul. Rather, this illusion of a separate, stable identity is created through experience. In other words, one "learns" to think of oneself as a separate entity as a result of experiences and the acculturation process. Through misidentifications such as "I am my thoughts," and by grasping at anything which maintains this mistaken identity, the individual splits the world repeatedly into an "I" and an "It" in attempts to maintain the security of a solid self-image.

This dualistic misperception that the individual exists as an entity separate from other entities emerges in one's experience through five stages called *skandhas*. In the first stage, the fictitious ego emerges out of ignorance manifested in dualistic thinking. This distorted perception (ego) continues to develop through four more stages of feeling, perception-impulse, conceptualization, and consciousness. The predispositions, tendencies and attitudes, which might be called "personality," are constantly being reborn moment to moment in the form of the five *skandhas*.

Although Jewish psychology acknowledges that persons exist as individual entities, separate from one another, less attention is given to the internal structure of personality than to the quality of interpersonal relationships people experience with one another and with God. What appears to matter most of all is "the stuff in between." This is a social-psychological perspective expressed by the Jewish philosopher-poet, Martin Buber.[9] Buber asserted that the fundamental ontological category for understanding reality and human life is not "substance," "experience," or "process," but "relation." The core of Judaism is relational—humans' relationships with God and with each other. Moreover, the self emerges from relationships, and there is no authentic "I" apart from a "Thou."

Although this relational emphasis is central, Jewish psychology is also holistic, and there are both dimensions and elements which give personality its structure. The dimensions are behavioral, cognitive, affective, intentional and moral, and the commitment to struggle for holiness. The structural elements include the self, the soul, the process of struggle, relationships, and the opportunity for their repair *(t'shuva)*. Jewish theory of personality structure could be characterized as a relational, self-theory. The self emerges from relationships with God and with other people, and apart from these relationships, the self or personhood of the individual cannot emerge.

The concept of the "soul" in Jewish psychology connotes the dual inclinations to do evil *(yetzer hara)* or to do good *(yetzer hatov)*. These predispositions seem to function both as structures and motives. One's personality is constructed from the choices and decisions one makes about how to live with respect to these good and evil dispositions. Consequently, personality is a construct with a moral dimension, and life is essentially a continual moral struggle of anxious choices between good and evil. Good and evil are defined by the Torah. To do evil is to sin. *t'shuva* is the way of atonement for one's sins. Reconciliation (atonement) requires repentance, forgiveness, and restitution. Obedience to divine commandments *(mitzvot)* gives personality its stability, continuity, and integration, hence both the moral and psychological structure to personal life.

Christian humanism offers an explicit self-theory of personality. The self is construed as a multidimensional unity, which defines the uniqueness of the whole person in relation to others. Distinct from Buddhist psychology, the human self is presumed to be a real, created, separate identity. The self is the structure through which the multiple dimensions of experience are integrated, unified, or synthesized. The self encompasses all dimensions; it symbolizes the oneness, totality, and unity of personality structure. This self is phenomenal, that is, a part of one's experience, central to it, part of it, yet also a real, autonomous reality that transcends and influences all dimensions of experience, including what one thinks, feels, intends, and does, and how one relates.

Unlike the somewhat hierarchical notion of "layers" and "sheaths" in Hindu psychology, Christian humanism adopts the social and spatial metaphor of "dimensions" as coordinates by which to map the individual self. Thus, the healthy self is the unifying whole of six dimensions of experience: biological, psychological, social, moral, spiritual, and historical. Synonyms for the self are the individual or person.

By speaking of personal life and personality structure as the unity of multiple, interacting dimensions, Christian humanism emphasizes the essential unity of the personality over any hypothesized divisions, although simultaneously affirming the uniqueness of each individual. Moreover, whatever conflicts that exist among these dimensions can be reconciled and must be reconciled without the destruction or absorption of one dimension by another. The reconciling agency is the self, that is, the person as a whole. All people are called to become liberating agents of reconciliation.

As with Christian humanism, Muslim psychology affirms a real self. All human beings have a common origin, the *nafs* (self or "living entity"). The self is an integrated whole of biological, psychological, and spiritual domains of life granted by the divine Creator. Its three major components of body, mind, and spirit interact with one another to form a whole person. The self (personality) is viewed as a complex and multifaceted unity. When body, mind, and spirit are integrated as God has intended for human life, the individual is called *nafs wama sawwaha.*

In the chapter on Muslim psychology, the term "mind" is used to express the psychological dimension. The mind exercises executive functions, and it serves as the agent of action and thought. Moreover, the mind mediates between the biological and spiritual components of the personality.

Consciousness of God is the defining attribute of the human spirit. The more one is conscious of God, the greater the chance that one will be blessed with spiritual endowments and illumination. Affirmation of the Oneness of God revealed by the prophet Muhammad is the essence of Islam. Only God is One. All other realities have a polar nature. For example, human being is characterized by male and female poles.

Similar to the Jewish notion of dualistic predispositions, Muslim psychology teaches that individuals are born with the potentials for both God-consciousness and moral failings, and the freedom to choose between good and evil. However, they are born without any original sin. Humans have an inherent moral capacity to differentiate between good and evil. Whether they actualize one or the other is a matter of choice and decision.

The basic psychological components of the mind in the Muslim theory of personality structure are intelligence, will, and emotions. These three components suggest a tripartite model of the mind parallel to the tripartite model of the self (body/mind/spirit). Of the three mental components, the will is primary because it is the capacity to choose and to make decisions. This capacity is the one human attribute that differentiates humans from other animals. In its explicit emphasis upon the will, Muslim psychology seems more similar to Christian humanism than to other religious psychologies. It shares with Jewish psychology an appreciation for human freedom and the importance of decisions and relationships.

In Muslim psychology, the "heart" serves as a metaphor for emotions. The heart also connotes an innate wisdom and intuitive way of knowing reality apart from observations through the five senses. Intuition is similar to a sixth sense, and a source of spiritual knowledge. The "heart" also symbolizes the center of human personality, that internal place where humans meet God. In this respect, the heart seems to function analogously to the concept of *Atman* in Hindu psychology as a realm within the person in which the human and the divine are connected or united. In Muslim psychology, the heart is a place of vision, understanding, and remembrance of God, but also the place of doubt, denial, and unbelief. The heart's intuitive and affective functions appear to operate within both the psychological and spiritual domains of human personality. To know someone, we must know what is in their heart.

Personality Dynamics

Personality dynamics are that portion of personality theory that explains human movement and motivation, action, and change. It is a broader concept than the notion of psychodynamics in psychoanalytic theory. Numerous terms have been used to allude to the dynamic quality of human life and personality: instincts, drives, desires, dispositions, traits, inclinations, needs, motives, strivings, goals, anticipations, expectancies, incentives, and reinforcers. In both personality theory and clinical psychology, these terms have replaced older concepts of "demons," "humors," "instincts," and to some extent the concept of "will."

Just as secular theories of personality address the question of personality dynamics in multiple terms, there is also variability among the religious theories of personality presented here. Hindu psychology postulates a variety of motives, which are related to the three different layers within personality structure. The biological motivation for survival belongs to the gross layer of personality structure, psychological motivation to the subtle layer, and spiritual motives are associated with the causal layer. Moreover, motivation is related to four additional aspects:

1. the stage of intellectual development,
2. identification with a particular sheath predominant in one's self-concept,
3. inner control issues, and
4. the level of awareness of the causal body.

Key concepts in understanding motivation are innate tendencies, attachment, identification, and desire.

In one sense, Hindu theory might be characterized as a psychology of desire. The desires for pleasure and worldly success will not yield human happiness. As ultimate concerns, both result in disillusionment. Serving one's community (as in a religion of duty) is a more noble desire, but only as a progressive step toward the final goal of union with the Supreme Soul. The desire for liberation from finitude, ignorance, and suffering is what humans truly want. Hindu psychology makes the startling claim that we can have what we want through the divine merger.[10]

In addition to the central concept of desire, Hindu motivational theory postulates three innate tendencies: *sattva* (good and truth), *rajasa* (energy and activity) and *tamasa* (ignorance and delusion). These tendencies function like motives to energize and direct human behavior. Development of the intellect is essential to the self-regulation of all types of motives.

The more spiritual one's attachments and identifications, the more likely one is motivated to achieve authentic humanity, and the ultimate goal of life, which is self-realization—union with Brahman. Awareness of the spiritual aspect within oneself, namely the bliss sheath, is essential to attain higher levels of functioning.

In Buddhist psychology, humans are described as motivated by three primary life forces: greed, hatred, and delusion. These motivational forces lead to behaviors that are centered in the illusory ego, and they function to protect and promote the ego. The basic motivating forces for all egocentric behavior are the pursuit of pleasure and avoidance of pain. If these are the fundamental human motives, all of which lead to a self-centered life, the Buddhist view of human being seems to be rather negative. Humans appear to be driven by insatiable desires, hence the inevitability of frustration and suffering. The good news is that Gautama the Buddha identified the way to end such suffering.

Key concepts in the Taoist psychology of personality dynamics include the energy of life *(chi)*, temperament *(jing)*, and spirit *(shen)*. Strivings consistent with Taoist principles include natural simplicity, spontaneity, harmonious action, virtue, and balance of *yin* and *yang* polarities.

In the Jewish psychology presented in this volume, the most fundamental personality dynamics are the dual, constitutional predispositions to do good *(yetzer hara)* and to do evil *(yetzer hatov)*. However, human choices in favor of one or the other appear to be the determining factors in character formation. Individuals can be motivated extrinsically by religious promises of reward and threats of punishment, or intrinsically by genuine commitments to Judaic values. They are also motivated to find meaning in life. Striving to bring holiness into the world through obedience to the *Torah* seems to be a paramount motivation in Jewish psychology.

According to its second proposition, Christian humanism supports a voluntaristic and teleological theory of motivation: purpose is paramount and conscious strivings count. Christian humanism relies primarily upon the concept of "will" or "the experience of willing" to affirm that people are both energized to act and directed to act toward a particular goal. The concept of will is used to express both unconscious wishes and conscious decisions. It presumes enough freedom to make finite choices, sufficient rationality to make discriminating and moral judgments about alternatives, the capacity to envision a future determined in part by one's present decisions, and the ability to bring about outcomes one intends through conscious commitments and selected actions. Human needs are also described in all six dimensions of life, but an emphasis upon choice and striving toward goals makes this theory of personality dynamics both voluntaristic and teleological. Moreover, the accent upon the future over the past makes this a future-oriented psychology of hope. As noted previously, however, optimism is a characteristic of all religious theories of personality. They are agreed that people can change.

Muslim theory about both personality structure and dynamics is comprehensive by virtue of its incorporation of all four types of causes: material, efficient, formal, and final causes. Both bodily needs and spiritual aspirations are affirmed. The primary motivating force, as well as the ultimate purpose of life, is striving to experience the Oneness of God *(Tawhid)*.

Muslim theory asserts that God instilled in humans a thirst for knowledge as an innate drive. Attaining the knowledge of good versus evil is both essential and possible. Moreover, because they are also born with the ability to discern good from evil (a cognitive and intuitive ability), humans are accountable for their actions. Being born also with the freedom to make choices and decisions makes humans the noblest of creatures.

In their strivings toward justice and the good *(Jihad)*, humans experience a constant struggle between their primal and pleasure instincts (including the attendant feelings of anger, jealousy, pride, and greed), and their more subtle spiritual urges, which are transcendent and enduring. This emphasis upon the human struggle between one's good and evil predispositions is found also in Jewish psychology. Moreover, consistent with both Jewish and Christian psychologies, personality dynamics include repentance and forgiveness, which both express and transform one's attitudes and behaviors.

Personality Development

Developmental theories provide a way to think about the dynamics of change and transformation, while simultaneously appreciating issues of equilibrium and continuity through time. Stage theories of development attempt to describe predictable changes in individuals through the life cycle in largely formal terms. Their approach to personality is nomothetic, that is, a descriptive outline of general features and patterns of growth applicable to all people.

In Hindu anthropology, personality development of the individual *(Jiva)* is governed by the impact of both prevalent religious beliefs and cultural practices expressing these beliefs. A central belief is that human development is influenced by the fundamental laws governing all reality, summarized as dharma. These dharma prescribe how people should think, feel, and act; what they should believe, value, and decide; and how they should structure their personal and collective lives for meaningful survival. Dharma is esteemed by Muslims as sacred teaching, as the *Torah* is by Jews and the New Testament is by Christians.

Applied to particular areas of life, Dharma becomes *Samaj-dharma* (social religion), *Varna-dharma* (prescribed social roles) and *Ashram-dharma,* which depicts developmental stages, goals, and tasks appropriate to various age groups. Performance of the tasks appropriate to each stage is essential to satisfactory adjustment and optimal growth. This notion seems similar to the epigenetic principle affirmed by Erik Erikson in his theory of stages in the human life cycle.

Just as individuals differ from one another, so they move through a variety of stages in the course of their life. Following the stage of being a student, one becomes a householder, and eventually retires. Retirement is not the final stage, however. The final stage is the state of *sannyasin,* defined by the *Bhagavad Gita* as "one who neither hates nor loves anything."[11] Following one's education and the satisfactory performance of social roles as spouse, parent, and citizen, the healthy individual is to extend his or her attachments to concern about the welfare of one's community, and to engage in spiritual practices such as meditation to achieve self-realization. The ultimate goal of human development is spiritual.

Buddhist psychology postulates a stage theory of human development. In addition to the five stages in the development of an illusory ego, the individual is presumed to experience six different states in the Wheel of Life *(Samsara):* striving for pleasure, distrust, pursuit of an ideal, the state of instinctual gratification and ignorance, the acquisitive state, and the state of aggression. These states are not chronological stages, since we can cycle through all of them in the course of a day as well as over a lifetime. However, the dynamic quality of these psychological states or stages suggests that human development is construed in motivational terms. A theory of motivation underlies the Buddhist theory of human development.

The theory of human development in Taoist psychology is guided by the ideal of the Sage personality type. The five main characteristics of the Sage personality are humbleness, flexibility, adaptability, persistence, and acceptance. Personality development is presumed to occur through stages defined less by chronological ages than by the quality of one's experiences and one's engagement with life. Personality development does not end with the attainment of adulthood. One becomes a Sage only when all distinctions between one's self and all the rest of nature have disappeared, that is, when the individual has become one with Tao.

According to Jewish psychology, the quality of relationships is pivotal in human development. I-Thou relationships are more conducive to healthy development than I-It relations, though the latter may be necessary and instrumental to human functioning. From early relationships a consciousness of the "I" as a separate entity takes form. This sense of identity is not illusory (contra Buddhist psychology). A real individual self sees, listens, thinks, feels, intends, and relates. The moral development of character is central in Jewish thought. Obedience to *mitzvot* is the means made possible by a redemptive I-Thou relation with God.

The development of character is central in Christian humanism. The cardinal virtues are faith, hope, and love. As a self-theory of personality, the development of the self is also central. Three major themes of the development of the existential self are faith formation, the moral development of character, and spiritual transformation and growth into a new spiritual identity through spiritual disciplines, which cultivate spiritual gifts bestowed by the Holy Spirit. Faith formation and character formation are both prerequisites for spiritual transformation into a more liberating life as an agent of reconciliation.

The influence of both nature and nurture are affirmed in Islamic theory about personality development. The equal emphasis placed upon both heredity and environment seems compatible with contemporary biosocial and developmental theories of maturation. Distinct stages of psychological development were not articulated in the chapter on Islamic psychology within this book, but spiritual development is presumed to occur in stages.

In addition to heredity and environment, a third factor, which is decisive for human development, is the will of God. The whole purpose of human existence in Islam is the moral achievement of submission to the will of Allah. Moral development presumes that humans are responsible agents of God to whom they ultimately return as the Creator of all goodness. The Five Pillars of Islam prescribe the pathway for moral development and guide spiritual development as well. These pillars are God consciousness, five daily prayers, fasting from dawn to sunset during the Islamic holy month of Ramadan, paying a 2.5 percent tax on one's savings and possessions in excess of one's needs for the benefit of the community and the poor, and making a pilgrimage to Mecca.

Three stages (and types) of spiritual development are described in Islamic psychology: a life of passion, a life conscious of evil and resistant to it, and a satisfied life of bliss, contentment, and peace that comes from knowing that in spite of one's failures in this world, one will return to God. Forgiveness and grace are affirmed in Muslim psychology, as they are in Jewish and Christian psychologies. These experiences are central to both spiritual development of the individual, and to just and harmonious social relations.

Individual Differences

The developmental approach to personality is nomothetic, that is, a descriptive outline of general features and patterns of growth applicable to all people. Occasionally neglected in such theories are the significant individual differences in rates of growth, and particular life sequences, events, and stories. A developmental approach needs an ideographic perspective to highlight the uniqueness of each and every individual and their individual differences.

Hindu psychology affirms that several factors contribute to individual differences: universal laws (dharma), heredity, environment, one's stage of life, one's station in life, the layer of personality developed, current personality traits, and the individual's level of conscious effort. Each individual is presumed to develop a unique personality, which in turn impacts future feelings, thoughts, decisions, actions, and the accumulation of new karma, hence one's ultimate liberation *(moksha)* from the cycle of multiple reincarnations.

Hereditary factors, present needs, and environmental factors interact to create individual differences. These three universal factors are present in varying degrees in individuals, and they lead to different motives and traits. Although each individual is unique, the universal soul *(Atman)* in all persons and at all stages of life is the same because it is part of the one Supreme Soul, Brahman. Paradoxically, people are both unique and the same. The most important determinant of individual differences is insight, particularly spiritual insight. Once insight emerges, no personality determinant or individual feature blocks spiritual growth and fundamental change.

In recognition of individual differences, Hindu psychology provides a variety of pathways *(yogas)* to spiritual insight and self-realization. For the more reflective personality, there is *jnana-yoga,* the way to God through knowledge. For more affective types, there is *bhakti-yoga,* the way to God through love. For action-oriented individuals, there is *karma-yoga,* the way to God through service and good works. For the more experimentally inclined, there is *raja-yoga*, the way to God through psychophysical exercises such as meditation. All pathways are valid; all lead to union with Brahman.

Comparable to other religious psychologies, Tantric Buddhism recognizes individual differences in the expression of personality. Five principles of Buddha nature, known as "buddha families" are the basis for distinguishing five personality types or styles: The logical style *(varja)*, the expansive style *(ratna)*, the passionate style *(padma)*, the active style *(karma)*, and the meditative style *(buddha)*. A person could identify primarily with one of these styles, all of them, or partially with several. Each family is associated with both a style of neurosis (a state of confusion) and a style of sanity. These distinctions could serve as a basis for differential diagnoses of mental disorders, particularly different types of neurotic adjustments.

Taoist psychology recognizes individual differences in the level of one's life energy *(chi)*, in temperament *(jing)*, and in spirit *(shen)*. Individuals vary in their developmental stages and in the degree to which they live according to the basic tenets of Taoism: natural simplicity, spontaneity, harmonious action, virtue, and *yin-yang* principles. They vary according to whether they are mindful of the present, past, or future. They are different in terms of their levels of intuition and in their degree of unity with the Tao. Some are similar to the Sage personality characterized by humbleness, flexibility, adaptability, persistence, and acceptance. Although suffering is to some degree an inevitable part of life, people suffer in varying degrees according to the multiple causes of suffering.

An important basis for individual differences in Jewish psychology relates to the varied manner in which Jews observe the *mitzvot*, the divine commandments. These commandments delineate most aspects of human behavior and relationships. Jews differ in how consistently and completely they adhere to the *mitzvot* concerning their relationship with God through ritual and with one another in personal relationships and in commercial dealings. Variability in the type and quality of one's relationship with God and others is central to any explanation of individual differences.

In Christian humanism variability in the quality of one's conscious relationship with God in Christ is considered primary in explaining individual differences. Nevertheless, individual differences also exist in all six dimensions (biopsychosocial, moral, spiritual, and historical), and in their relative dominance and organization within an individual and across time. Within the psychological dimension, individuals differ according to which domains are prominent: cognitive, affective, conative, behavioral, or relational styles. For example, some individuals feel more than they think, and some act without thinking.

The divergent dimensions become convergent within the mature self-structure as complementary aspects rather than conflicted elements. The healthy self-structure synthesizes polarities among dimensions, hence we may speak of the self as the unity of its multidimensional experiences. A classification of personality types or traits becomes possible based upon the unique organization of the dimensions and domains of experience within the self-structure of different individuals.

Muslim psychology recognizes that different people attain different levels of spiritual existence, and diversity in all creation is presumed to be a part of God's creative plan. In addition to cultural and national diversity, God bestows individual differences upon humans in capabilities, wealth, social status, power, family and knowledge. Differences in rank and preference are presumed to be divinely ordained in a manner that is somewhat similar to the Hindu idea of different stations in life based on the law of karma. The rights and responsibilities of different age groups are also different, commensurate with their developed capacities. These differences, however, are secondary to the degree of one's attainment of righteousness expressed in both ethical living and religious devotions grounded in one's consciousness of God.

Human Distress/Psychopathology

The therapeutic recommendations derived from religious theories of personality are grounded in their respective diagnoses of the human condition. Each theory presents an answer to the question of human suffering, and provides an explanation for human misery, including the form of suffering described under the Western rubric of mental disorders.

Hindu psychology suggests that the chief cause of human distress is ignorance *(avidya)*. Ignorance prevents the development of a vital balance between the three principles and practices which promote health and happiness, and which reduce distress: truth, nonviolence, and self-restraint. Along with insatiable desires and selfish actions, ignorance leads to attachments to sense experiences that create illusions *(maya)*, which divorce one from the Supreme Reality. One succumbs to misidentifications, dualistic thinking, and to a variety of addictions. The resulting bad *karma* destines one to the misery of repeated cycles of birth, death, and rebirth across multiple lifetimes. Without insight into the totality, unity and universality of the all-pervading Supreme Spirit, Self-realization is impossible. Without Self-realization, distress is inevitable. Self-realization consists in the conscious union with the one Supreme Reality, which is characterized as Infinite Being, Infinite Consciousness, and Infinite Bliss *(sat, chit, ananda)*. The deepest human desires for limitless being, limitless knowledge, and endless joy are found in unity with Brahman, the Godhead. Since Brahman is manifest within each individual as *Atman,* self-realization is the awareness that what we truly want we already possess within our own being.

The Buddhist explanation of distress is grounded in the first two of the Four Noble Truths: The reality of suffering, the origin of suffering, the cessation of suffering, and the end of suffering via the middle path. The realism of Buddhist psychology is evident in its affirmation that pain is unavoidable, suffering is inevitable, all life is *dukkha*. There is the suffering associated with sickness and injury, the aging process, and eventual death. There is the suffering one experiences being tied to what one dislikes, and being separated from what one loves. To these forms of natural suffering individuals add self-created pains ("double negativity"), exemplified in the dynamics of panic attacks and by interpersonal relations characterized by aggression and vengeful counterattacks. The good news is that people can eliminate the unnecessary suffering caused by double negativity "by letting go of holding onto ourselves." The eightfold middle path describes the way to end unnecessary suffering by attaining an indestructible state of awareness which enables one to become fully human.

The causes of human suffering are many and varied according to Taoist psychology. These have been summarized in a set of propositions. Akin to the first noble truth of Buddhism, Taoism affirms that suffering is a natural part of life. It occurs particularly when we separate ourselves from nature and its cyclical patterns; when we deny our internal self and place too much attention on external chaotic conditions. Ultimately, suffering is the result of imbalance between *yin* and *yang* principles. Human misery occurs when we lose our sense of safety and spontaneity, when we interfere with *wu wei* and push to get things done rather than letting ourselves follow our natural rhythms and the rhythms of those around us. People suffer when they are not mindful of the present, and live instead in the past or future. People suffer when their attachments to things become more important than developing spiritual strength and meaningful relationships with others and with nature. Misperceptions are additional causes of suffering, along with misplaced faith in technology and materialism as the solutions to all human difficulties. Suffering occurs when we become rigid, unyielding, and unwilling to change; when we create and nurture negativity; and when busyness and complexity are preferred over stillness and simplicity.

A central theme of Jewish psychology is that human distress is the consequence of something amiss in relationships. When something has gone awry in one's relationships with God or with other people, one is more inclined to give way to one's own innate, evil predisposition, which is expressed in various forms of idolatry and licentious behavior. Both existential anxiety and existential guilt are implicated in the development of psychopathology. Making the wrong moral choices is also implicated. An unrepentant heart and the experience of meaninglessness are additional etiological factors.

Christian humanism adopts a multidimensional view of the etiology of human distress, and emphasizes spiritual-ethical-historical dimensions. The main cause of human distress is alienated relationships which need to be reconciled with God, self, and others. The symptoms, diagnosis, and etiology of human distress are all viewed from a multidimensional perspective consistent with the basic notion of the multidimensional unity of life.

The variety of symptoms in all dimensions reflects a common characteristic: multiplicity without unity in personality structure and functioning. The essential multidimensional unity of life is existentially distorted, resulting in a compromise of true humanity, and an ambiguous life. The individual becomes alienated from one's true self, from others, and from God. The symptoms of distress and dysfunction reflect personal disintegration and alienation. Some suffering is inevitable because human life is an existence estranged from essence. The result is a fragmented life of conflict and distress.

The correlate of the multidimensional unity of life is a multidimensional diagnosis of the human condition and personal life. In addition to the biopsychosocial dimensions, the other three existential dimensions need to be taken into account in any case formulation (spiritual, moral, and historical dimensions). The common condition evident in all three is estrangement, experienced respectively in the spiritual, moral, and historical dimensions as unbelief, hubris, and an ambiguous life. Turning away from God, toward oneself, one experiences an ambiguous life estranged from God, self, and others.

Estrangement (alienation) is partially the consequence of the abuse of freedom, expressed as a repudiation of one's dependence upon God and manifest in selfish pride. This is the universal condition of sin. The common effects are self-deception and human misery. This is not to say, however, that all mental suffering is due to sin. But neither is the fundamental etiology ignorance, desire or attachment per se, nor a misidentification of one's true self with the conscious ego; rather, the fundamental human problem is the pretense to divinity, expressed in one's turning away from God (unbelief) toward a life centered in self (hubris), and resulting in ambiguity and suffering.

In Muslim psychology, health and illness, comfort and distress, ecstasy and suffering are the essential polarities of the dialectical nature of human life. God has equipped humans with the ability to deal with pain and suffering. The choices an individual makes in life either aggravate the negative conditions or restore positive states of being. Even when negative conditions (such as a terminal illness) cannot be removed, suffering is not meaningless because it is also construed as a form of atonement. Accepting one's pain and suffering with the belief that it is part of God's plan brings a person closer to salvation.

Summary of Personality Theories

The previous discussion reveals both multiple similarities and several differences among religious theories of personality. These similarities and differences are evident in their respective theories of the structure, dynamics, and development of personality, and in their views about individual differences and psycho pathology. These personality theories are important because they serve as the foundation for the religious theories of psychotherapy to which we now turn.

THEORIES OF PSYCHOTHERAPY

In this section we will explore some important points of convergence among religious psychologies with respect to their influence on the theory and practice of psychotherapy. After highlighting several general points of convergence among perspectives, we will sharpen our focus and look more carefully at some important areas that reveal distinctions among them. These distinctions have differential impacts on the practice of therapy. We will explore how different religious perspectives influence the stance of the therapist as an authority and expert, inform our understanding of the self and relationships, and guide the therapist's engagement with the client's suffering. Finally, we will present a brief description of two transpersonal models used within psychotherapy that integrate many of the religious principles and practices presented in this volume: An early integrative model (Assagioli's psychosynthesis) and a more recent one (Wilber's Spectrum model). Discussion of these latter two models should not be taken as an endorsement of a particular, integrative approach, but as an illustration how these integrative models have common roots in many of the religious principles and practices described in proceeding chapters. Future efforts at integration will be enriched by these same roots from both Eastern and Western religious traditions.

Impact of Religious Traditions on Psychotherapy Theory and Practice: General Points of Convergence

There is significant common ground among the traditions described in this volume as they are applied to the theory and practice of psychotherapy. However, overlapping areas of philosophy, common perspectives on distress and healing, and common values regarding healing relationships may create an impression of convergence that collapses when brought into the practical world of a psychotherapy experience with a particular therapist and client who have distinct religious orientations. Differences may arise only when we penetrate beneath these generalities to find how they translate into the practice of therapy in a very specific case application. In this section we will first highlight some significant points of convergence that arise in these religious perspectives on psychotherapy, and which appear to be expressed in the practice of therapy illustrated in the authors' discussions of the common case illustration.

Several significant points of convergence are described by psychologists from the respective religious traditions presented in this book. These include the following:

- Religious principles and practices function as the principles and practices of psychotherapy.
- Religious traditions encourage a multidimensional perspective on psychotherapy that emphasizes spiritual life and development while attending to biopsychosocial factors.
- Each religious tradition provides a framework and a methodology useful for deepening the phenomenal awareness of the client within psychotherapy.
- The purpose of psychotherapy is always integrally related to spiritual strivings and spiritual development.
- Therapists from each religious tradition perceive the person of the client as embedded in a larger network of relationships.
- Psychologists from each religious tradition value and incorporate subjective experience.
- Religious psychologists address the dimension of time.

Religious Principles and Practices Function As the Principles and Practices of Psychotherapy

The principles developed within each religious tradition serve many purposes, and significant among them is their use as comprehensive guidelines for living and grappling with the common struggles of human existence. Consequently, religious principles and practices can be viewed as therapeutic. Hindu philosophy offers the *Bhagavad Gita* as the source of principles for living, for solving human problems and for spiritual growth. The spiritual treatises that underlie contemplative Taoism, such as the *Tao te Ching*, support a similar set of principles for understanding daily living and how to cope in times of struggle and distress. These sacred texts connect religion to human experience; moreover they provide a basis for value judgments and decision making that inform the perspective expectations of the therapist and establish the context for the therapy itself.

Buddhism carries the authority of its tradition through instructions about its spiritual principles and through the practice of its spiritual disciplines. The spiritual framework provides guidelines for daily living, for grappling with common human struggles, and for progressive spiritual awakening. For example, the concept of a "Buddha nature" or "basic sanity" that lies beneath ordinary consciousness is brought into the lived experience of individuals through their consistent practice of meditation. That a reduction in psychological stress may result from this spiritual practice demonstrates how spiritual practice and psychotherapy can share a common objective and beneficial outcome (and, indeed, may be functionally the same thing).

Within the Western religious tradition, the sacred texts of Judaism, the *Torah,* the *Talmud* and the *Kabbalah* are the sources for the principles informing psychotherapeutic practice. As applied in these texts, the profound principle of covenantal relationships demonstrates a strong connection between religious perspective and actual psychotherapeutic practice. Indeed, as will be explored further in this section, the Judaic perspective on covenantal relationships appears to be fundamental to the professional values of nearly all Western psychotherapy practice, particularly the value placed on the therapeutic relationship.

Christian humanism affirms how the teachings drawn from the historical life of Jesus revealed through scripture, particularly through the Synoptic Gospels of the Holy Bible, provide guidance for ordinary human life and struggles. The life, message, and ministry of Jesus are ciphers for the meaning of human suffering and illustrate how religious values guide life decisions. Jesus is the human model of the reconciled life with God and others. A more reconciling life is the ultimate goal of Christian humanism and the goal of psychotherapy informed by this liberal Christian tradition. Inspiring stories and religious parables contained in scripture help inculcate the morality of a liberating covenant of reconciliation, especially within human relationships, including the therapist-client relationship.

As the primary scripture of Islam, the *Quran* offers a set of spiritual principles that guide the daily life practices of its adherents, and it identifies principles and metaphors that inform the theory and practice of psychotherapy within this tradition. Pursuing knowledge of God and self through an extensive process of examination of mind, feeling and intuition is an essential spiritual practice and thus provides a spiritually based rationale for psychotherapy.

Religious Traditions Encourage a Multidimensional Perspective on Psychotherapy That Emphasizes Spiritual Life and Development Although Attending to Biopsychosocial Factors

The dialectical engagement between body, mind, and spirit is emphasized in each contributor's account of his or her particular tradition, with the possible exception of the more unitive description of an inseparable psyche posited within Taoism. Within Taoism, biopsychosocial factors are considered nondivisible and inseparable from spirit. Yet the Taoist psychologist attends to the importance of the quality of interaction between heart and mind, which suggests a dialectical relation. It is through the nature and quality of the heart-mind connection that spiritual energy resides and finds expression. Consequently, although Taoism describes spiritual reality as an inseparable web of life, selected aspects of this whole may at times become a more specific focus of therapeutic attention. This is illustrated by the comments on the utility of centering the mind and working with the connection between mind and heart as an important step in the process of psychotherapy.

In both Christian and Muslim traditions the mind and spirit are vehicles for spiritual realization, sometimes described as apprehending the "will of God." Christian humanism and Islam appear to place the mental facility of cognition as the mediator between body and spirit, and they identify cognitive strategies useful for reinforcing spiritual engagement and connection. Examples include the study of scripture and theological reflections. Western monotheistic traditions emphasize the importance of the mind in acquiring knowledge of both their transforming truths and spiritual values as well as knowledge of God, self, and others summarized as spiritual wisdom. The attention given to volition and choice within psychotherapy emphasizes the conative aspects of mental functioning. It is interesting to note how the process of "willing," often neglected in otherwise multidimensional theories of psychology, is revivified through monotheistic perspectives.

The layered and nuanced dimensions of the spiritual path described within Buddhism and Hinduism facilitate the search for "wholeness" or "undividedness" within the self, which spiritualizes the therapeutic goal of self-actualization. Buddhism and Hinduism present a complex series of pathways, stages, and levels related to spiritual development. These traditions emphasize a spiritual maturity that is a multidimensional coherence of physical, emotional, and mental aspects of human experience reflecting and underlying spiritual unity.

Each Religious Tradition Provides a Framework and a Methodology Useful for Deepening the Phenomenal Awareness of the Client Within Psychotherapy

Hinduism and Buddhism have been valued particularly for the "spiritual technologies" they offer as adjuncts to Western psychotherapy. In fact, accessing the eightfold path within Buddhism or one of the many yogic disciplines within Hinduism is facilitated by a variety of meditation practices, some of which have been incorporated for some time into many Western psychotherapies. This Western incorporation has often isolated the technique from its spiritual and cultural context, and consequently, the spiritual dimension of the practice has been lost and the technique misunderstood or misapplied. Yet despite the corruption of this spiritual practice by some Western therapists, meditation as an adjunct to psychotherapy has grown in use as it has demonstrated effectiveness in helping clients do exactly what the advocates of Eastern traditions said it would do: help to quiet mental chatter, to still recursive thought, to calm anticipatory anxieties and fears, and to heighten awareness. These effects are generally therapeutic.[12]

The Taoist practices to achieve mindfulness and awareness correspond to the more complex elaborations articulated within Buddhism and Hinduism.

Stripped of the trappings of Eastern culture and religion, these Taoist practices have also frequently found their way into Western psychotherapeutic practice.

Curiously, many Western psychotherapists are more aware of the psychotherapeutic value of the "spiritual technologies" of Eastern religion than those advanced by monotheistic religious perspectives and practices within Western culture. Judaism, for example, advocates prayer as a powerful medium of healing. Christian humanism incorporates the Catholic tradition of contemplative prayer as a healing medium, and in some instances may encourage the practice of scriptural reading and contemplation within psychotherapy with Christian clients. In addition, the Muslim's attention to ritual prayer engages the physical, mental, and spiritual dimensions of its adherents, as does meditative chanting and breathwork—all useful adjuncts to psychotherapy within that tradition.

It is evident from these chapters how therapists from each religious tradition use a wide array of other psychological theories, techniques and approaches drawn from the secular world of psychotherapy. Nevertheless, these religiously oriented therapists apply the spiritual principles from within their tradition to define the purpose and process of therapy. The amalgam of assorted other theories and techniques drawn from secular psychology are used within the coherent framework of that spiritual tradition, not apart from it.

Purpose of Psychotherapy Is Always Integrally Related
to Spiritual Strivings and Spiritual Development

Each contributor describes from a biopsychosocial and spiritual perspective how the life concerns of the client are related to his or her fundamental spiritual development. The Islamic therapist works with the client's life issues to attend to the attainment of a "satisfied soul" and trust in God. The Christian humanistic therapist works with a client toward the ultimate goal of a more liberating life and reconciling relationships with God and other people. The Jewish therapist guides the client toward a deeper experience of personhood and more meaningful I-Thou relationships with others.

In the Eastern traditions the client's distress is presented as an opportunity for detachment from illusion (Buddhism), for aligning with a Supreme Self from which one is consciously separated or alienated (Hinduism), or for restoring balance and harmony to a life out of sync with the natural rhythms of the universe (Taoism). Within each of these traditions the life concerns of the client are viewed as nonpathological expressions in the service of a much larger and more profound spiritual quest.

Therapists from Each Religious Tradition Perceive the Person
of the Client As Embedded in a Larger Network of Relationships

In discussing the common clinical case, the Muslim therapist suggests self-care as a religious duty, and includes the client's relationship with her husband in a wider definition of what such self-care entails. She also calls for the inclusion of the client's husband in therapy, as does the therapist from a Christian-humanist perspective. The Jewish therapist sees the importance of her client's enhanced personhood being affirmed by forming increasingly authentic relationships in her life outside therapy. The Hindu priest "therapist" facilitates a changed engagement between the client and the mother from whom she's estranged. The Buddhist therapist also calls for conjoint work between client and her husband. The family system is affirmed as important to the therapeutic enterprise within these varied and sometimes differing religious perspectives.

Whether in service of a "reconciling relationship," a relational "covenant," or a "Supreme Self," therapists from each of these traditions place individual healing in the wider context of relationship and community. The Holy Other of monotheistic religions calls together a "people" as a community of believers—the people of God. The believing therapist participates in that community, and affirms its value to clients who share a similar belief. Even apart from the communal experience of relating to a deity, the Buddhist therapist recognizes a call to an awakened self in loving and compassionate participation in the communal web of all life. Similarly the Taoist therapist views separation from self, others, and the natural world as the very source of suffering itself: reconnection with a larger system is the road to healing. Biopsychosocial health and spiritual growth lie always within a larger relational context. In this sense, religious psychologies are conceptual.

Psychologists from Each Religious Tradition Value
and Incorporate Subjective Experience

There are other important areas of convergence among these traditions beyond those previously cited. For example, the contributors formulate their approach to psychotherapy by closely attending to the subjective experience of the client. This suggests that, irrespective of tradition, these psychologists adopt a phenomenological perspective rather than an external frame of reference in their work. Each therapist brings into his or her therapy aspects or elements of his or her tradition that share compatibility with the subjective experience of the client. In doing so they differ from more secular therapists by applying religious perspectives and practices within a single coherent tradition, but probably with differing points of emphasis in work with different clients. Religious psychologies are experiential theories of human functioning and healing.

Religious Psychologists Address the Dimension of Time

Religious psychologies all recognize that humans experience life in the present, bracketed by the past and future. Although there are some differences in emphases, all of these theories acknowledge the influence of the *past.* In this regard, they all adopt a historical perspective. The past may be limited to one's personal life history, to one's history as a people (Western religions), or extended to past lives of all individuals expressed in the concept of life cycles (Taoism) and reincarnation (Hinduism, Buddhism). These theories provide answers to the existential questions of the origins of life as clues to understanding what makes life uniquely human. Eastern psychologies construe individuals as the many manifestations of the One ultimate reality, whereas Western religions speak of human nature created by God in the divine image. In either case, history provides insights into both identity and destiny.

The different perspectives on time contribute to different approaches to psychotherapy. One would expect to find some convergence regarding how time is perceived on the part of psychologists practicing within an Eastern tradition, and this is reflected in their therapeutic approaches. The Buddhist and Taoist perspectives seem especially "here and now" oriented, whereas psychologists writing from a Christian humanist and Muslim perspective appear to accent the future. Yet these differences are a matter of emphasis and not categorical contrasts.

Psychologists from traditions emphasizing a *present* time orientation tend to deemphasize psychopathology and the removal of behavioral symptoms. However, this does not preclude therapists from within Buddhism, Taoism and Hinduism from availing themselves of specific approaches related to behavioral change, including occasional use of cognitive-behavioral strategies with clients. In addition, psychodynamic themes of early life experiences, unconscious motivation, anxiety, and defense have been integrated with religious psychologies.[13] They take seriously the temporal discussion of human experience.

Distinctions Arising Among Traditions

The previous discussion highlights several commonalities among religious theories of psychotherapy. In this section we note some of the unique aspects that differentiate them. Within each religious perspective the ultimate goal of therapy includes the restoration of the client to a harmonious relationship with the central tenets and realities affirmed in that tradition. Where important religious tenets differ, their distinctions influence the theory and practice of psychotherapy.

To explore further distinctions among traditions we will reflect on certain areas of therapeutic engagement addressed in each theory of psychotherapy, augmented with the specific application described in the common clinical case addressed by each author. Here we want to go beyond general comparisons to highlight some of the subtle distinctions in the practice of therapy that reflect differences in religious perspectives and spiritual practices. Of course, we have only one author representing each tradition. Consequently differences in the application to the theory and practice of therapy cannot be extrapolated as definitive distinctions among traditions. Nonetheless these distinctions can be used as starting points for a fruitful dialogue among religiously oriented therapists, and they are offered in that spirit.

In this comparative analysis we will attend to the following areas: the authority and expertise accorded the therapist; the construct of self; the construct of relationship; and the engagement with suffering. In each area we will look at how each tradition appears to influence the therapist's perception of a common client and that therapist's therapeutic engagement with that client.

Distinctions Regarding the Role of the Therapist As Authority and Expert

Differences appear among religious perspectives that influence how a therapist facilitates change in therapy. These are related to differences in the spiritual authority carried by the person of the therapist among these traditions. Differences also occur in how the self of the client is understood and accessed. Moreover, differences appear in perspectives and approaches describing how the therapist helps the client find answers to life's vagaries, perplexities, and dilemmas.

Viewing differences only as the result of a schism separating Asian religions (Hinduism, Buddhism, Taoism) from monotheistic religions (Judaism, Christian humanism, and Islam) misses the complexity of both overlaps and distinctions, and results in an invalid comparative picture. For example, the question of spiritual authority is delineated most carefully within the Hindu tradition. The therapist that appears in the author's case illustration is the priest, who functions as teacher, confessor, and nurturer. This accords with the Hindu personality theory that posits a Supreme Self as the ultimate identity of the phenomenal self. The spiritual authority vested in the priest helps to form a relationship with the "client" that expresses a Hindu understanding of this essential spiritual identity between one's personal self and the Supreme Self. Thus the role of the therapist-priest is grounded within the spiritual tradition and cultural heritage in contrast to a more secular and individualistic context that is more typical of Western approaches. The theory of therapy identifies the various levels within the self-system to which the therapist (or priest, in this case) must form a relationship. Within this web of relationship the priest relates as parent, wisdom figure, spiritual guide, and model of inner authority. In the case history, the formal therapeutic relationship is primarily a spiritual and paternal one: empathic, compassionate, and more formally as defined by the role of the priest in this tradition.

Within Buddhism and Taoism the question of the therapist's authority is not as clearly defined. The Buddhist therapist views the self differently than his Hindu counterpart. According to Buddhism, the egoic experience of self reflects attachments, illusions, and distortions. The client's current conflict and personal distress result from these illusions and attachments, and particularly the illusion of a separate self. The therapist understands that "basic sanity" lies beneath the client's conscious ego and experience of distress. The therapist carries no special spiritual authority, but is personally dedicated to the compassionate awakening of his client as a part of his own responsibility for right action. Indeed, developing the wisdom and compassion necessary to helping others puts his client on the path to becoming another resource in humanity's continuing enlightenment.

The Buddhist therapist who empathizes, confronts, and instructs, is also a sojourner on the path of unfolding awakening. Within the context of a "natural hierarchy," the Buddhist therapist is a fellow traveler, perhaps a more experienced one, but not of substantially higher standing than his distressed client. Influenced by this tradition, the relationship expressed by the therapist is a vehicle for his client's experience of "basic goodness" or "basic sanity," which is the fundamental structure of reality and human experience.

In Taoism, spiritual authority is manifested only through the quality of presence or "being" of the therapist. The phenomenal self is understood to be inseparable from the larger web of all life (the Tao), including the life of the therapist. In contrast to Hindu psychology, but similar to Buddhist psychology, there is no "personality," only life. A therapy focused on developing awareness of distortions in thought and feeling aims toward balance and harmony with life and the universe as a whole.

Monotheistic traditions base spiritual authority on God's self-revelations in historical events, scripture, and experience as interpreted through religious tradition and human reason. These traditions are closer to the Hindu perspective regarding how spiritual authority is formulated, but not in how that authority is applied. For example, the Judaic doctrine of religious conveyance can be expressed through the experience of a covenantal relationship between the therapist and her client. This is an expression of the more fundamental reality of God's covenant, and it can be viewed as paralleling the experience of "loving compassion" pivotal to the therapeutic relationship within Buddhism and Taoism. A similar parallel can be found in Christian humanism, wherein God's act of reconciling love in Jesus as the Christ is the rationale and enabling act of grace for establishing a reconciling relationship between therapist and client, and between the client and his or her significant others.

Distinctions Regarding the Construct of Self

Within monotheistic traditions the self is separate and complete, neither an illusion nor a distortion of a fundamental self-reality. Again, this is closer to the Hindu notion of an individual soul *(jiva)* than to Buddhism or Taoism.

This distinction is an especially vital one when we consider how a client is to receive answers to the questions that arise in the dilemmas of life. Within monotheism, answers lie in access to the important spiritual truths articulated in reasoned interpretations of spiritual texts, and in experience of the healing power of liberating relationship of reconciliation with God. This does not mean relating only to external sources of wisdom and compassion. Accepting divine forgiveness and acting in accord with the "will of God" allow the estranged self to be reconciled, and to experience divine, inner wisdom. To add further complexity, contemporary existential perspectives with roots in both Judaism and Christianity contemplate a source "in between," postulating an experience of authority and wisdom that resides within the relational space with a divine other (including another human being)[14] and also authority and wisdom residing through the experience of caring for another as an ethical imperative.[15] That these latter perspectives put a human face on God is explicit in the Jewish notion that God acts in human history through such events as the Exodus, and in the Christian claim of God's self-revelation in Jesus of Nazareth received by faith as the Christ.

Eastern religious traditions view the self as inseparable from other selves. This perspective appears to influence a less pathologizing, less symptom-oriented psychotherapy than is found in monotheistic traditions. Absent a separate and distinct "personality" there can be no pathology attributed to an individual, only symptoms expressing distortions or illusions covering the underlying reality of oneness. This perspective, identified particularly by the Buddhist and Taoist contributors, draws healing wisdom and understanding from the client's experience of that underlying, unitary reality. We recognize some overlap between traditions in this area. For example, we find intuitive understanding an important source within the Muslim client's search for understanding just as it is for the Taoist client. But we suggest a relationship between an emphasis on individuality and a consequently greater focus on pathology influenced by monotheism.

In our view, the case discussions demonstrate some further interesting distinctions regarding how the conceptualization of self influences the therapy with the client. We suggest, for example, that within the Eastern traditions, the psychologist applying a Hindu perspective incorporates a more active and instructional process of therapy then the Taoist or Buddhist psychologist. Moreover, we suggest that within the monotheistic traditions, the

Jewish psychologist emphasizes the "being" of the client in distinction to the more goal-oriented and problem-focused approaches of the psychologists from a Christian humanist or Islamic perspective.

These are subtly drawn distinctions, certainly arguable and offered tentatively. Yet the use of such measures as goal setting, goal-attainment scaling, and behavioral-contracting evidence a stronger psychotherapeutic focus on the activities of the client in Western traditions than are illustrated by psychologists from Eastern religious perspectives. These techniques engage the volition of the client, support conscious choices, and affirm behavioral changes that strengthen the client's experience of a more distinct and unique self. An Eastern approach appears to be less concerned about strengthening the individual "ego" of the client and would be less likely to use these techniques because they strengthen an attachment or illusion from which one must be liberated in order to experience the underlying truth realized within an embedded and possibly hierarchical system of relationships.

We have suggested that an Eastern religious accent on the unitive, universal Self contrasts with a stronger monotheistic emphasis on individuality experienced by unique, separate selves. We wonder how we would proceed to verify the essential "truth" of either perspective. In the words of St. Ignatius, the truth of one's individual experience of life can be a "disconsoling" one. It is to such a separated soul that the liberating experience of reconciliation is addressed. The quintessential Western value of freedom involves the experience of will and choice, and that in turn requires an experience of individuality. To mitigate the agony and alienation resulting from individual separateness, self-transcendence through relationship is required.

The Western therapist within a monotheistically oriented culture knows well the experience of separation, and the wishes and fears that attend it. The therapeutic relationship between client and therapist provides both a model of liberation and transcendence and (if all goes well) an experience of a reconciling relationship in therapy that transcends the experience of separation. One is released from aloneness, but not from individuality. An I-Thou relation is emphasized over any merging of separate identities into oneness. By contrast, in Eastern traditions the truth of one's ultimate interrelationship, one's fundamental connectedness to all of being, is affirmed in the experience of Oneness in which the burden of an illusory ego-self is released. These very significant perspectives on one's identity and relationship of self with another, and on subtle shifts in the experiences that accompany them, warrant continuing dialogue.

Distinctions Regarding the Construct of Relationship

We see strong parallels between the relationship-oriented value base of Judaism and the Christian humanist focus on a reconciling life and relationships as the goal of psychotherapy. In contradistinction to Buddhism and

Taoism, this relational emphasis preserves and enhances the individuality and "personhood" of the client. The movement from estrangement to reconciliation that describes the major thrust of the Christian religious experience is also a metaphor for the process of psychotherapy. Self-integration, self-transcendence, and a dynamic, reconciling engagement with others are expressions of lived religious experience and outcomes of a productive psychotherapy. This perspective offers the life of Christ as the *imago Dei*, which serves as both metaphor and practical guide to the Christian humanist therapist. An expanded focus occurs as the therapeutic goal moves from personal reconciliation to engagement as an agent of reconciliation in society. This social focus complements the Jewish emphasis on service to others. Both Christian and Jewish theories construe psychotherapy as a movement toward goals that point beyond the consulting room. Yet the activism projected is an individual effort at social change, and this emphasis differs from Eastern religious experiences of the "web of life" in which one is embedded and from which one is inseparable.

Both the Jewish and Christian contributors support the view that the psychotherapeutic relationship is an authentic realization and revelation of God's transforming power. The dynamics of therapy are generated within a very personal and interpersonal context: an I-Thou relation and the transforming experience of reconciliation both depend on the agency of a particular and individual human being. Significantly, in the therapeutic experience of the transforming I-Thou relation, the client's individuality is not lost, but rather channeled to serve higher spiritual purposes.

Although there are striking similarities in these monotheistic perspectives, there are also distinctions. For example, the Judaic focus on the covenantal relationship based on the *Torah* becomes in the Christian-humanist perspective, a covenant based uniquely in the person of Jesus as the Christ. These distinctions describe how and from where a Holy Other impacts the transforming power of authentic and graced relationships. A contemporary theme of Judaism suggests that God resides in the face of the other and in the fulfillment of *mitzvot* or in commandments that "maintain the divine-human bond."[16] Christian humanism suggests that one finds God's compassionate and transcendent love in liberating experiences of reconciliation, one form of which is the authentic therapeutic relationship. The human response of living a more liberated and reconciling life becomes increasingly the object of psychotherapy supported by this perspective.

The view of the therapeutic relationship in Muslim psychology appears less covenantal than Judaic conceptions, but equally attentive to the individual client's needs and life concerns. The Islamic therapist attends to the client's constructs of self and other, working toward her client's greater self-awareness through self-examination informed by Islamic truths. The therapist's own relationship with Allah and the tenants of Muslim faith are engaged in the service of the client through encouragement, verbal reinforcement, and recommendations of specific religious practices like prayer and meditation. Although the case illustrations are not isomorphic descriptions of the style of all therapists from these particular religious traditions, we note in the Muslim view of the therapist's role as a spiritual guide is at points similar to the role presented by the Hindu therapist/priest.

Distinctions Regarding Engagement with Suffering

The value-base described herein as a uniquely Jewish contribution to psychotherapy has informed the theory and practice of Western psychotherapy since its inception. Relationship as a covenant between therapist and client is described (as indeed, Buber described it)[17] as an unfolding knowing of the other into an "I-Thou" relation. The process of therapy is formulated in terms of the dynamics of the shared human experience of parenting, as both religious metaphor and as the necessary human obligation to care for another. The therapist's obligation to care for the other, and the responsibility to act on the client's behalf is emphasized in this tradition. Caring for the other includes forming a relationship with the client's inner-experience of pain and suffering. Suffering is embraced as a significant and meaning-filled experience.

These points of emphasis in the Jewish religious tradition find familiar themes within the history of psychotherapy, particularly the psychodynamic therapies that arose from the value base of Judaism and which continue to formulate an explication of meaningful suffering through contemporary existential theory and practice. The dictum of responsibility for another, and the obligation to the care for others as both a fundamental requirement of life and as a preordained obligation to one's Creator, is expressed in the writings of the Jewish existentialist, Emmanuel Levinas.

Levinas was the student of both Heidegger and Buber, and carries the doctrine of "care" to the radical conclusion that selfhood is realized only in actively engaging one's greater concern for another. Levinas suggests that we become human only when we engage the suffering of another, and find in that engagement the true face of God. Levinas advances an obligation for care that illuminates and crystallizes the more opaque roots of Western psychotherapy.

All religious psychologists express genuine care about their client's suffering. But there are distinctions between them in the meaning attached to suffering and the therapist's subsequent engagement with it. For example, a Jewish psychotherapy promises no ultimate liberation from human suffering, but penetrates into the nature of suffering to affirm its meaning and value as a self-transcending and self-affirming experience. This contrasts with the Christian humanist position that affirms healing of some suffering in and through the experience of graced forgiveness and reconciliation.

Finding the *meaning* in suffering as the Jewish therapist advocates is not the same as helping clients *overcome* their suffering, which is one of the goals of a Christian humanist therapist. One might argue that although the perspective of Christian humanism favors a more hopeful psychotherapy, that perspective may at times provide less of a fit to the actual lived experience of a client suffering an irreversible fate.

The common case illustration provides some interesting examples of these differences. In her discussion of the case, Elaine Hartsman speaks to the possible underlying meaning of the client's suffering. The client's experience of suffering associated with the conflict with her mother, and with her feelings of obligation in relation to her continued care, may not be entirely resolved through the normal resolution of guilt and anxiety. Rather, penetrating into the underlying meaning of suffering opens a window to important life choices and to unfolding awareness about the transformational possibilities within the "I-Thou" relation between this adult daughter and her aged parent. Hartsman concludes that the reciprocal encounter between therapist and client, in which the therapist is open to the impact of the client's pain, also influences significantly the clients engagement with her parents and with other significant relationships in her life. Finding one's humanity strengthened through engaging the suffering of another echoes the Judaic philosophers cited previously.

In presenting his Christian humanistic commentary on the case illustration, Paul Olson describes the experience of "compassionate confrontation" as a significant mechanism of therapeutic change. His description of a bio-psychosocial perspective includes an emphasis on the subjective experience of the client's life and current experience. Olson's critique of the discourse analysis of the case is that the client's experience of guilt was deemphasized in favor of a more cognitive focus on the client's self-judgments and assumptions that guided her process of decision making (a staple of cognitive-behavioral approaches to psychotherapy). Penetrating into value conflicts as an experience of "conscience" moves closer to the client's experience of self-alienation and suffering related to self-worth. Depression is viewed as a consequence of powerlessness and related despair. In this tradition, hope is a therapeutic mechanism in relieving suffering and despair, reinforcing the experience of the "liberating freedom" characteristic of the reconciling life.

The differences noted between Judaic and Christian humanism may be a springboard for fruitful dialogue about the meaning and experience of suffering and hope within human experience. The themes of suffering and hope are powerful points of relation for the psychotherapist. Both therapists bring to their work important cultural patterning on the meaning of suffering, and on the possibility of liberation from despair. The religious therapist's construal of psychotherapy as "soul work" would be strengthened by fruitful dialogue that engages our deeper reflection on these two dynamics of suffering and hope within any psychotherapeutic encounter.

The Jewish and Christian humanist contributors present an overlapping emphasis on the role of personal sin and guilt. From the Christian humanist perspective, sin is the consequence of an alienated life, an "unreconciled" life, an ego-dominated life. The Christian view that healing or reconciliation is facilitated through compassionate confrontation in the context of a Spirit-centered therapeutic relationship is compatible with the Jewish tradition. The goal of therapy is the restoration of relationships in a more reconciling life characterized by wisdom, compassion, and courage, qualities emphasized in both Greek and Judeo-Christian traditions.

Although there may be no final cure for suffering in the Judaic application, the Christian humanist points to the curative or healing effects of a liberating experience of reconciliation. The Islamic contributor also affirms the hope for restoration to wholeness. Zehra Ansari suggests that suffering finds it's resolution through the Muslim instruction to place one's trust in God's justice, and in practices from the Quran that "overcome anxiety and sadness." The practice of meditation is also introduced to "overcome" experiences related to the pain and suffering of the client. Underlying beliefs supporting guilt and unworthiness may be alleviated through self-knowledge. Spiritual knowledge, prayer, and meditation are used in conjunction with other techniques such as deep breathing, progressive relaxation, and imagery to facilitate the client's experience of wholeness beyond the experience of her guilt, anxiety, depression, and struggles with self-worth.

According to the Hindu contributor, Asha Mukherjee, the client's suffering places her on a path to self-development and further spiritual realization. In the case formulation Mukherjee provides, the distressed client is engaged through subjective reassurance and encouragement to contact her inner spiritual resources (the Brahman within). The priest's compassionate attention facilitates her inner-opening and consequent emotional relief. The client notes a shift in her experience of distress, and she continues to reach toward both the outer source of assurance found in the person and instruction of the priest, and within herself as she becomes increasingly able to sustain outer guidance and her own inner resources.

There is no liberation from the suffering self in this narration. This case formulation suggests that improved social relationships are only a partial resolution of the client's suffering. The Hindu therapist supplies no immediate solution to the client's distress; rather, the therapist is the source of nurturing engagement so that the spiritual principles and insights can be increasingly internalized and sustained. Further resolution comes from a continued nurturing engagement with the therapist and a corresponding inner acceptance of, and sustained connection with the spiritual principles articulated through spiritual teaching. In this tradition the selected teachings evoke and reinforce the client's experience of inner-compassion, acceptance, and essential divinity. Suffering and distress fade over time as the inner experience of acceptance stimulates a more compassionate perception of outer relationships. Self-knowledge is formed less from directly engaging the mind than from a more intuitive, but disciplined inner-unfolding.

Suffering is accorded legitimacy within Buddhism as an inevitable consequence of life. But, as Scott Kamilar notes, necessary suffering is complicated by the unnecessary suffering resulting from the process of our struggle to eliminate it. This struggle results in the formation of an "egoistic attachment," which is a significant focus of therapy with the client described through the case illustration. The Buddhist therapist helps his client to embrace suffering rather than resist it, so it can be gently released as evidence of her "basic sanity." The client's connection with her "basic sanity" or "Buddha nature" is experienced as her own basic goodness, and it is this insightful experience that occasions the release of her attachment to suffering. However, this client continues to work with her experience of her mother's pain through the application of a specific practice *(tonglen),* which engages her compassion without personalizing it through further egoic attachment.

In this comparison among perspectives, we note an interesting parallel between the Buddhist perspective on suffering and that acknowledged within Judaism. These contributors bring into the therapeutic context traditions that acknowledge suffering as an essential reality of existence, and work within their traditions to mitigate its unnecessary consequences. This emphasis on engaging the existential experience of the suffering client would seem to be a distinction from the manner in which spiritual knowledge is used to relieve suffering in the Hindu tradition, spiritual reconciliation to reduce suffering in Christian humanism, and spiritual principles regarding intuition, intelligence, and knowledge are used to resolve suffering in Islam.

That Taoist psychology takes suffering seriously is evident from the discussion in Lynne Hagen's chapter on the etiology of suffering. The causes are multiple and suffering is considered a natural part of life. Suffering is real, not illusory. In her discussion of the clinical case, Hagen critiqued the DSM diagnosis as a label that did not fully appreciate the reality of the woman's suffering, including her anticipatory grieving over the eventual loss of her mother. Moreover, the woman's busyness and negativity about her past and present situation, and the imbalance of *yin* and *yang* principles in her life, needed to be changed for more lasting relief of her suffering. Although the client's suffering of depression was alleviated, the case did not appear to achieve the ultimate goals of Taoist therapy: recovery of her genuine self, development of the client's intuitive ability, recognition of the cyclic nature of life, and living according to its natural rhythms. These goals imply that living in harmony with the Tao alleviates suffering beyond the salutary effects experienced by discovering its meaning.

Religion, Psychotherapy, and Transpersonal Psychology

The theories of personality and psychotherapy presented in this book are explicitly spiritual or religious theories. Yet, even the more secular history of psychotherapy comprises an interweaving of religious and psychological traditions that has resulted in the development of Western psychodynamic psychotherapy. For example, the practice of psychotherapy advocated by Freud, although a-religious if not antireligious in its content, was nonetheless grounded in the value base of the Judeo-Christian tradition that dominated the culture of Freud's day. Freud's abiding respect for his patient's underlying experience, even as that experience was in conflict with the mores of his contemporary Victorian society, could be seen through the lens of the relational convenance of Freud's Judaism. Jung added several contributions, especially his construct of a "religious impulse" that lies within the human psyche, and which became a seminal principle within his psychology. In his autobiography Jung describes how he overcame the small and constricting God of his childhood to uncover a numinous divinity within each person whom he encountered as a patient.[18]

Eastern religious perspectives on health and healing have had much to offer the Western psychotherapist, and these perspectives converge in some contemporary practice settings. One noteworthy example is the psychotherapy that blends modern existential notions with Buddhist and Yogic principles, sometimes referred to as "existential-contemplative" psychotherapy. The principles of contemplative psychology and psychotherapy associated with the Naropa Institute of Boulder, Colorado, offer another contemporary example. Recent writings, especially those integrating Buddhist perspectives into Western psychodynamic frameworks, are further illustrations of integrative approaches to psychotherapy. Two noteworthy examples can be found in the work of Epstein[19] and Kawai.[20]

These integrations of Eastern and Western perspectives into a psychospiritual framework have a much earlier history than the Western psychological tradition. These have remained outside the mainstream of Western, particularly American, psychological and psychotherapeutic theory, perhaps because they failed to fit the prevailing positivistic models of science requiring experimental verification. Until recently, the latter models excluded phenomenological methodologies that systematically tap deeper human experiences. Consequently, they have neglected religious or spiritual *experiences* in favor of more quantifiable human *behaviors*. As illustrated in the chapters of this book, Eastern and Western spiritual perspectives offer us rich, textured theories about the structure and experience of the self, although simultaneously they add both interpersonal and transpersonal dimensions and perspectives. Some of these theories lend themselves to phenomenological exploration that would further the knowledge base of psychotherapy.

Two contemporary models of integrating the spiritual dimension into psychotherapy are mentioned here as additions to the variety of "transpersonal" theories illustrated in the other chapters. These are Assagioli's psychosynthesis and Wilber's spectrum model. We offer these models as illustrations without endorsement.

Psychosynthesis: An Integrative Psychology and Psychotherapy

An integration of Eastern and Western psychospiritual frameworks was proposed as early as 1910 by the Italian psychiatrist, Roberto Assagioli, called "psychosynthesis."[21] Psychosynthesis is a comprehensive approach to understanding human development within an evolutionary context. It reflects Assagioli's abiding interest in the "higher aspects" of human nature. Assagioli had an integrative mind, synthesizing the work of Freud (with whom he studied), Jung (with whom he collaborated), and a variety of humanistic existentialists including William James and Abraham Maslow. He combined these with spiritual disciplines drawn from Buddhism and Hinduism, the Kabbalistic tradition with Judaism and the mystical tradition within Christianity.

Assagioli postulated core concepts or "principles" to describe his conceptual integration of perspectives and practices rooted in the traditions identified above. The study of psychosynthesis includes his extraction of Freud's drive theory in conjunction with Jung's conception of human spiritual needs and the process of transformation in the psyche. Moreover, he incorporated Maslow, Frankl, and other existential psychologists' perspective on the nature of the self and self-experience. In addition, his integration included Christian and Jewish religious perspectives and contemplative Buddhist perspectives and practices. His model of psychospiritual development is heavily influenced by Kabbalistic and Hindu views on the nature of the self. His concept of a "higher Self" parallels in many ways the "supreme Self" *(Atman)* of Hindu spiritual teachings. Assagioli created an integration of all of these traditions, which yielded experiential principles of human life and development, with all its attendant opportunities and crises.

Assagioli's original formulation used the term psychosynthesis to distinguish it from the prevailing psychoanalysis of his time. His choice of the particular descriptor psychosynthesis reflected his primary interest in exploring what Maslow, a kindred spirit, was to call the higher reaches of human nature. Assagioli viewed Freud's drive theory as only one rudimentary point in an evolving and increasingly spiritualized development of the human psyche. He wanted to formulate through concept, framework and method how a higher, more spiritual organization of the personality might be viewed and achieved.

Assagioli generated a psychological framework that elaborates a "higher unconscious" with more positive contents than the Freudian conception of the unconscious dominated by sexual and aggressive instincts. Indeed, much of Assagioli's focus pivoted around the identification and explication of strategies and methods drawn from Buddhist and yogic sources to amplify the workings of higher consciousness. He contended that higher consciousness unfolds as naturally in human development as any other aspect of consciousness. In this sense, psychosynthesis can be seen as the theory and practice of conscious alignment with the natural unfolding process of "higher unconsciousness" within and between individuals.

The model of the human psyche Assagioli developed through his explorations was grounded in the experience of the individual. He viewed the individual psyche in relationship to a higher unifying center of consciousness, and developed a series of approaches to help his patient develop, mature, and increasingly experience his or her higher possibilities. Similar to each of the religious traditions espoused in this volume, Assagioli saw human existence as essentially a spiritual enterprise that required spiritual knowledge and unfolding self-awareness. Yet he was careful in drawing a distinction that contained his work within the domain of psychology.

Psychosynthesis does not attempt in any way to appropriate to itself the field of religion and of philosophy. It is a scientific conception, which is neutral toward the various religious traditions and the various philosophical doctrines, excepting only those that are materialistic and therefore deny the existence of spiritual realities. Psychosynthesis does not aim, nor attempt to give a metaphysical nor a theological explanation of the great mystery—it leads to the door, but stops there.[22]

From his early work in 1911 to the time to his death in 1975, Assagioli continued to elaborate and refine his perspective. More of an integrator and incorporator than inventor, Assagioli continued to search out relevant concepts and techniques from Eastern and Western traditions to incorporate into his comprehensive and overarching perspective. He knew it was in the nature of his task that his work would not, indeed could not, be concluded; this was not possible when one is working with an unceasingly unfolding, evolutionary process. From contemporary eyes it appears that Assagioli's very openness to the continual development of his theory led to a system that was neither complete, tight, nor polished. He felt that any closed, authoritarian stance lead to dogmatism and the eventual dissolution of his perspective. A more critical view contends that psychosynthesis, by dint of its evolutionary openness, has too much room for fanciful, less credible notions, and can become a hodgepodge of stratagems and techniques without a solid unifying framework. The uneasy tension between these evaluations has characterized the continued evolution of psychosynthesis during the quarter century since Assagioli's death.

Presently, Assagioli's perspective continues to be developed and refined principally through an international network of practitioner/theorists who apply psychosynthesis and its attendant methodologies in work within mental health practice, within educational settings, in organizational and management practice settings, and within alternative approaches to spiritual growth and healing. The psychosynthesis approach reaches mental health professionals, educators, pastoral counselors, and organizational and management professionals through training programs sponsored by a network of independent centers and training institutes in the United States, Canada, the United Kingdom, and across the continent of Europe.

Psychosynthesis presents an evolutionary model of human growth. To contrast the psychosynthesis perspective with other related perspectives, we need to reiterate the existential basis of this approach, and its theoretical and historical connection to significant aspects of the work of Sigmund Freud and Carl Jung and some of their contemporaries. Other important crosscurrents exist within Buddhism, Hinduism, the Christian mystical tradition, and the Jewish Kabbalistic tradition.

A few examples will illustrate how both monistic and monotheistic spiritual traditions influence psychosynthesis theory and applications. First, applications in psychosynthesis of the process of disidentifying from the contents of consciousness echo Buddhist practice. Second, the manner in which will, choice, and decision are understood in psychosynthesis finds parallels in Buddhism, Yogi practices drawn from Hinduism, Islamic spiritual principles, and Western philosophic traditions expressed in Christian perspectives, such as Duns Scotus' view that the nature of the soul is will. Patanjali's *Yogi Sutras,* and D. T. Suzuki's writings on the significance of the will in Zen Buddhism (e.g., "The Will is the man himself and Zen appeals to it")[23] are both used by Assagioli to buttress his view of the universal primacy of the will. Indeed, the life story of the Buddha himself is cited as an example of the relationship between the application of the will in service to others and one's personal enlightenment project. In fact, Assagioli suggests that the life of the Buddha is "the highest and fullest example of the will to meaning."[24]

Continuing Integrations: Wilber's Spectrum Model

Perhaps the most intriguing theory describing a complementary approach comes from the massive legacy (twenty volumes and counting!) of the transpersonal theorist Ken Wilber.[25] Wilber's work is among the most read and most quoted material within transpersonal psychology at the present time. His massive integration of Eastern and Western psychological and spiritual perspectives provides a detailed and comprehensive theoretical structure. His careful delineation of a stage-based model of evolving consciousness shares important ground with Assagioli's integrative model.

There are also important differences in the level of detail incorporated into these two models. For example, in his writing Assagioli is not committed to any particular stage theory of development, something strongly identified by Wilber. Borrowing from stage-based models of other developmental theorists, Wilber describes a "ladder" theory of human development through progressive stages of growth. In more recent writing, Wilber's "spectrum model " of development has itself been incorporated into a psychosynthesis approach[26] to add detail necessary to describe important shifts in the experience of self-identity, particularly in relation to the experience of trauma.

Wilber's model is also an amalgam of Eastern and Western perspectives, and that indeed is one of its similarities to a psychosynthesis perspective. Assagioli often skips over theoretical elaboration to describe particular applications with greater detail. Examples include his description of the value and uses of music in therapy and healing, his citations of others' work related to the impact of mental imagery on brain function, and his translation of what might be viewed as a *vipissan*-oriented process of meditation. Assagioli is lean on theory and long on application, underscoring the significance he places on individual application to specific situations. His pragmatic approach is drawn from a somewhat rudimentary theory, and we notice how the fact that many paths can lead to the same goal is of little concern to him. By contrast, Wilber carefully constructs the specifics of the path in relation to the goal. An example is his elaboration of specific stages in progression from prepersonal to transpersonal development in his spectrum model of consciousness. His model is comprehensive, yet without detailed application to clinical practice.

Thus the field of transpersonal psychology offers Assagioli, the clinician, contrasted with Wilber, the quintisessential theorist. Assagioli's model of psychosynthesis is a system for healing and for learning rather than for abstract theoretical understanding. His perspective, although existentially drawn, parallels the Buddhist concept of attachment (clutching to positive experience to avoid suffering) as a general characteristic of human experience. Wilber's more neatly categorized stages of development, which unfold epigenetic ally through the life span, is well fortified by level of detail, but was also inspired by a similar Buddhist perspective. These two approaches resonate in their comprehensive perspective on human experience, their presentation of the layered complexity of human life, and their common regard for spiritual unification as the ultimate goal of the human journey.

With the addition of the theories of Assagioli and Wilber to the preceding chapters, the reader has been presented several models that integrate the spiritual dimension into theories of personality and the practice of psychotherapy. In one sense, all of these approaches could be construed as transpersonal, since they share a perspective on human experience beyond both personal and interpersonal points of view. Self-transcendent dimensions of experience are affirmed in these theories as both real and therapeutic.

Several models of spiritually oriented approaches to personality and psychotherapy have been presented to encourage the reader to feel the freedom to articulate one's own unique integration of spiritual strivings and religious convictions into clinical practice with religiously oriented clients. Our own attempts in this chapter to note some similarities and differences among these approaches have been intended as encouragement for respectful and informed dialogue among clinicians of various religious persuasions. This dialogue has just begun. We look forward to further contributions from religiously oriented psychologists who are liberated from the silence imposed by a narrow definition of scientific psychology. From our perspective, no psychological theory can claim to be scientific that ignores the reality and relevance of the spiritual dimension of life. The biopsychosocial model that dominates contemporary applied psychology must be transcended to incorporate spiritual, moral, and historical perspectives in order to advance psychology as a genuinely *human* science.

Researching the Psychotherapeutic Efficacy of Spiritual Principles and Practices

Our review of material in the preceding chapters has identified some interesting areas in which further research would advance the theory and practice of psychotherapy grounded in the spiritual wisdom of the world's magnificent religions. Some religious insights and spiritual principles can be subjected to rigorous study through certain qualitative research methodologies. For example, we believe that phenomenological and heuristic research methodologies can be constructed to explore how religious concepts influence a client's experience of therapy. Such research can explore religious experience in a manner consistent with the cultural contexts in which those principles and practices are applied. The results of such research would enrich the general practice of psychotherapy beyond the limited scope of much current applied research. In fact, because religious and spiritual principles and practices speak to the heart of human experience, to issues surrounding the purpose and meaning of human life, the questions that are generated from the exploration of these principles and practices are of ultimate value to the study and practice of psychotherapy.

A research agenda for spiritual approaches to psychotherapy might include the following:

- A phenomenological/heuristic exploration of the relationship between the concept of self and one's experience of self-identity in clients from Eastern and Western religious traditions.

- A phenomenological inquiry into the dynamics and meaning of suffering and hope approached from monistic and monotheistic perspectives.
- A qualitative analysis of the experience of reconciliation within one's self and the dynamics of reconciliation in healing relational wounds.
- A phenomenological exploration of the experience of grace and its relationship to healing.
- The experience of forgiveness and its implications for individual and relationship therapy.
- A descriptive study of the meaning of central religious constructs using the Semantic Differential with various populations.
- Process research to evaluate the mechanisms of change postulated by religious theories of psychotherapy.
- Outcome research to assess the effectiveness and efficiency of religiously based interventions.

NOTES

1. Barbour, I. (1966). *Issues in science and religion*. New York: Harper and Row, p. 172.

2. See Ashley, D. and Orenstein, D. (1990). *Sociological theory: Classical statements*. Boston: Allyn and Bacon, pp. 12, 28, 30-31, 95-96, 119, 128-129, 131-132, 173, 272, 296, 398.

3. Emmons, R. (1999). *The psychology of ultimate concerns: Motivation and spirituality in personality*. New York: Guilford Press, pp. 8-14.

4. Browning, D. (1987). *Religious thought and the modern psychologies: A critical conversation in the theology of culture*. Philadelphia: Fortress Press.

5. For the distinctions among material, efficient, formal, and final causes, see Rychlack, J. (1981). *Introduction to personality and psychotherapy*. Boston: Houghton Mifflin, pp. 2-6.

6. For a phenomenological description of the sense of the holy, see Otto, R. (1923/1950). *The idea of the holy: An inquiry into the non-rational factor in the idea of the divine and its relation to the rational* (trans. By J.W. Harvey). London: Oxford University Press.

7. Allport, G. (1968). *The person in psychology: Selected essays*. Boston: Beacon Press.

8. James, W. (1902/1958). *The varieties of religious experience: A study in human nature*. New York: New American Library.

9. Buber, M. (1937/1958). *I and Thou*. New York: Collier Books/Macmillan Publishing, pp. 3-5, 18, and 27.

10. Smith, H. (1991). *The world's religions*. New York: HarperSanFrancisco, pp. 12-22.

11. Ibid., p. 53.

12. Emmons, M. and Emmons, J. (2000). *Meditative therapy: Facilitating inner-directed healing*. Atascadero, CA: Impact publishers. A useful guide for clients

is LeShan, L. (1974). *How to meditate: A guide to self-discovery.* New York: Bantam Books; Andresen, J. (2000). "Meditation meets behavioural medicine," in Andresen, J. and Forman, R. *Cognitive models and spiritual maps.* Bowling Green, OH: Imprint Academic, pp. 21-26.

13. Examples include Collins, G. (1988). *Christian counseling: A comprehensive guide.* Dallas,TX: Word Publishing; Pruyser, P. (1968). *A dynamic psychology of religion.* New York: Harper and Row; Tournier, P. (1965). *The meaning of persons: Reflections on a psychiatrist's casebook.* London: SCM Press; Brazier, D. (1995). *Zen therapy: Transcending the sorrows of the human mind.* New York: John Wiley and Sons; Epstein, M. (1999). *Going to pieces without falling apart: A Buddhist perspective on wholeness.* New York: Broadway Books.

14. Voegelin, E. (1990). Equivalences of experience and symbolization in history. In Voegelin, E. (1990). *Collected works of Eric Voegelin, Vol. 12.* Baton Rouge, LA: Louisiana State University Press, p. 119.

15. The theme of one's personal responsibility to the other as an absolute spiritual requirement or primary obligation of "being" extends beyond Heidegger's earlier focus on "sorge" or "care" in Martin Buber's formulation of the I-Thou relation. Buber's student, Emmanuel Levinas, has taken the primacy of one's obligation to the "face of the other" beyond Buber's relational structure. For further discussion, see Hand, S. (Ed.) (1989). *The Levinas reader.* Cambridge: Blackwell, pp. 59-74.

16. Levinas, E. (1989). "Ethics as first philosophy," in S. Hand (Ed.). *The Levinas reader.* Cambridge: Blackwell, p. 75.

17. Buber, M. (1958). *I and thou.* New York: Scribner, pp. 37-72.

18. Jung, C. G. (1965). *Memories, dreams, reflections.* New York: Random House, pp. 56-83, 327-359.

19. Scott Kamilar refers to psychiatrist Mark Epstein's integration of Buddhist principles and practices into psychotherapy. Epstein continues that integrative effort in his second volume. See Epstein, M. (1999). *Going to pieces without falling apart: A Buddhist perspective on wholeness.* New York: Broadway Books.

20. Hayao Kawai is a Japanese psychologist and Jungian analyst who created a unique integration of Western psychoanalytic theory into a Buddhist cultural context. See Kawai, H. (1996). *Buddhism and the art of psychotherapy.* College Station, TX: Texas A & M University Press, pp. 7-35.

21. Roberto Assagioli wrote two volumes detailing his theory of psychosynthesis and its applications to clinical practice. These are: *Psychosynthesis* (New York: Penguin, 1965) and *The act of will* (New York: Penguin, 1973). A posthumously published collection of Assagioli's writings was also issued in 1991, entitled *Transpersonal development.* Hammersmith, London: Crucible.

22. Assagioli, R. (1965). *Psychosynthesis: A manual of principles and techniques.* New York: Arkana/Penguin Group, pp. 6-7.

23. Assagioli, R. (1973). *The act of will.* New York: Penguin, p. 236.

24. Ibid., p. 111.

25. Wilber, K. (1995). *Sex, ecology, spirituality.* Boston: Shambala. This volume contains a detailed elaboration of Wilber's spectrum model of consciousness. An updated (2000) and concise overview of Wilber's work integrating models of consciousness is Wilbur, K. (2000), *Integral psychology.* Boston: Shambala.

26. Firman, J. and Gila, A. (1997). *Primal wound: A Transpersonal view of trauma, addiction, and growth.* Albany: SUNY press.

Index

Abdulati, Hammudah, 340
Abraham, 211-212
acceptance
    and Buddhism, 100-101
    and Christianity, 302, 312 n. 68
    and Hinduism, 55, 68
    and Islam, 330, 333
    and nature, 145-146
    and Taoism
        and action, 152-153
        and change, 163
        as focus, 145-146, 180
        and mindfulness, 144
        and Sage, 165
        of self, 155-156, 162, 180,
            192-193
accommodation, 31-32
accountability. *See* responsibility
achievers, 171
action
    and Buddhism, 90-91, 92, 128, 133
    Hindu view, 46, 81 n. 36
    and Judaism, 228-229
    in Taoism, 144, 152-154, 180 (*see*
        also wu-wei)
acts
    and Buddhism, 88, 95, 107, 372
    of God (Christianity), 285
    and Hinduism, 22, 39
    and Islam, 327, 328, 339, 340
    in Judaism, 216, 217, 223, 224
    in Taoism, 141
adaptation
    Christian view, 293
    and reconciliation, 288
    and Taoism, 163-164, 169, 171, 192
        (*see also* flexibility)
addictions, 20
Adler, Alfred, 277
affirmation, 228, 233
afterlife
    and Buddhism, 64
    and Confucius, 64

afterlife *(continued)*
    and Hinduism, 20-21, 64
    and Judaism, 221-222
    and Taoism, 147
aggression, 89, 93
aging, 159
agitation, 182, 198
Al Ghazzali, 334, 335, 341
Alcoholics Anonymous, 104, 117, 127
alienation
    and Christianity
        causes, 384
        and distress, 260, 262, 269-270
        Tillich view, 310 n. 45
    and Hinduism, 389
    and Taoism, 145, 160, 390
Allport, Gordon, 254, 308 n. 20, 322 n.
        165, 368
altruism, 297
ambition, 168
analysis, 160-161, 172, 178-179. *See*
        also categorization;
        psychoanalysis; therapy
anger
    against parents, 120
    and body, 113
    and Buddhism, 93, 94, 98, 100-101
    and Islam, 341, 349
Ansari, Zafar Afaq, 335-336
anxiety
    and body, 113
    and Buddhism, 94, 107
    existential, 83 n. 68, 229, 264-265
    Frankl view, 232
    and Hinduism, 20, 57, 59
    and Islam, 349
    and Judaism, 229
    May view, 227
    and meditation, 122
    moral, 297
    neurotic, 264-265
    panic, 96-97
    performance, 187
    and Taoism, 154

appearance(s)
  and Taoism, 142, 166, 175
  of therapist, 103
Asad, Muhammad, 333
Assagioli, Roberto, 277, 402-404, 405
assertiveness, and Buddhism, 101,
      109-110
assumptions, 2-3, 109
asthma, 122
Atisa, 114
Atman, 375, 402
atonement
  and Islam, 343
  and Judaism, 223
attachment
  Hindu view, 54, 80 n. 33, 82 n. 57
  Taoist view, 183-184
  Wilber view, 405
attitudes
  in Hinduism, 28
  judgmental, 131, 153, 174, 183-184
  of Krishna, 45
  of therapist, 271-272
authenticity
  and Buddhism, 110
  and Christianity, 309 n. 35
authority
  and Buddhism, 393
  and Confucianism, 148
  and Hinduism, 393
  and monotheistic religions, 393
  and Taoism, 147, 393
awareness. *See also* mindfulness
  in Buddhism, 103, 106, 107-108,
      111
  and Christianity, 265
  and Hinduism, 38, 41, 50, 51, 60
    in therapy, 76
  of patterns, 131
  and Taoism, 142, 155, 158-159, 189

Baker, Richard, 98
Bakkan, David, 217, 237
balance
  and Christianity, 287
  and Hinduism, 58
  and Islam, 340, 344, 348
  and Taoism
    and concentration, 191-192
    as goal, 172, 178, 180, 389

Barbour, Ian, 270, 361
Barkham, M., 12, 292
Bateson, Gregory, 104, 127-128
behavior
  and Hinduism, 59
  and Islam, 333
  versus experience, 402-403
behavior contracting, 395
behavioral therapy, 131-132, 391
behaviorism, 102, 360-361, 372
Bergin, Allen, 280
Bhagavad Gita
  background, 23-24
  and death, 55, 57-58
  and egoism, 40
  ideal human being, 65, 66
  and therapy, 43-47, 56-63
  and *Upanishads,* 28
bhumis, 106-109
big picture, 111
biofeedback, 345
biopsychosocial model
  and Christianity, 156, 288-289, 352,
      360
  as commonality, 360, 406
  future, 406
  and Islam, 352
  and Taoism, 156
blessings, 341-342
bliss
  and Buddhism, 91
  and Hinduism, 23, 39-40, 48
  and Islam, 341
blood pressure, 122
bodhichitta, 87
bodhisattva, 106-109, 118
Bonheoffer, Dietrich, 287
Borg, Marcus, 250, 307 n. 15
boundaries
  and Judaism, 220
  and Taoism, 179, 182-183, 193
Bowlby, John, 225
Brace, Kerry, 225
Brahman
  and anxiety, 59
  attributes, 321 n. 150
  and Christianity, 286
  concept, 19, 21-23
  etymology, 321 n. 150
  and individuals, 29

Brahman *(continued)*
  merger with, 38
  and purification, 29, 37
  and spiritual cleansing, 37
  trust in, 73, 77
Brahmins, 25, 34
Brazier, David, 113, 117
Buber, Martin
  on affirmation, 233
  on guilt, 228
  on obligation, 408 n. 15
  on relationships, 227, 233-234, 373
Buddha. *See* Siddhārtha Gautama
Buddhism. *See also* Zen Buddhism
  and Christianity, 124-125, 286-287
  and cognitive-behavioral therapy,
    131-132
  and cybernetic epistemology,
    127-128
  egocentricity, 89-90
  and goals, 87, 95, 98
  and God, 85, 123
  and Hinduism, 125
  and individual differences, 93-96,
    381
  and Judaism, 123-124, 238-239
  koans, 116-117, 366-367
  and narrative therapy, 130-131
  and Native Americans, 125-126
  noble truths, 96-98
  paths, 86-87, 98, 105-109
    eightfold, 109-111
  personality theory, 88-96
  psychological states, 91-93
  and psychosynthesis, 404
  and psychotherapy, 126-127, 386,
    388
  scripture, 87
  and Taoism, 125, 195, 196
  and trance, 128-129
  Wheel of Life, 90-91, 378
Bultmann, Rudolph, 250
Burton, Arthur, 261

calm, 61, 68, 157, 198
case study
  Buddhist approach, 132-135
  Christian approach, 290-304, 398
  Hindu approach, 70-79

case study *(continued)*
  Islamic approach, 352-354
  Judaic approach, 239-243
  Taoist approach, 197-200
categorization
  and Buddhism, 101-102, 109
  of disorders, 161 (*see also*
    diagnoses)
  and Taoism, 150-151, 158-159
causality
  and Islam, 332, 333
  similarities, 364-365
  and Taoism, 141-142, 151-152
centeredness, 181-182, 191-192, 311
    n. 61
change
  Christian view, 261, 266-271, 292
  Hindu view, 41-43, 51, 67
  similarities, 362-363
  in Taoism
    achieving, 199
    and centeredness, 192
    controlling, 145, 153
    and goals, 185
    personality structure, 158-159
    and therapy, 174, 176
    yin and *yang,* 163
chanting, 59
charity, 347
child, mind of, 155, 166
China, 87
Chodron, Pema, 87, 99
choice. *See* decisions
cholesterol, 122
Christian humanism
  and grace, 281
  and Jesus, 282, 289-290
  personality structure, 373-374
  and pluralism, 281, 282-283, 285
  propositions, 248
  and psychotherapy, 289-290, 387,
    389
  and suffering, 398
  therapist-client relationship,
    267-270, 294-295, 297, 393
Christian Humanistic Therapy (CHT),
    290-304
Christianity. *See also* Christian
    humanism
  background, 247-249

Christianity *(continued)*
  and Buddhism, 124-125, 286-287
  cardinal virtues, 254
  Catholicism, 257, 285-286
  and God, 257-258, 269
    in case study, 301-302
    concept of, 285
    covenant, 238
    and love, 269
    spirituality, and, 257
  grace, 265, 268, 281, 284
  and guilt, 228, 278
  and Hinduism, 63, 285-286
  imago Dei, 288, 299, 312 n. 67, 396
  individual differences, 258-259,
    381-382
  and Islam, 238, 284
  and Judaism, 238, 283-284
  liberal, 306 n. 12
  personality theory, 250-259
  Protestantism, 257, 321 n. 148
  and relativism, 281
  religionless, 287
  scriptures, 249-250, 253, 277
  and Taoism, 287
Chuang-tzu, 161, 167, 170
clarity, 105, 106, 109, 133
cleansing. *See* purification
client-centered therapy, 13, 271, 352
clients. *See also* therapist-client
    relationship
  focus, 13
  Hindu view, 49
  problems of, 117
  and religion, 9-10, 11, 349
  symptom recording, 113-114, 131
clinical intuition, 143
clinical practice. *See* therapeutic
    practice
cognitive activities, 28
cognitive therapy
  and Buddhism, 103
  and Taoism, 179-180, 199
cognitive-behavioral therapy
  Christian-based, 280
  and eastern religions, 131-132, 391
  and Islam, 352
coins, throwing, 150
comfort, 144
commandments. *See* rules

community, 390. *See also* society
comparisons, between religions
  distress, 382-384
  motivation, 375-378
  personality development, 378-380
  personality structure, 370-375
  relationships, 395-397
  self, 187, 220, 394-395
  suffering, 397-401
  time, 391
compassion
  and Buddhism, 87, 105, 115-116,
    118
    in case study, 134
  and Christianity, 267, 295-296, 301
  and Hinduism, 48, 55
  religions stressing, 64
  and Taoism, 145, 155, 179
  and therapist-client relationship,
    393, 398
competition, 42
concentration, 111, 191-192
conceptualization
  in Buddhism, 89-90, 101-102, 109
  in Judaism, 123
  and Taoism, 142, 170
conflict(s)
  and Hinduism, 39, 42
  and Islam, 353
  and Taoism, 141
  work-related, 110
Confucius, 64, 148
confusion, 129
congeniality, 42
congruence, 110
connections. *See also* relationships
  in Hinduism, 53
  in Judaism, 232
  in Taoism, 160, 192-193, 195, 198,
    390
conscience, 298
conscious mind
  and Buddhism, 129
  and Christianity, 254
consciousness
  and Buddhism, 90
  and Christianity, 264
  of God (Islam), 329, 374
  purposive, 127-128
  and Taoism, 145

constructionist therapy, 130-131
contemplative psychology, 401
contemplative Taoism, 147
contentment, 23, 37, 66
context, 103-104, 111, 134
contracting, in therapy, 395
contrasts. *See* comparisons, between
    religions
control
    and all approaches, 362
    and Judaism, 228-229
    self-, 32, 39
    and Taoism, 171, 184, 186
conversational strategy, 294
cooperation
    Hindu view, 42
    religions stressing, 64, 65
    and Taoism, 145, 174, 193
countertransference, 111, 272
couples, in case study, 119, 296, 354,
    390
courage
    and Buddhist therapy, 105, 133
    and Christianity, 267, 300, 312 n. 71
    and Judaism, 231
covenant, with God, 217-220, 238, 283,
    393
crises, 171
critical theory, 6-7
criticism, 92, 118
Csikszentmihalyi, M., 144
cultural determinism, 292
Cupitt, Don, 286
cybernetic epistemology, 127-128
cycles, 147, 191, 199. *See also yin-*
    yang polarity

Dalai Lama, 114, 123-125
death, 54-55, 57. *See also* afterlife
decisions
    and Christianity, 253, 270-271, 279,
      293-294
    of clients, 9
    and Hinduism, 61
    and Islam, 335, 337, 374
    and Judaism, 216, 228-231
    similarities, 363, 367
    and values, 9
deconstruction, 130-131

defense mechanisms
    and Buddhism, 96-97, 100-101, 109
    and Taoism, 194
deities, 19, 24, 92. *See also* God
DeMartino, Richard, 126
deMello, Anthony, 124
depression. *See also* case study
    and Buddhism, 122
    Hindu-based therapy, 70-79
    and Taoism, 198-200
desire
    in Buddhism, 89, 90-91, 94-95, 376
    in Hinduism, 39
    and Taoism, 172, 182-183
destiny. *See also* determinism
    and Christianity, 268
    and Taoism, 164
detachment
    and Buddhism, 389
    and Hinduism, 46, 49-50, 54, 60
determinism, 292
Dewey, John, 49
dharma
    and personality development, 35,
      378
    and self-actualization, 55-56
    and society, 33
    and unity, 28
    and yogas, 22
diagnoses
    and Buddhism, 102, 109
    and Christianity, 259-260, 272
    and Islam, 344-345
    and Taoism, 161, 197
dialogue, 14-15
discipline
    and Buddhism, 105, 107, 110
    and Islam, 335, 347
discourse analysis, 12-14, 301
distress. *See also* suffering
    and Buddhism, 96-98, 382-383
    and Christianity, 259-261, 383-384
    and Hinduism, 38-40, 48, 56-57,
      382
    and Islam, 343, 344, 384
    and Judaism, 227, 383
    similarities, 363-364
    and Taoism, 167-173, 196, 383
divine intervention, 338
divine principles, 338

Doherty, William, 312
double negativity, 96-97, 100-101, 109,
    131
dualism
    in Buddhism
        of ego, 89, 108, 110, 372
        and knowledge, 108
        mind-body, 102
    in Hinduism, 40, 66
    in Islam, 329, 332, 343
    in Judaism, 219-220, 221-222
    mind-body, 102
    in relationships, 219-220
    similarities, 365-366
    in Taoism, 156-157 (*see also yin-*
        yang polarity)
Duns Scotus, John, 404
duty. *See dharma;* obligation(s)

effort, right, 110-111
ego
    and Buddhism
        definition, 97
        duality, 110
        emergence, 89
        and goodness, 134
        and identity, 88, 105, 372
        and meditation, 111
        and mindfulness, 106
    and cybernetic epistemology, 127
    and group therapy, 121
    and Hinduism, 40, 46
    and Islam, 344
    and Taoism, 125, 155-156
    and trance, 129
    and yoga psychology, 310 n. 53
egolessness, 97-98, 108
electroencephalograms (EEGs), 111,
    112
Elkadi, Ahmed, 344, 347
emotions. *See also specific emotions*
    and Buddhism, 100-101, 127, 134
    and Christianity, 274
    felt meanings, 315 n. 100
    in Hinduism, 28, 58-59
    and Islam, 332-333, 337, 341, 375
    and Taoism, 161, 191
empathy, 13, 17 n. 20

energy
    and Buddhism
        and emotions, 98, 100, 101
        and healing, 107, 108, 110
    and Christianity, 293
    and Taoism
        of life, 371
        of opponent, 153
        pervasiveness, 142, 151
        positive versus negative, 184, 199
        and wisdom, 166
enlightenment, 87
environment. *See also* individual
        differences
    and Buddhism, 95-96, 103-104, 134
    for emotions, 127
    Hindu view, 34, 42, 68
    home and work, 103-104
    and Taoism, 143, 145
envy, 95
Epstein, Mark, 91, 113, 126-127, 401
equanimity, 61, 68, 157, 198
Erickson, Milton, 128-130
Erikson, Erik
    developmental theories, 256
    epigenetic principle, 378
    personal integrity, 70
estrangement. *See* alienation
ethics, 9, 22. *See also* values
evil. *See* good and evil
existential psychology, 227-229, 230,
    394
existential-contemplative
        psychotherapy, 401
Exodus, 212, 224, 302, 394
experience(s). *See also* attachment
    and Buddhism, 102, 104-105, 164,
        372-373
    and Christianity, 255-256, 258, 265
        and CHT, 291-292
    and Islam, 352
    and psychology, 288, 289, 322 n. 165
    and Taoism, 143, 156, 160, 187
    truth of, 395
    versus behaviors, 402-403
externalization, 101

faith
    and Buddhism, 89
    and Christianity, 254, 255, 268

faith *(continued)*
 and Islam, 341, 342
family
 and Buddhism, 119, 120, 130
 and Islam, 349
family therapy
 and Buddhism, 104, 120
 and cybernetic epistemology, 127
Faruqi, I. and L., 333-334, 335
fasting, 347
feeling, 89
felt meanings, 315 n. 100
flexibility
 of Hindu therapy, 46, 60, 61
 and Taoism, 162-163, 171, 173,
  190-191
focus, 13, 144
form, 89
Fowler, James, 256
Fox, David, 232
Frankel, Ellen, 221
Frankl, Viktor
 and Assagioli, 402
 Holocaust experience, 230, 231
 on relationships, 224-225, 227
 on suffering, 232
freedom
 Buddhist, 87, 116-117
 Christian
  and decisions, 270, 292
  and reconciling personality, 312
   n. 68
  and religion validity, 282
  and repression, 265
  and sin, 261, 263
  Tillich view, 311 n. 61
 Hindu, 21, 59, 60, 79 n. 12
 and individuality, 395
 and Islam, 374 *(see also under* good
  and evil)
 and Judaism, 223
 similarities, 362-363
Freud, Sigmund
 and Al-Ghazzali, 357 n. 55
 and counterwill, 252
 drive theory, 402
 and *Kabbalah,* 217
 and religion, 236-237, 401
Fromm, Erich, 126

future
 and Buddhism, 108
 and Christianity, 254, 273
 research, 280-281
 and Taoism, 144, 145, 187

games, 92
Gandhi, Mahatma, 82 n. 61, 83 n. 62
Garfield, Sol, 280
generosity, 106-107
genuineness, 162
Gestalt theory, 59, 67, 314 n. 91
goal orientation, 395
goals. *See also* motivation; striving
 and Buddhism, 87, 95, 98
 and Christianity, 254, 262, 273-274
 and Hinduism, 31, 32, 49-50
 and Islam, 339, 352-353
 and Judaism, 217, 236
 and Taoism, 144, 172, 185, 189, 196
goals, therapeutic
 Christian humanist, 261-263,
  268-270, 279-280, 303-304
 Hindu, 49
 Islamic, 352-353
 Judaic, 236
 Taoist, 180-181, 196
God. *See also* will, of God
 and Buddhism, 85, 123
 and Christianity
  case study, 301-302
  concept of, 285
  and love, 269
  and spirituality, 257
 covenant, 212
 and Hinduism, 21, 24-25, 41, 66-67
 and Islam
 consciousness of, 329, 374
 covenant, 238
 monotheism, 284, 325, 333-334,
  336
 and psychotherapy, 345-346, 353
 and spiritual development, 341-342
 and Judaism
  covenant, 237
  and *mitzvot,* 216-217, 223, 396
  monotheism, 212
  and personality, 217-220
 similarities, 365-366
 and Taoism, 142

good and evil. *See also* virtue and vice
   and Buddhism, 115, 134
   and Christianity, 260
   and Hinduism, 24-27, 66
   and Islam
      Al Ghazzali view, 341
      heart role, 336
      jihad, 337-338, 374
      knowledge role, 335
      Satan, 335, 336, 356 n. 38
   and Judaism, 221-223, 228, 373
Gospels, 249
grace
   in Christianity, 265, 268, 281, 284
      in case study, 297
   in Islam, 341
gratitude
   and Buddhism, 119
   and Islam, 341
group therapy
   and Buddhism, 121
   and Taoism, 200
growth. *See* personal growth
guilt
   and Buddhism, 133, 134
   Christian view
      in case study, 297, 298
      and healing, 398-399
      Heidegger view, 228
      and salvation, 278
   and Islam, 339, 399
   and Judaism, 228, 399
   and parent-child relationship, 240,
      297, 298
gurus, 61

habit, 113, 372
   addictions, 20
Haddad, Yasser, 341
halacha, 216
Hanh, Thich Nhat, 106
happiness
   and Hinduism, 23, 65
   and Taoism, 142, 144, 168
hardship, 338
harmony, and Taoism, 151, 169,
     177-178
Hartman, Robert, 66
Hathout, Hassan, 327, 334

healing
   Buddhist, 105-109, 394
   Christian view, 263-266, 269, 301
   Islamic view, 343-345
   Taoist, 156, 394
health, 262
health maintenance organizations
     (HMOs), 266
heart
   and Islam, 335-336, 344, 349, 375
   and Taoism, 192-194
Heart Zones, 345
Heidegger, Martin, 228
Helminiak, Daniel, 309 n. 35
heredity. *See* individual differences
Heschel, Abraham J., 219, 222
Hinduism. *See also* therapeutic process;
     therapy, theory of
   afterlife, 20-21, 64
   Atman, 375, 402
   and Buddhism, 125
   and Christianity, 63, 285-286
   and death, 54-55, 57
   deities, 19, 21-23
   divine incarnations, 24-27, 67
   and duty, 22, 28
   freedom, 21, 59, 60
   and God, 21-22, 24-25, 66-67 (*see*
     also Brahman)
   good and evil, 24-27
   human beings, 25, 34-38, 68
   and individual differences, 34-38,
     60-62, 69, 380
   and Judaism, 228-230
   karma (*see* karma)
   Kshatriyas, 25-26, 33, 34
   personality theory, 53-54, 392
   and psychosynthesis, 404
   and psychotherapy, 386
   purification, 19-20, 21, 37
   scripture, 23-28 (*see also Bhagavad
     Gita*)
   self, 22-23, 80 n. 21, 195, 394
   self-realization, 29, 39-40, 55-56,
     371
   society, 33-34 (*see also dharma*)
   spirituality, 29, 32-33, 39-40, 50
   and Taoism, 195
   and time, 24, 67, 68
   and unity, 28, 40, 41-42, 46, 48, 67

Hinduism *(continued)*
　worldview, 19
　yogas *(see yogas)*
history, 302, 394
Hobson's model, 294
Hoff, B., 155, 170
holding environment, 127
holistic approach, 368. *See also* healing
Holocaust, 284
honor, 341-342
hope
　and Christianity, 254, 277-278, 299, 398
　and Islam, 343, 354
　and Taoism, 168
Hsien Taoism, 147-148
human nature, 367. *See also imago Dei;* self
humanism, 306 n. 9. *See also* Christian humanism
humility, 161
humor
　and Buddhism, 110-111
　and Taoism, 156, 196
hypnosis, 128-130

I Ching, 150
ideals, 92
identity
　and Buddhism, 88, 105, 372
　and Christianity, 257, 373
　and Hinduism, 31
　and Judaism, 215, 221, 225
Ignatius, Saint, 395
ignorance
　in Buddhism, 89, 92
　in Christianity, 63
　in Hinduism, 35-36, 38-40, 63, 382
illusion
　and Buddhism, 389
　and Hinduism, 37-38, 39, 49-50, 81 nn. 36, 38
　and Taoism, 171
imagery, 345, 353, 405
imago Dei, 269, 288, 299, 312 n. 67, 396
impulses, 172
inculturation, 285-286

individual differences
　and Buddhism, 93-96, 381
　and Christianity, 258-259, 381-382
　and freedom, 395
　and Hinduism, 34-38, 60-62, 69, 380
　and Islam, 342-343, 382
　and Judaism, 225-227, 381
　and Taoism, 160-161, 196, 381
inner life, 14
insight, 37
insomnia, 97, 122
Integrated approaches
　Assagioli model, 401-404
　Wilber model, 404-406
integrity, 70
intellect
　in Buddhism, 89-90, 92, 93-94
　in Hinduism, 28, 31-32
　in Islam, 334-335
　in Taoism, 153
intention
　and Buddhism, 109
　and Christianity, 252
　and Judaism, 217
intuition
　clinical, 143
　and Islam, 335-336, 344, 349, 394
　similarities, 367
　and Taoism
　　authentic living, 162
　　definition, 143
　　distractions, 169
　　interconnectedness, 195
　　knowing Tao, 146
　　as therapy approach, 175
　　yin and *yang,* 184
Iqbal, Mohammed, 336
Islam
　beliefs and practices, 327-330, 339-340, 346-350
　and Christianity, 284, 327-328
　God *(see under* God)
　history, 326, 329
　and individual differences, 342-343, 382
　jihad, 337-338, 340, 354
　and Judaism, 238, 327-328
　personality theory, 332-343, 350-351

Islam *(continued)*
    prohibitions, 331, 348
    prophets, 327
        Muhammad, 284, 326, 338, 340
    and psychosynthesis, 404
    and psychotherapy, 387
    ritual, 327, 341, 346
    scripture, 327-328, 340, 347
    sects, 331
    state and religion, 330
    and women, 330-331
Islamic Medicine, Institute of, 344

Jalalú Din As-Suyuti, 344
James, William, 402
Japan, 87
jealousy, 95
Jeevan-mukta, 21
Jesus
    Christian humanist view, 282-283
    and God, 257-258
        kingdom of, 247-248, 252,
            268-269
    and knowledge, 63
    and meditation, 276
    and sin, 263
    and Tao, 287
    in theology, 304 n. 4
jihad, 337-338, 340, 354
jiva, 28-29
Job, 232-233
Judaism
    and Buddhism, 123-124, 238-239
    and Christianity, 238, 283-284
    Exodus, 212, 224
    and God, 212 *(see also* God;
        mitzvot)
    Golden Calf, 227
    and Hinduism, 63, 238-239
    history, 211-214
    and individual differences, 225-227,
        381
    and Islam, 238
    Job, 232-233
    Kabbalah, 123, 214, 215, 217
    personality theory, 216-227
    and psychotherapy, 387, 389, 395
    ritual, 217, 218
    scripture, 213, 214-215, 216

judgmental attitude
    and Buddhism, 131
    and Taoism, 153, 174, 183-184
judo, 153
Jung, Carl, 401, 402
justice
    and Hinduism, 26
    and Islam, 337-338, 339
    religions stressing, 64, 283

Kabat-Zinn, Jon, 113, 120
Kabat-Zinn, Myla, 120
Kabbalah, 123, 214, 215
    in psychotherapy, 217, 402
kalpas, 24
Kamilar, Scott, 400
karma
    in Buddhism, 88-90, 95, 372
    in Hinduism, 19-20, 39, 79 nn. 5, 9
Kawai, Hayao, 401
Kitamori, Kazo, 287
knowledge. *See also* intellect; intuition;
        wisdom
    in Buddhism, 108
    in Christianity, 63
    in Confucianism, 64
    in Hinduism, 22, 27-28, 63
    and human potential, 337
    in Islam
        historic legacy, 328
        religious, 348
        self-, 348-349, 352, 399
        types, 334-335
        versus desire, 340
    in Judaism, 216
    in Taoism, 142, 147, 185, 194
koans, 116-117, 366-367
Kohlberg, Lawrence, 256, 273
Kohlenberger, J. R., 249
Korea, 87
Kornfield, Jack, 113, 114
Krishna
    background, 23-24, 26, 82 nn. 57,
        59, 60
    flexibility, 61-62
    and self-realization, 55-56
    as therapist, 43-47, 70
Kshatriyas, 25-26, 33, 34
Kulkarni, S. D., 56
Küng, Hans, 269

language
    in case study, 291, 294, 301
    and discourse analysis, 301
    religious, 14
    Semantic Differential, 15
Lao-tzu, 156, 157, 190
Lazarus, Arnold, 260, 261
Lester, Andrew, 277-278
letting go
    and Buddhism, 97
    and Hinduism, 73, 77, 82 n. 57
    and Taoism, 182-183
Levinas, Emmanuel, 397, 408 n. 15
Lewin, Kurt, 65, 278
liberation. *See* freedom
Lieh-tse, 170
life, reverence for, 369-370
lifestyle
    Adlerian analysis, 277
    Buddhist, 110
    Christian, 251, 262, 277
    Hindu, 33-34
    Islamic, 331, 341, 342, 348
    similarities, 363
    Taoist, 147, 185
limits
    and Christianity, 299-300
    and Taoism, 182-183
Linehan, Marsha, 131
listening skills, 272
logic
    in Buddhism, 93-94
    in Taoism, 184-185
Logotherapy, 224-225
lojong, 114-116
loneliness, 154
lotus analogy, 54
love
    Christian
        acts of, 277, 284
        and God, 285
        and healing, 301, 302-303
        and motivation, 254
        and therapeutic relationship, 268
    Hindu, 48, 55

Macquarrie, John, 323 n. 185
Maddi, S. R., 88, 336
Madill, A., 12, 292

Mahabharata, 28
Maimonides, 230, 236
Manu, Swayambhu, 55-56
Maritain, Jacques, 289-290
Maslow, Abraham
    and Assagioli, 402
    and Christianity, 255
    and Hinduism, 53, 55, 65-66, 76
materialism
    and Buddhism, 90-91, 92-93, 108,
        110
    and Hinduism, 21, 30-31, 54, 81 n.
        38
    and Islam, 332
    and Taoism, 169, 170-171
May, Rollo
    on meaningfulness, 224, 230-231
    on relationships, 220, 224, 225, 227,
        233
    throwness, 228-229, 231
maya. See illusion
meaningfulness
    for Christianity, 283-284
    for Frankl, 232
    and Islam, 339
    for Judaism, 224-225, 227, 230,
        242-243
    in psychosynthesis, 404
    similarities, 367
    and suffering, 398
meanings, felt, 315 n. 100
mediators, 67, 366, 374
medication, 239, 291, 353
meditation
    in Buddhism, 95, 103, 106, 111-118
    and Christianity, 276-277, 300, 317
        n. 114
    in Hinduism, 22, 23, 65, 72-76
    in Islam, 346, 353, 399
    physiological effects, 111, 112, 122
    in psychosynthesis, 405
    in Taoism, 142, 154, 182
    and therapy, 131, 388
    and Westerners, 114
memory(ies)
    and Buddhism, 102
    and Christianity, 273
    and Taoism, 160, 188
Merton, Thomas, 124

Messiah
  and Christianity, 238, 247, 284
  and Judaism, 214, 284
metaphor, 294
middle way, 98
migraine, 122
mind, 374-375, 388. *See also* intellect;
    knowledge
  of child, 155, 166
  and Islam, 334-335
  and Taoism, 192-194
mind training
  Buddhism, 114-116, 134
  Taoism, 182-194
mindfulness
  in Buddhism, 106, 107, 111, 112
    in therapy, 113, 134
  in Taoism, 144-146, 187-188
mirroring, 118
misfortune, 165. *See also* suffering
mitzvot
  and case study, 241
  and choice, 226, 229-230
  and God, 216-217, 223, 396
moderation
  and Islam, 340, 348
  and Taoism, 185
modesty, 155
moksha (nirvana), 20, 35, 64
money, 110
monotheism
  and authority, 393
  and Christianity, 283, 284, 285
  and Islam, 284, 325
  and Judaism, 212, 283
  and mind, 388
  and self, 394
moral ideal, 311 n. 66
morality
  and Buddhism, 107, 110, 134
  and Christianity, 256, 265, 273,
    296-298
  and Hinduism, 60, 64
  and Islam, 335, 339-340, 379-380
  and Judaism, 379 (*see also mitzvot*)
  and psychotherapy, 312 n. 75
  similarities, 364
Moses, 212, 302
motivation. *See also* goals; striving
  and Buddhism, 376, 378-379

motivation *(continued)*
  and Christianity, 252-255, 292-293,
    377
  comparisons, 375-380
  and Hinduism, 31-32, 39, 48,
    375-376
  and Islam, 336, 377-378
  and Judaism, 216, 223-224, 376-377
Muhammad
  as founder, 326
  on *jihad,* 337-338, 340
  on knowledge, 348
  as prophet, 284
Murata, Sachiko, 335-336
muscle tension, 122
music, 405
mysticism, 402

Naikan, 119
Nanak, Guru, 83 n. 77
Narada, Sage, 61
Naropa Institute, 124, 401
narrative therapy, 130-131
Native Americans, 125-126
nature
  sensitivity to, 146, 147, 150-152,
    153
  and simplicity, 150-152
  and suffering, 168
  yin-yang polarity, 157
needs. *See also* materialism
  for affirmation, 228, 233
  and Christianity, 254-255, 292-293
  and Hinduism, 21, 30-31, 54
  and Islam, 332-333, 337
negativity, 171, 173-174, 183-184, 199
negotiation, 294
neuroses, 115
New Testament, 249, 253
Niebuhr, Reinhold, 288
nirvana
  in Buddhism, 87
  in Hinduism, 20, 64
nonviolence
  and Hinduism, 39, 61-62
  religions stressing, 64, 65
normativism, 363-364
nothingness, 156-157

objectivity, 367
obligation(s), 241-242, 273, 296, 397.
    See also rules
Oglesby, William, 277
Old Testament, 249
openmindedness
    and Buddhism, 101-102, 109
    and Taoism, 143, 144, 162, 167, 170
optimism, 100-101
order, 151-152
otherness, 89
OUM, 81 n. 35
outcome measurement. *See* therapy,
        evaluating
overachievers, 171

pain. *See* suffering
pain management, 113, 115
panic attacks, 96-97
Pannikar, Raimundo, 285-286
paradox, 366-367
paramitas, 106-109
paranoia, 92
parenting
    and Buddhism, 120, 130
    and therapist-client relationship, 397
Parr, V. E., 187
passion
    and Buddhism, 89, 94-95
    and Islam, 332-333
passivity, 98
Passover, 224
Patanjali, 404
patience
    and Buddhism, 107
    and Hinduism, 77
    and Taoism, 165
patterns
    in Buddhism, 131
    in Gestalt theories, 314 n. 91
    in Taoism, 142, 184-185
peace
    and Hinduism, 23
    Islamic view, 325, 339, 341, 347
    and Taoism, 144, 145, 147, 151, 175
perception-impulse, 89
perfection, 19-20
performance anxiety, 187
persistence, 165

personal growth
    Christian view, 255
    in psychosynthesis, 404
    similarities, 369-370
    and Taoism, 173, 178
personal integrity, 70
personality
    definition, 88
    and situations, 182
    and spirituality, 2-3
    styles of (Buddhist), 93-96
personality development
    in Buddhism, 91-93, 378-379
    Christian view, 255-258
    in Hinduism, 33-34, 378
    in Islam, 338-342, 379-380
    in Judaism, 225, 379
    in Taoism, 161-167, 379
    Wilber model, 405
personality dynamics, 375-380. *See
        also* action; change;
        motivation
personality structure
    and Buddhism, 88-90, 372-373
    Christian humanist, 373-374
    and Hinduism, 28-31
    and Islam, 374-375
    and Judaism, 373
    similarities, 370-375
    and Taoism, 371-372
personality theory. *See also* similarities
    Buddhist, 88-96
    Christian view, 250-259, 278, 308
        n. 22
    Hindu, 52-56, 392
    Islamic, 332-343, 350-351
    Judaic, 216-227
    Taoist, 157-167
pessimism, 81 n. 38
phenomenology, 13-14, 390
phobias, 122
physical body. *See also*
        biopsychosocial model
    and Hinduism, 28
    and Islam, 353
    and Taoism, 158, 159
physical causes, 290-291
physical objects, 107
physiological effects, 122
Piaget, Jean, 31-32

pilgrimage, 347
pleasure
    Buddhist view, 376
    Hindu view, 20
    Islamic view, 332, 340
    Taoist view, 192
pluralism, 8
Podvoll, Edward, 103-104
Polster, Erving and Miriam, 220
positive regard, 68
positive thinking, 100-101
postmeditation, 116
posttraumatic stress, 122
potential, 107, 339
power
    and Buddhism, 108
    and Taoism, 154
powerlessness, 117, 127
praise
    and Buddism, 118
    and Taoism, 183
prarabdha. See providence
prayer
    and Christianity, 277, 300, 389
    contemplative, 389
    and Islam, 327, 342, 354
preconceptions, 170
presence, unconditional, 176-179
present moment. *See also*
            experience(s); future
    and behaviorism, 391
    and Buddhism, 102, 104-105
    Christian view, 273, 299
    and Taoism, 119, 145, 156, 170, 172
present-mindedness, 186-188
pride, 263, 340
problem solving
    and Islam, 353
    and Taoism, 182, 189-190
process research, 281
promises, 26
providence, 46
psychoanalysis
    and Buddhism, 126-127
    and Taoism, 179
psychology
    Hindu, 41-50
    religious-scientific, 3
    religious versus secular, 369
    transpersonal, 402-406
    versus religion, 5, 8

psychopathology. *See* distress
psychosis, 104
psychosynthesis, 402-404
psychotherapy
    and Buddhism, 85, 99-109, 113-114
    Christian views, 261-263, 270-271,
        300, 312 n. 75
        theonomous, 268-269, 314 n. 88
    existential-contemplative, 401
    and Hinduism, 56-63
    history, 401
    integrated approaches, 401-406
    Islamic view, 343-345
    and Judaism, 231-235, 395
    and meditation, 113-114
    and moral responsibility, 312 n. 75
    religious impact, 385-391
    similarities, 385-391
    and spirituality, 2-3, 300
Puranas, 28
purification, 19-20, 21, 37, 59
purpose, 9. *See also* meaningfulness

questioning, 198-199
Quran, 327-328, 340, 347

Rajasa, 35
Ramayana, 28
rapport, 271-272
rational-emotive therapy, 352
rationality, 147
Ratnagiri, 37-38
readiness
    Christian view, 273
    Hindu view, 49, 73
realism, 361
reality
    and Buddhism, 109, 394
    and Christianity, 267, 301
    Hindu view, 46, 49-50
    similarities, 367, 368-369
    and Taoism, 146, 192, 371, 394
reality therapy, 352
realms, 250-251
rebirth, 20, 21, 38
reconciliation
    and Christianity, 261-263, 268-270,
        279-280, 303-304

reconciliation *(continued)*
    as motivation, 255
    and psychology, 288
    and self, 374
    and Taoism, 287
    and transformation, 257, 396
Red Elk, Gerald, 125-126
redaction criticism, 14
relapse prevention, 275
relationships. *See also* connections;
        therapist-client relationship
    with appearances, 175
    and atonement, 223
    and Buddhism, 119, 390
    child-parent, 300 (*see also* case
        study)
    and Christianity, 238, 255, 265
    comparisons, 395-397
    hierarchical, 130-131
    and Hinduism, 41-42, 70-79
    in Islam, 238, 390
        in Judaism
        I-It and I-Thou, 219, 220, 225,
            233-234, 236
        and meaningfulness, 227-228
        and personality, 225, 373, 390
        Ruth and Naomi, 240
        with God, 217-220, 283
    May views, 220, 224, 225
    monotheistic views, 390
    mother-daughter (*see* case study)
    parenting, 120, 130
    and Taoism, 160
relativism, 281
relaxation, 345, 353
religion(s). *See also* comparisons,
        between religions;
        similarities; *specific religions*
    and clients, 9-10, 11, 349
    Freudian view, 236-237
    and psychotherapy, 385-391, 401
    significance, 323 n. 185
    Taoist view, 179
    versus psychology, 5, 8
    versus spirituality, 16 n. 1
renunciation, 87
repression, 100-101
research topics, 280-281, 406-407
responsibility
    for happiness, 168

responsibility *(continued)*
    and Hinduism, 46, 67
    and Islam, 329-330, 337, 342-343
    and Judaism, 228, 230, 241-242
    moral, 312 n. 75
    and Taoism, 168, 194
right absorption, 111
right effort, 110-111
right intention, 109
right mindfulness, 111
right morality, 110, 134
right speech, 109-110
right view, 101-102, 109
ritual
    and Islam, 327, 341, 346
    and Judaism, 217, 218, 226
    and Taoism, 147
ritualism, 64, 83 n. 77
Rogers, Carl
    on change, 271
    client-centered therapy, 13, 271
    and *imago Dei,* 312 n. 67
    person-centeredness, 69, 76
    self-concept theory, 68-69, 310 n. 47
    on therapists, 117-118
    and trust, 225
role functioning
    in Hinduism, 58, 59, 60, 81 n. 36
    May view, 220
Rorschach ink blots, 23, 150
Rossi, Earnest, 128-130
rules
    and Christianity, 300
    and Islam, 349
    and Judaism, 216, 217, 223
    and Taoism, 147, 151-152, 153-154
Rumi, 343
Rychlak, Joseph, 252, 253-254

Sages, 161-167
salvation
    and Christianity, 269, 278, 320 n.
        140
    Confucius view, 64
    and Hinduism, 50
    and Judaism, 214
sanity, 104-105, 106-107, 133
Satan. *See* good and evil
satisfaction, 70

Sattva, 35
Saucy, Mark, 250
Schindler, Alexander, 226
Schwietzer, Albert, 369-370
science, 3, 179
scripture
    Buddhist, 87
    Christian, 249-250, 253, 277
    Hindu, 23-28
    Judaic, 213, 214-215, 216
    Taoist, 149-150
    in therapy, 277
self
    Buddhist view, 88-90, 195, 393
    Christian view
        in CHT, 248
        development, 255, 379
        dimensions, 250-251, 258, 259,
            264, 266
        imago Dei, 269, 288, 299, 312 n.
            67
        and reconciliation, 373-374
        Wells view, 278
    comparisons, 394-395
    existential view, 227, 394
    Hindu view, 22-23, 80 n. 21, 195,
        371, 394
    Islamic view, 332-334, 351
    Judaic view, 220-221, 373, 379
    in psychology, 288
    in psychosynthesis, 402
    Rogers view, 227
    Taoist view, 160, 167, 195
self, ideal, 68-69, 310 n. 47, 311 n. 66
self-acceptance, 155-156, 162, 180,
    192-193
self-actualization
    Buddhist, 121
    and Christian, 255, 288, 309 n. 35
    comparisons, 371
    Hindu, 55-56, 65-66
    Islamic, 335
self-assertion, 27, 60
self-blame
    and Hinduism, 46
    and Taoism, 155
self-care, 353, 390
self-concept
    and Buddhism, 109
    Christian view, 268, 272

self-concept *(continued)*
    in case study, 291-292, 293, 297
    and Hinduism, 32, 68
    and self-ideal, 310
self-control, 32, 39
self-deception, 263
self-discovery, 186
self-esteem
    and Buddhism, 114
    Christian view, 272, 295, 300
    and Hinduism, 69-70
    and Islam, 349, 354, 399
    and Taoism, 182-183
self-ideal, 68-69, 310 n. 47, 311 n. 66
self-indulgence, 94
self-knowledge, 348-349, 352, 399
self-realization, 29, 39-40, 55-56, 378
self-righteousness, 108
self-sacrifice, 55
Semantic Differential, 15
sense enjoyment, 20, 21, 35, 39, 60
sensitivity, 155
separation, 395. *See also* alienation
service, to others
    and Buddhism, 105-106
    and Hinduism, 48, 64
    and Islam, 349
    and Judaism, 397
    and psychosynthesis, 404
sex, 332, 348
shamatha, 106
Shapiro, Deane, 123, 131
Shiites, 331
Shudras, 34
Siddhārtha Gautama (Buddha)
    Assagioli view, 404
    background, 85-86
    and Hinduism, 26-27, 125
    meditation advice, 110-111
similarities. *See also* comparisons,
        between religions
    and behaviorism, 360-361
    biopsychosocial model, 360
    dualism, 365-366
    existential themes, 367
    holistic approach, 368
    human freedom, 362-363
    normativism, 363-364
    optimism, 362
    and paradox, 366-367

similarities *(continued)*
  personhood, 369-370
  phenomenological perspective, 362
  psychotherapy, 385-391
  realism, 361
  spirituality, 368-369
  teleological, 364-365
simplicity
  and Christianity, 320 n. 145
  and Taoism, 150-151, 162, 185-186
sin
  and Christianity, 260-261, 278, 399
  and Islam, 339, 343
  and Judaism, 221-222, 223, 399
slogans, 116
social action, 277
social involvement, 277
society
  and Confucius, 148
  engagement in, 396
  and Hinduism, 33-34, 60
  and Islam, 330, 339, 342, 349
  Judaeo-Christian view, 283
  and Taoism, 162, 169
soul
  and clinical psychology, 288
  and Hinduism, 380
  Islamic view, 341
  in Judaism, 221-222, 228, 373
  in psychosynthesis, 404
  similarities, 369
sound therapy, 345
speech, 109-110. *See also* language
spirit, 333
spiritual direction, 16 n. 7
spiritual healing, 264-265
spirituality
  in Buddhism, 106-109
  and Christianity, 250-251, 256-257,
    268-270, 272-273 (*see also*
    imago Dei)
  and clinical psychology, 288
  and clinicians, 9
  and Hinduism
    ego-state analogy, 67-68
    enhancement of, 47, 50
    in human nature, 29, 32-33,
      39-40, 53-54
    and unity, 41, 42-43, 46, 48
    yoga, 79 n. 11

spirituality *(continued)*
  in history, 302
  and Islam, 333, 334, 341-342
  realm of, 2
  similarities, 368-369
  in Taoism, 179
  versus rationality, 83 n. 71
  versus religion, 16 n. 1
spontaneity, 151-152, 164
stages. *See* personality development
statements, selection of, 14-15
Stern, William, 308 n. 22
stillness, 171
Stone, M. H., 158
stress
  Christian view, 293
  Hindu view, 39, 42
  and Islam, 347, 349, 350
  and meditation, 113
  posttraumatic, 122
  and Taoism, 154
striving. *See also* goals; motivation
  and Buddhism, 92, 378
  and Islam, 328, 337-338, 341
  and Taoism, 189, 376
struggle
  and Islam, 337-338
  and Judaism, 217, 222, 228, 235,
    236
subject positioning, 13
submission, 325, 339, 344
suffering
  and Buddhism, 87, 96-98, 109-111,
    400
  and Christianity, 124, 260-261, 287,
    398-399
  client view, 11
  comparisons, 397-401
  and Hinduism, 19-21, 37, 64-65,
    399
  and Islam, 343, 344, 347, 399
  and Judaism
    and anxiety, 229
    and God, 219
    and guilt, 228
    in history, 214
    of others, 397
    as reality, 400
    and therapy, 232
  of others, 397

suffering *(continued)*
    and Taoism, 167-172
        acceptance, 165
        and balance, 196, 400
        and separation, 198, 390
        and yoga psychology, 310 n. 53
Sufi, 284
Sunnis, 331
superego, 341
surprise, 129
surrender, 117, 127
Suzuki, D. T., 126, 404
Suzuki, Shunryu, 97
symptoms
    and Christianity, 259
    of distress, 169, 172
    and mindfulness, 113-114, 131

Tamasa, 35
Tao te Ching, 125, 149
Taoism
    age of perfect virtue, 148-149
    basic tenets, 150-157
    and Buddhism, 125, 195, 196
    and causality, 141-142
    and change, 145
    and Christianity, 288
    and Confucianism, 148
    contemplative, 147
    essence, 145
    and God, 142
    and Hinduism, 195
    history, 148-149
    Hsien, 147-148
    and individual differences, 160-161,
        196, 381
    and intuition, 143, 146, 162
    levels of existence, 159-160
    and mindfulness, 144-146
    and nature, 146
    personality theory, 157-167
    and psychotherapy, 145, 386, 387,
        388-389
    ritual, 147
    scriptures, 149-150
    the Tao, 141-142, 146
    wu-wei, 152-154, 169, 176, 190-191
    yin-yang, 156-157, 163, 169,
        184-185

Tawhid, 333-334, 336
techniques
    and Buddhism, 101, 111
    Christian view, 276-278
    goal-oriented, 395
    and Islam, 345, 353, 399
    and Taoism, 175
technology, 170-171
telosponse, 253-254, 292
temperament. *See also* individual
        differences
    Hindu view, 34-38
    Taoist view, 159
theology
    and current situations, 6
    defined, 16 n. 6
    and psychology, 7
theonomous psychology, 268-269, 314
        n. 88
therapeutic practice
    Buddhist
        couples therapy, 119
        eightfold path, 109-111
        family therapy, 120
        group therapy, 121
        meditation, 111-117
    Christian, 271-278
    Hindu view, 47-50
    Islamic, 346-350
    Judaic, 236
    Taoist
        centering, 181-182
        emptying, 182-186
        grounding, 186-192
        mind-heart connection, 192-194
therapeutic process
    Hindu, 43-47, 71-79
    Taoist, 179-181, 196-197
therapist-client relationship
    Buddhist, 111, 130-131
    Christian humanist, 267-270,
        294-295, 297, 393, 396
    Hindu, 392
    Islamic, 396-397
    Judaic, 235, 242-243, 393, 396, 397
    and separation, 395
    Taoist, 178-179, 193
therapists. *See also* attitudes; values
    behavior, 117-118, 126
    Buddhist view, 103, 118, 390, 393

therapists *(continued)*
  Christian view, 271-278
  and clients, 111
  dress, 103
  Hindu view, 48, 49, 70-79, 392
  Judaic view, 234-236, 397-398
  and money, 110
  nonreligious, 4
  religious, 3, 8, 390
  Taoist view, 176-179, 180, 393
therapy. *See also* goals, therapeutic
  evaluating, 15, 274-275, 278-281
  growth-oriented, 99-100
  informal, 48
  length of, 180, 198, 266
  settings, 180, 200
  Taoist, 145, 169
  termination of, 78
  theory of
    Buddhist, 99- 109
    Christian humanist, 261-271
    Hindu, 41-43
    Islamic, 343-346, 350-351
    Judaic, 231-235
    Taoist, 173-176, 196
therapy-by-objectives, 274-275
Tibet, 87, 123
Tillich, Paul
  on courage, 312 n. 71
  on estrangement, 310 n. 45, 312 n. 67
  existential anthropology, 250, 311
    n. 61
  on gospels, 307 n. 15
  on reconciliation, 257
  on theology, 322 n. 169
Tilopa, 118
time
  and Buddhism, 107
  and Christianity, 266
  comparisons, 391
  and Hinduism, 24, 67, 68
tonglen, 114-116, 134
Towler, S., 167
trances, 128-129
transference, 272
transformation
  Christian view, 255-258, 261, 265,
    269
  of negatives, 171, 173-174
  and Taoism, 171, 173

Troeltsch, Ernst, 250
Trungpa, Chogyam
  on Buddhist styles *(yanas),* 87-88
  on ego, 89-90
  meditation technique, 112-113
  and Native Americans, 125-126
  on suffering, 96, 98
truth
  and Hinduism, 25-26, 35, 39
  individual views, 395
  Islamic view, 336
  and Taoism, 184
twigs, throwing, 150

unconditional presence, 176-179
unconscious
  Assagioli view, 403
  and Buddhism, 128-130
  Christian view, 254
  and Taoism, 150, 179
unity
  Buddhist, 102-103, 106, 394
  Christian, 259, 283, 292
  client and therapist, 111
  and Gestalt theory, 67
  Hindu
    and Brahman, 54
    as *dharma,* 28
    and mental health, 41-42
    and responsibility, 67
    strategies, 40
    therapeutic role, 48
    therapy, 78
    versus selfishness, 46
  and Islam
    of body-mind-spirit, 284
    of God, 330, 333, 336, 340
  of Judaic God, 219, 221
  of personality, 292
  Taoist, 195, 394
Upanishad, 28, 29-30, 52-56, 57

Vaishyas, 34
Vajrayana path, 87, 108-109
values
  and Christianity, 273, 277
  of clients, 9

values *(continued)*
    and Judaism, 224
    of Krishna, 45-46
    similarities, 364
Vatican II, 285
Vedas, 27-28
viewpoint, 101-102
vipashyana, 106
virtue, gathering of, 107
virtue and vice. *See also* good and evil
    in Buddhism, 114-115
    Christian view, 254, 257
    in Hinduism, 64
    and Islam, 336, 337, 341, 375
    in Taoism, 147, 154-157
Vishnu, 24, 25
visualization, 345

Walsh, Roger, 123
water, 146, 152, 162-163
Watts, Alan
    on Buddhism, 103, 117
    on Taoism, 146, 151, 153, 160-161
wealth, 32, 35. *See also* materialism
Wells, David, 278, 285
Welwood, John, 119
Westerners
    and anxiety, 227
    and meditation, 114
    and mindfulness, 187
    and Taoism, 146-147, 156
White, Michael, 101
Wilber, Ken, 404-406
will. *See also* decisions
    and Christianity, 252-255, 292-293
    and Islam, 333, 335, 343, 375
    in psychosynthesis, 404
    similarities, 363
will, of God
    and Christianity, 302
    Islamic view, 330, 338, 353, 379
Winnicott, Donald, 127, 225

wisdom
    in Buddhism, 95-96, 108, 129, 134
    in Hinduism, 65
    in Islam, 335-336
    in Taoism, 142, 145, 147, 166
women, 330-331
work
    and Buddhism, 103, 107, 110
    in Hinduism, 22
    Taoist view, 168, 169
workplace, 103
worldviews
    and discourse analysis, 301
    Hindu, 19
wu-wei
    and Buddhism, 125
    description, 152-154
    and suffering, 169
    in therapy, 176, 190-191

Yalom, Irvin, 121
yin-yang polarity, 156-157, 163, 169,
        184-185. *See also* cycles
yoga psychology, 79 n. 11, 310 n. 53
yogas
    and Brahman, 53, 58-59, 381
    description, 21-22
    and individual differences, 37, 58,
        380
    and purification, 37

Zen, 107-108, 125
Zen Buddhism
    and Christianity, 286-287
    and *koans,* 117
    meditation, 111-112
    origin, 87
    and personality structure, 372
    and psychosynthesis, 404
    and therapists, 118
Zen Buddhism and Psychoanalysis, 126
Zoroaster, 63, 64, 83 n. 74

T - #0455 - 101024 - C0 - 212/152/25 - PB - 9780789012371 - Gloss Lamination